Pearls and Pitfalls in Oral and Maxillofacial Surgery

Dina Amin · Hisham Marwan

Editors

Pearls and Pitfalls in Oral and Maxillofacial Surgery

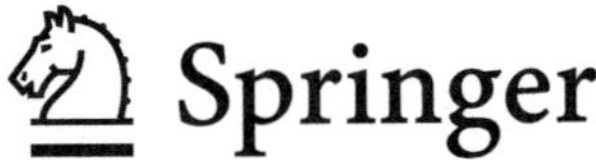 Springer

Editors
Dina Amin
Department of Oral and
Maxillofacial Surgery
University of Rochester
Rochester, NY, USA

Hisham Marwan
Department of Surgery
The University of Texas Medical Branch
Galveston, TX, USA

ISBN 978-3-031-47306-7   ISBN 978-3-031-47307-4   (eBook)
https://doi.org/10.1007/978-3-031-47307-4

This Springer imprint is published by the registered company Springer Nature Switzerland AG
The registered company address is: Gewerbestrasse 11, 6330 Cham, Switzerland

I dedicate this book to my daughter (Lana), who fills my heart with joy and survives my absence as I pursue my career. To my mother (Noor), who has given me enormous support and taught me the value of education and hard work. To my mentors who have, over the years, directly and indirectly, contributed to this work. Finally, I am grateful for all the struggles that I have faced in the past, as they have led to the achievements that I celebrate today.

—Dina Amin

*I am deeply indebted to God, then to my wife,
friends, teachers, and colleagues who
provided me the support and mentorship for
a successful surgical career and fulfillment
in my life.*

—*Hisham Marwan*

Preface

Pearls and Pitfalls in Oral and Maxillofacial Surgery is the first textbook of its kind in the field of Oral and Maxillofacial Surgery. It presents residents, fellows, and young surgeons with expert-level knowledge of surgical procedures. The inception of this book was 8 years ago when I (Hisham Marwan) was rounding on patients with my residents. Paul Lee, an astute Oral and Maxillofacial Surgery resident at that time, was preparing for his first operating room appearance. Dr. Lee and I discussed our thoughts regarding the absence of a concise textbook in our field that would outline how to perform a procedure efficiently and the steps required to avoid surgical complications. We both came up with the name "Pearls in Oral and Maxillofacial Surgery." Eight years later, I joined my colleague, Dina Amin, in editing this textbook. This textbook is for residents, fellows, and surgeons, who need a quick go-to read before the procedure.

Our target was to cover the most performed Oral and Maxillofacial Surgical procedures. During the process of creating the book, national and international surgeons who are experts in their respective fields were successfully recruited. The expert surgeons were asked to share their expertise on how to perform a specific procedure in an efficient approach and how they would avoid intraoperative and/or postoperative complications. The book covers topics including dentoalveolar, office-based sedation, pediatric anesthesia, craniomaxillofacial trauma, temporomandibular joint, head and neck oncology, reconstructive, craniofacial, facial cosmetics, and obstructive sleep apnea surgical procedures. All chapters have a similar design, including practical pearls and determinantal pitfalls. We hope readers will find this book indispensable to prepare for their day-to-day procedures.

Finally, we extend our gratitude to all the authors who invested their time and shared their expertise to develop this book. Without their support, we would not be able to create this book.

Rochester, NY, USA   Dina Amin
Galveston, TX, USA   Hisham Marwan

Key Features

- Over 28 high-quality illustrations demonstrating surgical anatomy and procedures.
- All chapters are written by surgeons who are experts in the chapter's topic.
- The book discusses the most commonly performed Oral and Maxillofacial procedures.

Acknowledgments

We want to acknowledge Victoria A. Mañón for her substantial contribution to this book. Victoria spent countless hours away from her newborn child to create the illustrations. Her high-quality and detailed illustrations speak out to readers, highlighting important detail fundamental to the surgical procedure. Furthermore, Dr. Mañón collaborated with expert surgeons in writing essential chapters in this book.

Dina Amin
Hisham Marwan

Contents

Part III   Craniomaxillofacial Trauma

Part IV   Head and Neck Pathology

Part I
Pearls and Pitfalls in Dentoalveolar Surgery

Chapter 1
Limitations and Indications of Coronectomy

Andrew Read-Fuller

Abstract Coronectomy, or partial odontectomy, is a technique used in dentoalveolar surgery to treat a mandibular third molar when complete removal of the tooth considerably risks injury to the inferior alveolar nerve (IAN). As IAN injury is one of the more feared complications in third molar removal, occurring in 1–5% of cases, coronectomy can appear to be an attractive option when there is radiographic evidence of an intimate relationship between the tooth roots and the IAN. However, the actual indications for coronectomy are relatively limited due to the sensitivity of the technique and the various complications that can result from the procedure. The purpose of this chapter is to review the indications, procedure, and complications of coronectomy.

Practical Tips

- Coronectomy is indicated if the following clinical criteria are present:

  - Surgical management of the third molar due to problems caused by its crown. For example, periocoronitis of the third molar and/or when the crown of the third molar causes a periodontal pocket on the distal aspect of the adjacent molar.
  - High risk of injury to the inferior alveolar nerve with complete removal of the tooth.

- Ankylosed roots are considered a relative indication for coronectomy.
- Consider angling the bur 45° inferiorly, aiming below the lingual cemento-enamel junction.

A. Read-Fuller (✉)
Department of Oral and Maxillofacial Surgery, Texas A&M University School of Dentistry, Baylor University Medical Center, Dallas, TX, USA
e-mail: readfuller@tamu.edu

D. Amin, H. Marwan (eds.), *Pearls and Pitfalls in Oral and Maxillofacial Surgery*, https://doi.org/10.1007/978-3-031-47307-4_1

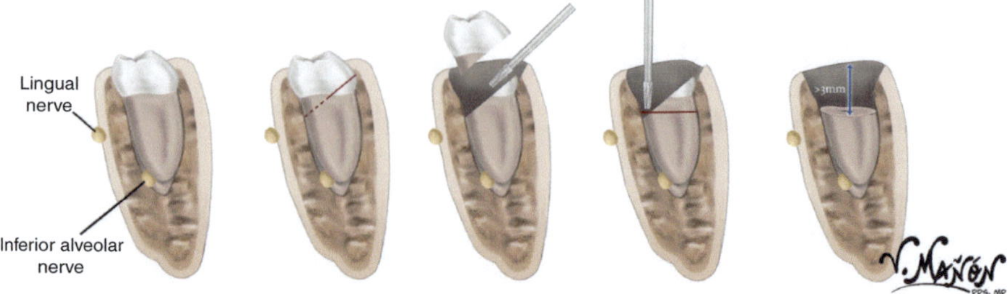

Fig. 1.1 Surgical sequence for a coronectomy. (Illustration courtesy of Victoria A. Mañón, DDS MBA MD)

- Avoid perforation of the lingual cortex and injury to the lingual nerve by sectioning ¾ of the crown and then fracturing the rest (Fig. 1.1).
- Ensure that there is at least 3 mm of distance between the alveolar crest and remaining roots and obtain primary closure.

Complications

- *Root migration*: Remaining roots can migrate in a coronal direction after crown removal (2–85%), leading to exposed roots that must be removed later (2–6%).
- *Infection*: The remaining root structure becomes infected, requiring removal (1–9.5%).
- *Lingual nerve injury*: During sectioning of the crown, the bur can perforate the lingual cortex leading to injury to the adjacent nerve (0–2%).
- *Inferior alveolar nerve injury*: Although the primary purpose of coronectomy is to avoid IAN injury, it still occurs in up to 9% of cases.
- *Incomplete soft tissue closure*: Dehiscence of the soft tissue overlying the remaining roots during the healing process and resulting in persistent exposure of root remnants. The inadequate vertical distance from the alveolar crest to the roots increases the risk of this occurring.

Pearls

- Use 701 or 702 burs to section the crown.
- Always apply Rood criteria when evaluating a third molar for extraction (darkening of the root, diversion of the canal, and/or interruption of the white line of the canal).
- Cone-been computed tomography (CBCT) may be used to confirm that removal of the roots would likely risk injury to the IAN.

- Do remove *all* enamel. The remaining enamel will prevent complete healing.
- Do remove enough tooth structure so that tooth remnants are at least 3 mm (some authors recommend at least 4 mm) below the alveolar crest. This is also required to ensure complete healing and prevent infection.
- Do take a radiograph immediately postoperatively as a baseline and obtain serial radiographs to monitor for any migration of the roots. (Root migration, when it occurs, is typically within the first 2–3 years following coronectomy and does not happen in every case).

Pitfalls

- Coronectomy is indicated when the risk to the inferior alveolar nerve (IAN) is anticipated (Fig. 1.2).
- Avoid injury to the lingual nerve by sectioning ¾ of the crown and breaking off the rest. Alternatively, place a retractor subperiosteally on the lingual and section completely through the crown.

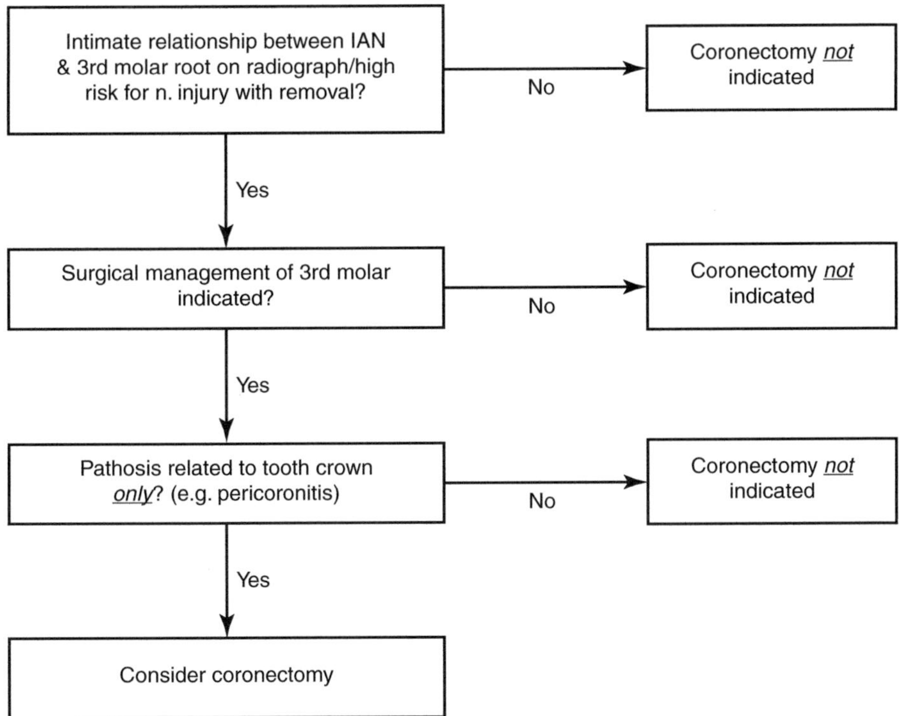

Fig. 1.2 Summary: decision tree for coronectomy

- Do not use coronectomy as a salvage procedure after a failed attempt at extraction and mobilizing roots. Mobile roots can increase the risk of infection or root migration.
- Do not perform root canal treatment (RCT) on the remaining root structure. This increases the risk of postoperative infection (87.5% infection rate with RCT).

Further Reading

Martin A, Perinetti G, Costantinides F, Maglione M. Coronectomy as a surgical approach to impacted mandibular third molars: a systematic review. Head Face Med. 2015;11:9. https://doi.org/10.1186/s13005-015-0068-7.
Pogrel MA, Lee JS, Muff DF. Coronectomy: a technique to protect the inferior alveolar nerve. J Oral Maxillofac Surg. 2004;62(12):1447–52. https://doi.org/10.1016/j.joms.2004.08.003.

Chapter 2
How to Avoid Injury to the Lingual Nerve

Hisham Marwan, Victoria Manon, and Dina Amin

Abstract The lingual nerve is a branch of the trigeminal nerve's mandibular division (V3). It carries general sensation to the anterior two-thirds of the tongue, lingual gingiva, and ipsilateral floor of the mouth. It also carries a special visceral sensation (taste) via the chorda tympani nerve. In addition, it carries the parasympathetic innervation to the submandibular ganglion. Injury to the nerve will result in significant morbidity for the patient. The patient will suffer from paresthesia of half of the tongue, resulting in difficulty talking, eating with drooling, and tongue biting. Moreover, the taste is usually impaired with a possibility of persistent metallic taste. Finally, xerostomia and reduction of saliva production are other morbidity if the nerve is injured.

After the lingual nerve branches from the mandibular nerve, it receives the chorda tympani nerve that transmits taste sensation to the anterior two-thirds of the tongue. At this level, it is usually located about 1 cm anterior to the mandibular foramen between the medial pterygoid muscle and the medial surface of the mandibular ramus (Fig. 2.1). At the level of the third molar, it runs superior to the mylohyoid muscle, and it can be at the level of the alveolar crest or higher in about 17% of the cases. Furthermore, the distance from the alveolar crest to the nerve at the level of the third molar is found to range between 2.28 and 3.01 mm. The surgeon should be careful with the atrophic mandible since the nerve will be near the ridge following bone resorption. Subsequently, the nerve will move anteromedially and run beneath the submandibular duct before it terminates at the ventral surface of the tongue. The purpose of this chapter is to explain how to avoid injury to the lingual nerve during routine dentoalveoloar procedures.

H. Marwan
Department of Surgery, The University of Texas Medical Branch, Galveston, TX, USA

V. Manon
McGovern Medical School, UTHealth School of Dentistry, Houston, TX, USA

D. Amin (✉)
Department of Oral and Maxillofacial Surgery, University of Rochester, Rochester, NY, USA
e-mail: dina_amin@urmc.rochester.edu

© The Author(s), under exclusive license to Springer Nature Switzerland AG 2024
D. Amin, H. Marwan (eds.), *Pearls and Pitfalls in Oral and Maxillofacial Surgery*, https://doi.org/10.1007/978-3-031-47307-4_2

Practical Tips

- Chemical injury to the nerve is characterized by a patchy area of paresthesia around the distribution of the lingual nerve. These chemical injuries are the most difficult to treat. Avoid high-concentration local anesthetic (4% Articaine) in performing lingual nerve blocks (Fig. 2.1).
- It is unnecessary to search for the lingual nerve during routine dentoalveolar procedures.
- During third molar surgery, careful design of the mucoperiosteal flap is paramount. Avoiding the incision on the top of the retromolar trigone will reduce the risk of lingual nerve injury (Figs. 2.2 and 2.3).
- Use a buccal hockey stick extension following the external oblique ridge. This extension will allow wider exposure, avoid the retromolar trigone, and minimize the stretching.
- The most common injury to the lingual nerve is neuropraxia. This is mainly resulting from excessive stretching on the lingual flap. Avoiding the lingual reflection of the mucoperiosteal flap, if possible, will eliminate the risk. However, a specific type of impacted third molar (deep vertical, horizontal, and lingually oriented mesioangular) will require careful subperiosteal reflection of the lingual flap. Overly aggressive stretching during reflection or removal of the impacted tooth will result in Neurapraxia, which can be permanent.
- In deep lingual impaction, the careful elevation of the subperiosteal lingual flap with the gentle placement of a Molt #9 or a Seldon to help retract the tissue is crucially vital. Carefully monitor the placement of the retractors to avoid compression injury to the lingual nerve.
- Another potential pitfall is sectioning the tooth. Since the lingual plate is very thin and the lingual nerve can be adherent to the plate, overzealous use of the drill during sectioning might result in transection injury, permanent paresthesia, and possible painful neuroma formation.
- It is always recommended to leave 2 mm of tooth structure close to the lingual plate. Subsequent use of hand instruments (e.g., straight dental elevator) to split the tooth structure will minimize the risk of lingual nerve injury.

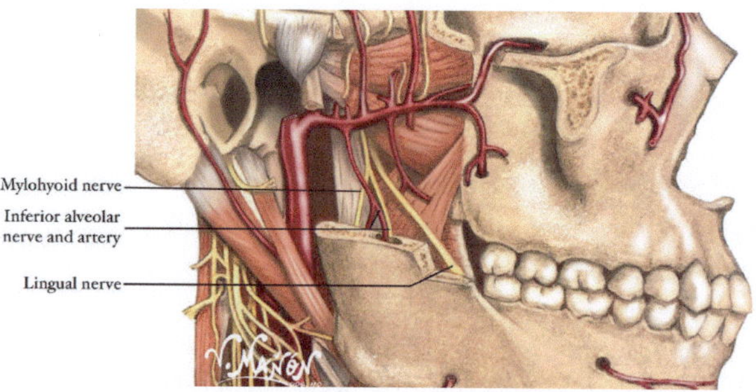

Fig. 2.1 Anatomy of the lingual nerve at the infratemporal fossa

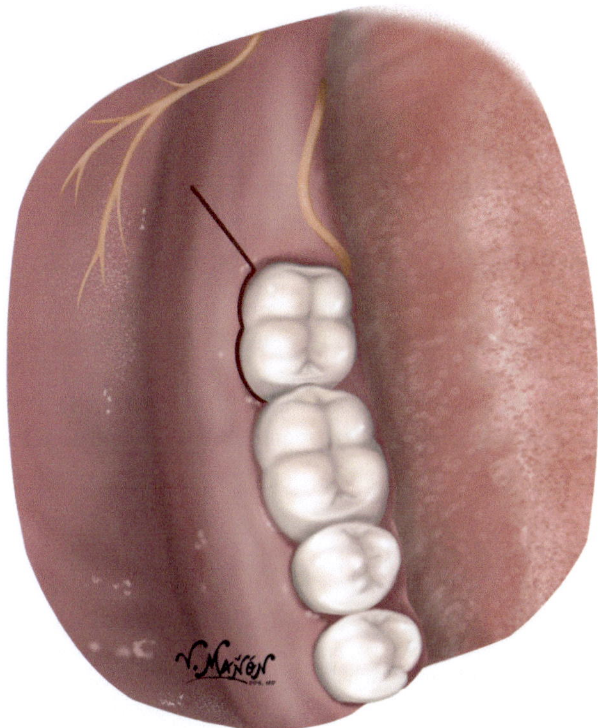

Fig. 2.2 Proper incision design to avoid injury to the lingual nerve

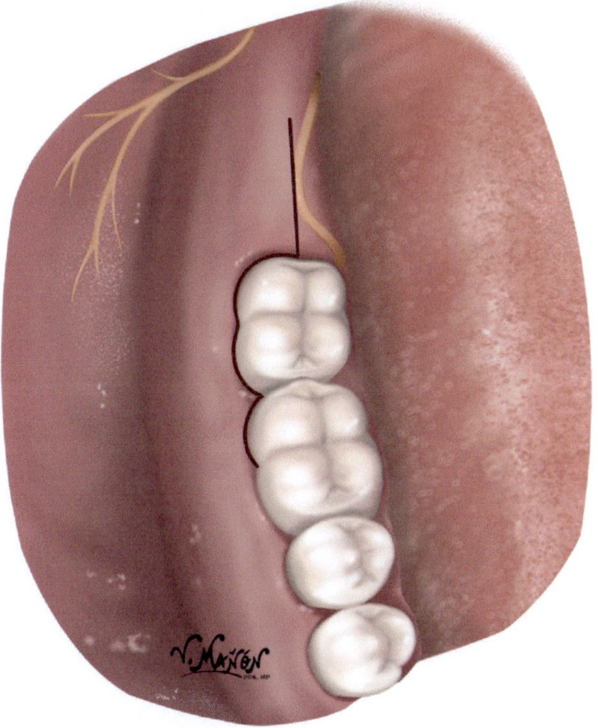

Fig. 2.3 Straight line incision at the top of the retromolar trigone will increase the risk of lingual nerve damage

Pearls

- Avoid high-concentration local anesthetic (4% Articaine) in performing lingual nerve blocks.
- Leave 2 mm of tooth structure close to the lingual plate.

Pitfalls

- Carefully monitor the placement of the retractors to avoid compression injury to the lingual nerve.
- Avoid overzealous use of the drill while sectioning the teeth, as it might result in transection injury, permanent paresthesia, and possible painful neuroma formation.

Further Reading

Kim SY, et al. Topographic anatomy of the lingual nerve and variations in communication pattern of the mandibular nerve branches. Surg Radiol Anat. 2004;26(2):128–35.

Pogrel MA, Renaut A, Schmidt B, Ammar A. The relationship of the lingual nerve to the mandibular third molar region: an anatomic study. J Oral Maxillofac Surg. 1995;53(10):1178–81.

Chapter 3
Practical Tips for the Surgical Management of Impacted Canine

Marianela Gonzalez, Christopher White, Palak Desai, and Dina Amin

Abstract Management of impacted teeth (except third molars) can be challenging. Proper diagnosis and treatment planning requires interdisciplinary care by an orthodontist, general dentist, and oral and maxillofacial surgeon. The most common impacted teeth are third molars (maxillary and mandibular), followed by maxillary canines, the maxillary second molar, mandibular second premolars, and mandibular second molar. The impacted maxillary canine is twice as common in females and three times more likely to be impacted palatally. The purpose of this chapter is to explain the pearls and pitfalls in managing impacted canines.

Practical Tips

- Localization of the impacted canine requires a visual inspection, digital palpation, and radiographic evaluation.
- Clark's Rule (SLOB rule) can be used to determine the impacted canine location (buccal vs. palatal). The SLOB rule is an acronym standing for "Same-Lingual Opposite-Buccal."

M. Gonzalez · C. White
Department of Oral and Maxillofacial Surgery, Texas A&M University, Baylor Medical Center, College Station, TX, USA

P. Desai
Allegheny Health Network, Pittsburgh, PA, USA

D. Amin (✉)
Department of Oral and Maxillofacial Surgery, University of Rochester, Rochester, NY, USA
e-mail: dina_amin@urmc.rochester.edu

D. Amin, H. Marwan (eds.), *Pearls and Pitfalls in Oral and Maxillofacial Surgery*, https://doi.org/10.1007/978-3-031-47307-4_3

- Three-dimensional (3D) cone-bean computed tomography (CT) scan is superior in determining the location of the impacted canine
- Management of the impacted canine can include (1) no treatment with regular clinical and/or radiographic observation, (2) extraction of the primary canine, (3) surgical extraction of the impacted tooth, (4) surgical exposure to aid eruption, (5) surgical exposure with eruption aided by orthodontic guidance, or (6) autotransplantation of the canine.
- Techniques for surgical exposure of impacted canine include (1) open surgical exposure, surgical exposure with packing and delayed bonding of the orthodontic bracket, and (2) surgical exposure and bonding of immediate bonding of the orthodontic bracket.
- The flap design is dictated by the impacted tooth's location, the mucogingival junction's relation to the crown, and the amount of available keratinized tissue.
- Consider using apically positioned flaps when (1) the crown is located apical to the mucogingival junction and/or (2) there are <2 mm of keratinized gingiva in the erupted area.
- When using the closed technique, suture the traction chain to the existing orthodontic hardware.
- Consider using the gingivectomy (open surgical technique) when (1) the crown is located coronal to the mucogingival junction and/or (2) there is ≥2 to 3 mm of keratinized gingiva in the erupted area.
- Expose only 2/3 of the clinical crown (enough space to bond the orthodontic bracket).
- If the bracket becomes detached following the bonding procedure, ensure that the area is completely hemostatic and that the tooth is dry before restarting the etch/bond procedure from the beginning.

Pearls

- The position of the impacted canine is important when deciding management options for the patient.
- The crown of the lateral root may be proclined when the canine is lying labial to the lateral incisor.
- The flap design is important to ensure periodontal health.

Pitfalls

- Avoid vertical releasing incisions on the palatally impacted canines.
- Avoid exposing the cementoenamel junction. Exposure of the root may lead to ankylosis, external root resorption, and/or long-term periodontal issues.

Further Reading

Alberto PL. Surgical exposure of impacted teeth. Oral Maxillofac Surg Clin North Am. 2020;32(4):561–70.

Becker A, Chaushu S. Surgical treatment of impacted canines. Oral Maxillofac Surg Clin. 2015; 27(3):449–58.

Chapter 4
Practical Tips for Full Arch Dental Implant Reconstruction

Kroum D. Dimitrov

Abstract Full arch dental implant rehabilitation has been extensively documented as a successful long-term fixed solution for patients with terminal dentition for both Jaw Arches. This process is marketed by many names such as All on 4, All on X, Implant Supported Immediately Loaded Fixed Denture, and/or Teeth in a Day. The optimal long-term success of this treatment requires a multidisciplinary, diagnostically driven treatment planning and execution between an oral and maxillofacial surgeon, a prosthodontist, and a qualified laboratory technician. Most of the surgical complications are related to traumatic removal of the terminal dentition, mishandling of the subperiosteal flaps, damage to inferior alveolar nerve (IAN) vascular bundles, inadequate enucleation, and curettage of the jaw infection present, loss of implants into the maxillary sinus, or not diagnosing oral pathological lesions in the pretreatment planning phase. Using original fixtures for the chosen implant system and new drills for the implant osteotomies is necessary to decrease the chance of bone overheating and not a perfect fitting of the prosthetic parts. Prosthetic complications will occur because of a too-conservative vertical reduction and irregular alveoloplasty of the jaw arches to allow for enough restorative space for the strength of the prosthesis and inadequate anterior-posterior spread of the implants, improper angulation of the implant axis to allow the emergence profiles of the multiunit abutments to come as close as possible to the mid arch of the prosthesis. A non-passive impression technique or forced denture fitting will cause unequal distribution of the implant forces. It may overload some of the implants during the healing time, causing bone loss and loss of implants in the long term. Perfect fit to all abutments and high rigidity within the framework is required, as it allows for even distribution of

K. D. Dimitrov (✉)
American Board of Oral and Maxillofacial Surgery, Chicago, IL, USA

National Dental Board of Anesthesiology, Chicago, IL, USA

International Association of Oral and Maxillofacial Surgeons, Chicago, IL, USA

American Dental Society of Anesthesiology, Chicago, IL, USA

Love Your Jaws Surgery Center/Miami's First Robotic Dental Implant Solution, Miami, FL, USA; https://www.loveyourjaws.com

D. Amin, H. Marwan (eds.), *Pearls and Pitfalls in Oral and Maxillofacial Surgery*, https://doi.org/10.1007/978-3-031-47307-4_4

loading forces and casting the implants during the healing phase. Preventing many of these complications can be achieved using the technological advances of Digitally and Prosthetically Driven Surgical treatment pre-planning, utilizing scanned denture Standard Tessellation Language (STL) files onto the cone-beam computed tomography (CBCT) surgical treatment plan, and precise implant placement using minimally invasive robotically assisted implant placement technology or pre-planned guided surgery with stents. Medically compromised patients, heavy smokers, and patients with suboptimal manual dexterity to care for their implants should not undergo this elective procedure because of the high chance of failure and peri-implantitis-associated complications.

Practical Tips

Preoperative

- Prosthetically Driven Virtual pre-surgical planning is required with a detailed review of the CBCT and digitized STL files of prosthesis implemented into the CBCT workup.
- Minimally invasive robotically assisted implant placement allows for direct visualization of the surgical sites and alveolar ridge with minimal soft tissue retraction.
- Using prefabricated stackable splints for bone reduction and implant placement is an option, but be prepared to revert to free-handed surgery of some implants since these stackable options are often too bulky and don't allow for direct visualization of the surgical sites for irrigation and placement with high primary stability.
- Patients with myofascial pain syndrome from chronic clenching and grinding need to be treated beforehand with Botox, behavioral therapy, and muscle relaxants because this habit will fail the implants. Request a new night guard be done after the prosthesis is delivered to protect from parafunctional overloading on the implants, abutments, and prosthetic breakage.
- Evaluate the Bedrossian zones carefully to ensure adequate bone at the premaxilla and bicuspid regions for tilted implant placement and mark the IAN anterior loops to avoid paresthesia to pre-plan the widest anterior-posterior spread of the implants.
- Select tapered active implants such as Nobel Active BioCare or Straumann BLX, with a min of 2 mm of circumferential bone.
- AP spread is defined as the distance between the most anterior implant to the most distal implant on each side. The distal prosthetic cantilever should be at most 1.5× the AP spread on the implants (Fig. 4.1).
- Model surgery must be done on the casts to determine the adequate amount of alveoloplasty necessary to hide the transition zone.

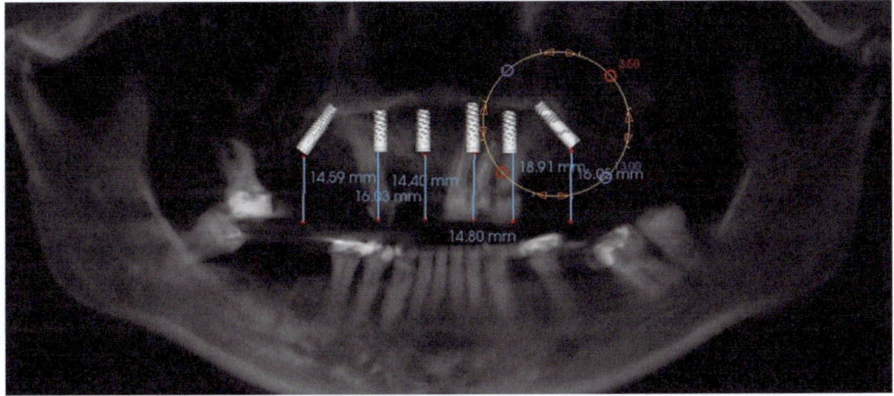

Fig. 4.1 Preliminary preplanning is done on the panoramic cut of the Pre-Operative CBCT

Fig. 4.2 Transitional prosthesis with included transition line/min bone reduction place for intraoperative reference, facial view

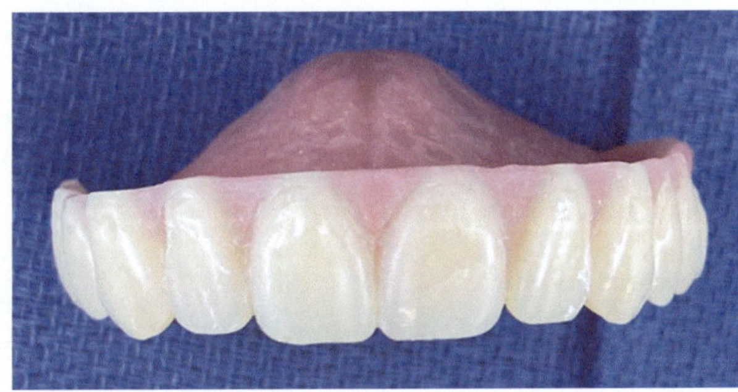

- Request from the laboratory technician a denture that has implemented transition line/bone reduction and implant emergence slot incorporated (Fig. 4.2).
- Well-fitting dentures are used for the edentulous patient to obtain the new occlusion. They should be scanned with radiolucent material (Triad Dualine) and six uniformly spherical markers attached to buccal and palatal areas of the denture with bite registration to ensure dentures are well seated. Scan the patient, scan the dentures separately, or obtain an STL file for your workup (Figs. 4.3, 4.4 and 4.5)
- The new smile line positioning needs to be established, and min 15–17 mm interocclusal space is required for adequate maxillary prosthesis material.
- The mandibular prosthesis will follow the maxillary occlusal line and needs min 13–15 mm of interocclusal space.
- Ensure clear communication between the surgical, restorative, and lab teams; everyone knows what implant parts they are responsible for bringing to the surgical case.
- Ensure that you have sharp new drills for implant osteotomies and that everyone on the team uses the correct, authentic implant parts. Usually, the surgeon is responsible for the Implants, Multi-Unit Abutments, and Whitecaps. The other

Fig. 4.3 Transitional prosthesis with included emergence slot for anterior implants for intraoperative reference. STL files can be generated and used for final CBCT planning

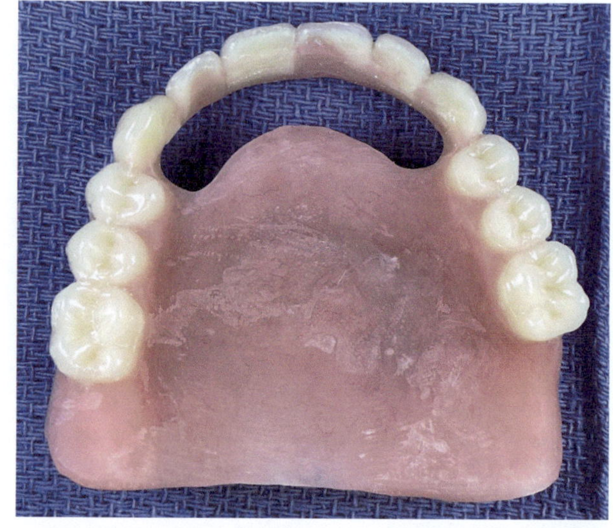

Fig. 4.4 Final implant CBCT plan with STL file of transitional prosthesis implemented and Yomi Bone link splint to be used for robotically assisted implant placements (Software Yomi Plan from Neocis, INC), lateral view

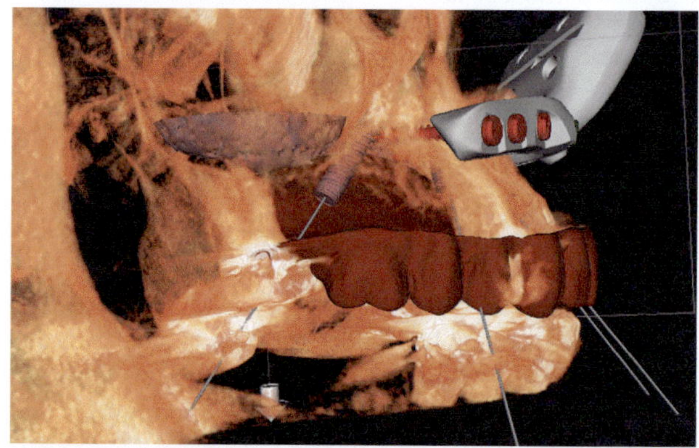

Fig. 4.5 Final implant CBCT plan with STL file of transitional prosthesis, showing transition line/ bone reduction plane implemented and Yomi Bone link splint to be used for robotically assisted Implant placements (Software Yomi Plan from Neocis, INC), frontal view

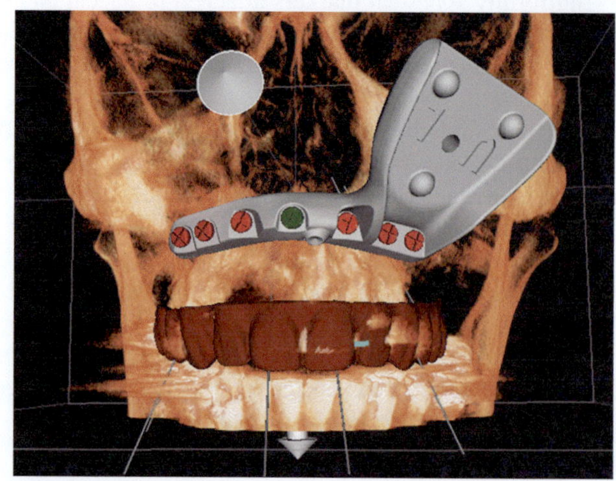

parts are supplied by the restorative doctor and the laboratory technician. Don't assume; communicate with all team members and ensure you have all authentic components days before surgery.

- When selecting the MUA, always use your digital workup for the best angulation. Also, have a backup of different angulations for the chosen implant platform in case a better one is necessary to obtain the best result clinically. Always select the shortest height of MUA, considering the thickness of the patient's gingiva.
- Decide on the safest anesthesia for the patient; if the dual arch is planned, the best is to have Naso endotracheal intubation. Single arches can be done safely with Open Airway General anesthesia, a well-designed throat curtain with 4 × 4 gauze, and a Sea sponge.
- Clinical stent/denture should be requested for both arched and will help you clinically confirm that your digital workup is accurate. Be ready to move implant positions at the time of surgery regardless of the preplan; this can be done easily intraoperatively using robotically assisted implant technology (Yomi, Neoscis, INC).
- Patient positioning for optimal comfort is critical as these cases can take up to 4 h for two arches, ensure the neck and lower back are well padded, and have no pressure points that can bother the patient in the middle of the surgical procedure.
- Ensure the patient has voided before surgery and has a diaper. If the case goes longer than 4 h, wake up the patient and make them walk to decrease the chance of DVTs.
- Selecting tapered and active implants (with cutting apical tips such as Nobel Biocare) is recommended. The tapered effect will decrease the chance of loose implants via apical migration, and active implants allow manual changing direction or angulation for the prosthetic emergence.
- Ensure everyone on the team will be at the correct time for the denture conversion; the restorative dentist and lab technician need to know when surgery will finish to start their work. Don't underestimate the time necessary to do the surgery perfectly.
- Avoid narcotics and over-sedation in these patients since they will need to be active during lab transition and loading the implants.

Intraoperative

- If minimally invasive robotically assisted surgery is planned, best is to minimize subperiosteal reflections only up to the area of the bone reduction plane. Recording the amount of vertical bone reduction clinically will help your lap technician mount the case on the semi-adjustable articulator (Figs. 4.6 and 4.7).
- If traditional splits are used or completely free-handed surgery, you will need to do a subperiosteal reflection of the maxilla bilaterally to expose piriform areas, maxillary buttresses, and open lateral sinus windows and for mandible complete

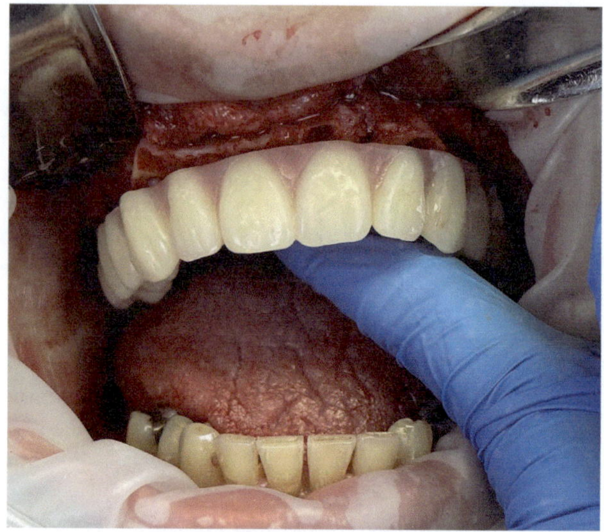

Fig. 4.6 Intraoperative clinical verification of transition line and bone reduction plane using the lap-made transitional prosthesis

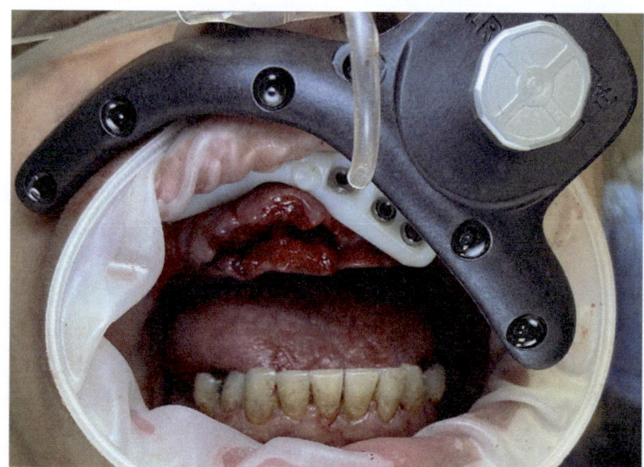

Fig. 4.7 Extraoral fiducial array connected onto Yomi Link bony supported Splint (Neocis, INC) with 18–20 mm screws from Stryker to perform the day of surgery scan and execute precise minimally invasive robotically assisted implant placements

subperiosteal dissection to visualize the mental nerve canals and loops to avoid placing the implants into these vital structures.

- Ensure clean subperiosteal dissection is carried on all flaps. Do not sacrifice any attached gingiva until the implants are placed and MUA and White caps are in and ready for closure. Do your best to suture by interdigitating the gingiva instead of amputating healthy keratinized tissue.
- Remove any malposed posterior molar teeth and third molars that are hyper-erupted before implant surgery, so you will have access to better angulate your tilted posterior implants, which will usually have 30° of multiunit abutments.
- Make the bone reduction with high-speed straight surgical handpiece with Laboratory Carbide Bur, Medium, Cross Cut, Barrel, 6 mm at 15,000 RPMs with seldom retractor protection of the palatal/lingual tissues.

- Avoid using rongeurs and bone files alone since the alveoloplasty will be a more irregular and higher chance of breaking vital bones necessary for implant stability and circumferential implant bone stock.
- Trust your digitally driven preplan and stents, but always verify clinically that your osteotomies and implant positioning are right on. Using robotic assistance, you have direct visualization of the surgical sites, while stackable guides can comprise irrigation, overheat the bone, and misplace implants if the guide moves. Be ready for free-handed implant placement if guides and stents are not usable. It happens more often than not; robotically assisted surgery is best and allows for intraoperative changes on the fly. Premade stackable guides do not allow for intraoperative implant position changes and will go in the trash.
- Keep a close eye on your assistant retracting with the Minnesota retraction around the mental nerves, as they can be crushed or cut solely from heavy retraction alone.
- If you are doing non-guided surgery, you need to make a sinus window and inspect the anterior sinus wall, so you can place your posterior tilted implants all into the bone of the anterior sinus wall.
- For mandibular full jaw reconstruction, always keep an eye on the level of the floor of the mouth since implants placed deeper than the anterior floor of mouth attachments will always have saliva pooling and a higher chance for long-term failure.
- If you are doing open-airway anesthesia, ensure you continuously change the throat curtain and use a new sea sponge as a double layer for secretions to accumulate.
- Laryngospasms from sections during the open airway general anesthesia surgery will set you back quite a bit.
- Measure and record the vertical amount of bone reduction; it will help your laboratory technician set up the casts easier on the articulator.
- Open tray impression coping technique is recommended because it allows for a stress-free impression and, therefore, less chance of pulling out less stable implants.
- Closed tray impressions are not recommended if your implants are on the low stability, less than 35NCM.
- Refer to pictures for prosthesis set up on open tray impression and denture transition execution (Figs. 4.8, 4.9, 4.10 and 4.11).
- Ensure the intaglio surface is cleansable, with no lab ridge but an oval and smooth surface and space for the patient to flush easily (Fig. 4.12).
- The passive fit of the prosthesis is essential so all implants share the same load and not overstressing/overloading some at the expense of others.
- When seating the prosthesis, start with the anterior implant at the correct torque for the prosthetic parts and then continue triangularly with the opposite, most distal, etc. (Figs. 4.13, 4.14, 4.15 and 4.16).

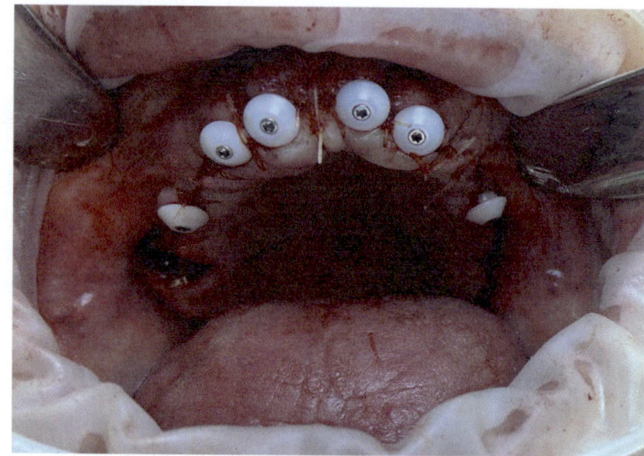

Fig. 4.8 Implants placed with multiunit abutments and white healing caps. Sutured primarily with minimal removal of attached gingiva. Select the shortest multiunit abutments for the patient's gingival thickness

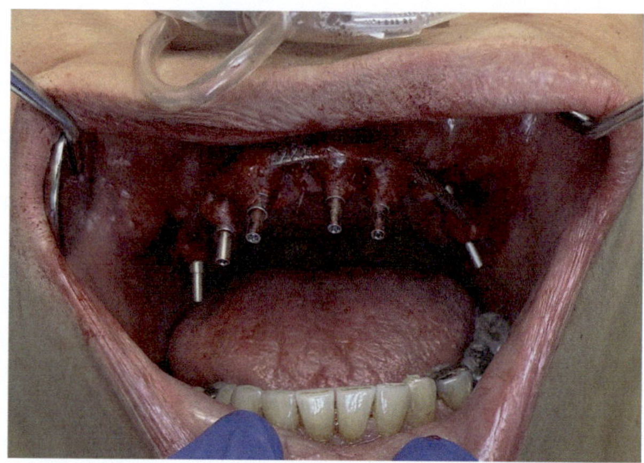

Fig. 4.9 Indirect technique for capturing all implants with minimal stress on implants. Shows open tray impression copings for multiunit abutments connected passively to bended universal plate strengtheners (Yates Motloid) with Pattern R (acrylic resin for patterns), salt and pepper technique

Fig. 4.10 Passive impression open tray technique has taken using Exa'lence Heavy Body Vinyl Polyether Silicone and Take 1 Advanced Base and Catalyst Putty Fast set and Gingifast Rigid for gingival space fill. The implant analogs are in place

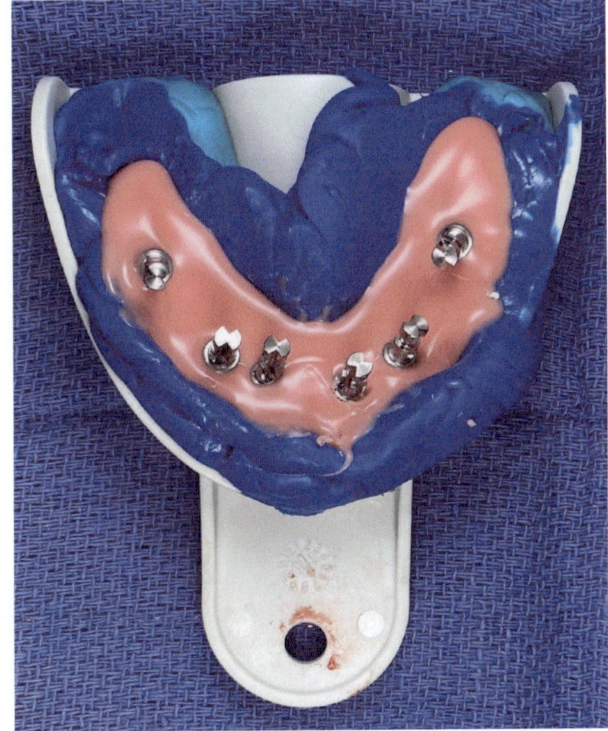

Fig. 4.11 Anterior two implants' temporary impression copings are connected with pattern resin to the prosthesis after clinically adjusting the denture position

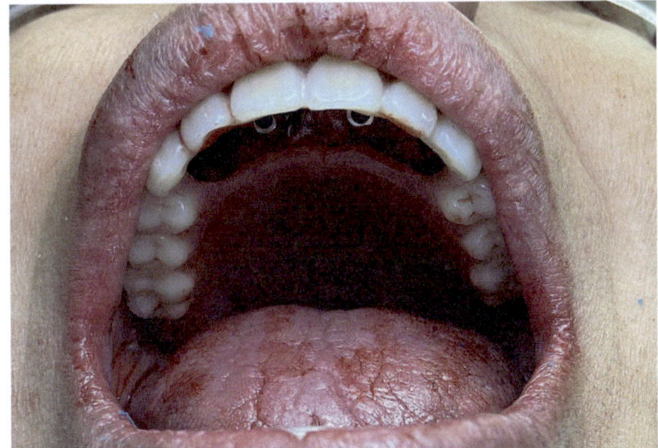

Fig. 4.12 Intaglio surface of transitional prosthesis showing the pattern resin temporary impression copings

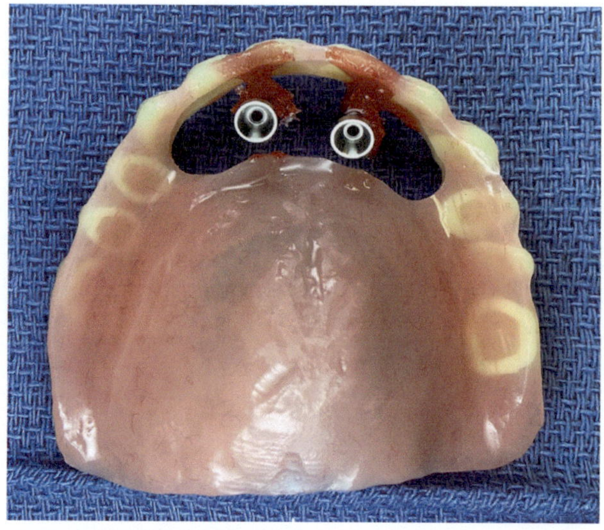

Fig. 4.13 Clinical bite registration is taken, and the case is mounted on a semi-adjustable articulator

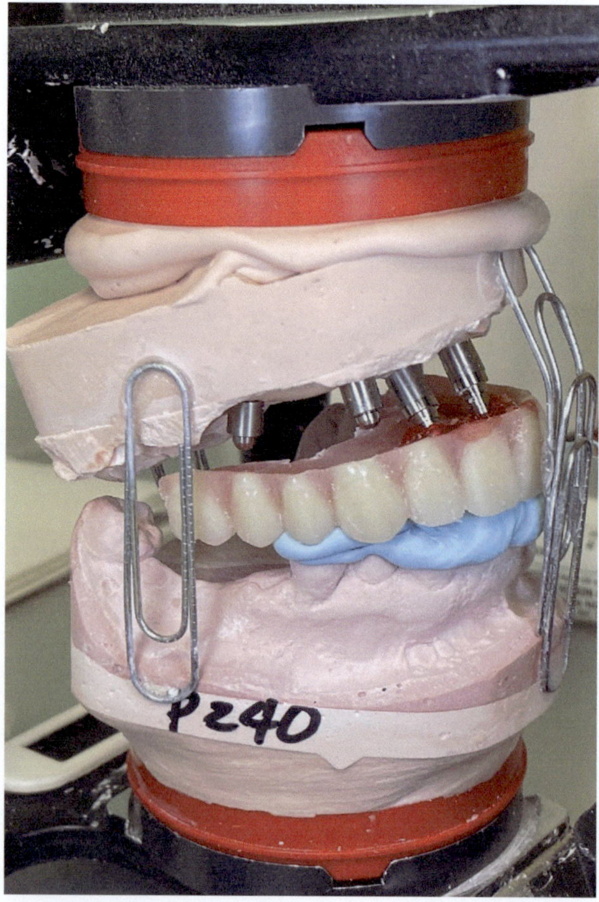

Fig. 4.14 Transitional prosthesis polished and intaglio surface made oval for cleanability

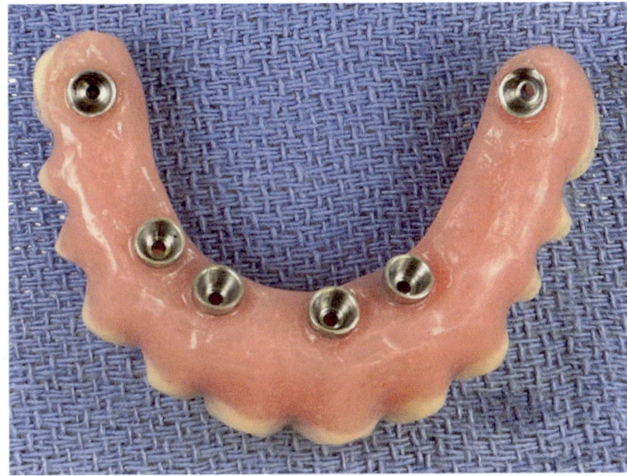

Fig. 4.15 The occlusal surface of the transitional prosthesis shows implant positions allowing enough material thickness for the transitional prosthesis to not break during the healing period

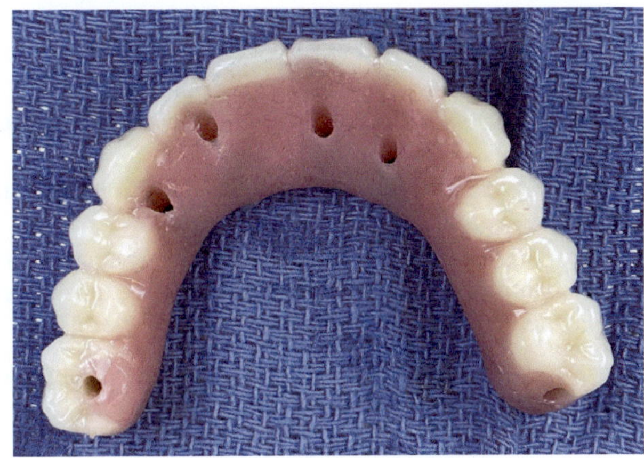

Fig. 4.16 Transitional prothesis smile on surgical day

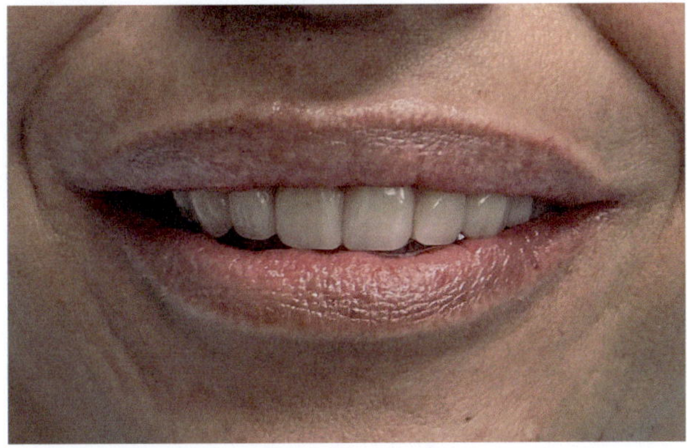

Postoperative

- Post-op CBCT should be obtained if robotic technology is not used for surgical implant placement. Otherwise, a panoramic X-ray is enough for an immediate post-op check (Fig. 4.17).
- Verify that the implant positions are as your preplan.
- Evaluate that your surgical execution plan went as planned and brainstorm where things could be improved for the next case.
- Patients can have paresthesia from retraction even if your implants are perfect and not impinging on the nerves.
- Paresthesia also can be from the prosthesis being bulky at the mental nerve exits. Diagnose the level of paresthesia accordingly with Neurosensory testing, steroids, and adjustment of the prosthesis if impinging of tissues.
- Advise patients to keep a liquid diet until the first post-op check.
- The patient needs to have equilibration with the prosthodontist on weekly bases.
- Hygiene with gentle rinsing with Peridex under the denture and saltwater rinses for the first 2 weeks. Start using a water pick on the lowest setting with Peridex and hydrogen peroxide rinse once you have seen surgically that the mucosa has closed completely 2–3 weeks after surgery.
- You can use tranexamic acid mouthwash to rinse under the flaps for post-op bleeding.
- Request a soft night guard for the transition and final prosthesis, especially in patients with a clenching/grinding habit.
- See your patients regularly after surgery, continue to reevaluate their hygiene, and continue to educate them on hygiene; otherwise, the implants can fail just like their natural teeth failed.

Please review the two case of full mouth rehabilitation (Figs. 4.18, 4.19, 4.20 and 4.21).

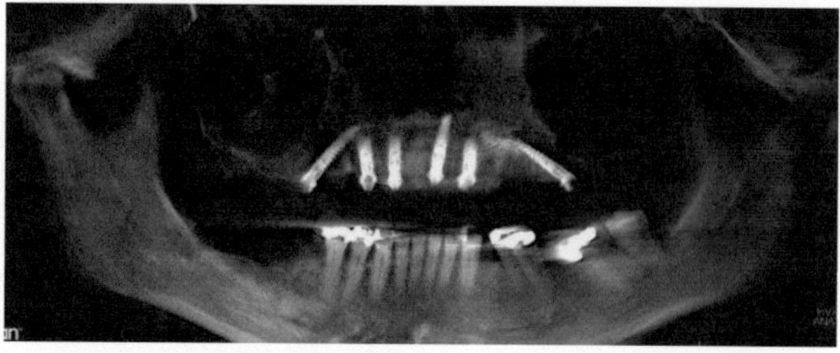

Fig. 4.17 Post CBCT scan day of surgery

Fig. 4.18 Upper and lower full-arch reconstruction with a day of surgery transitional prosthesis delivery

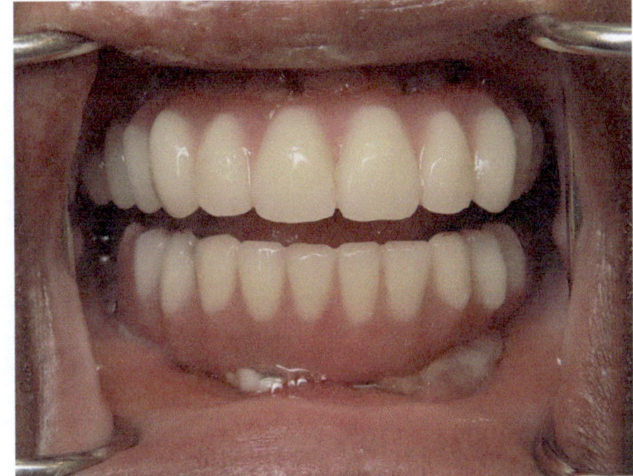

Fig. 4.19 Upper and lower full-arch reconstruction with a day of surgery transitional prosthesis delivery

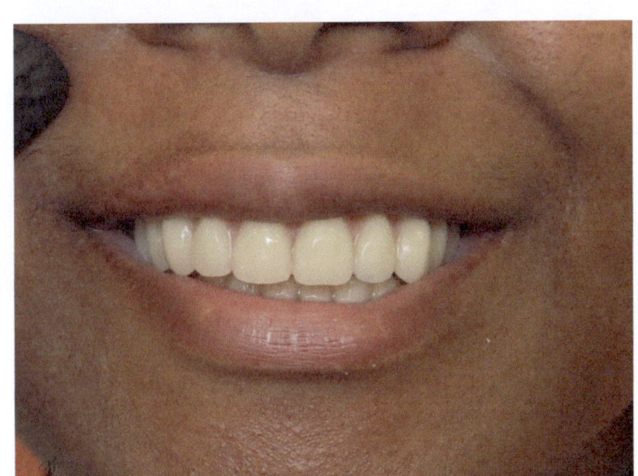

Fig. 4.20 Mandibular partially edentulous patient

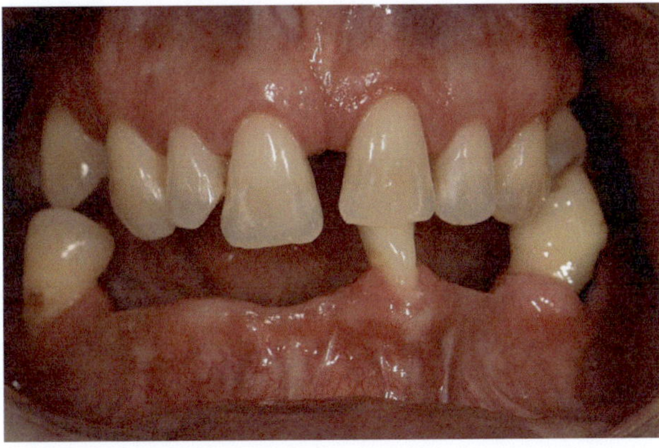

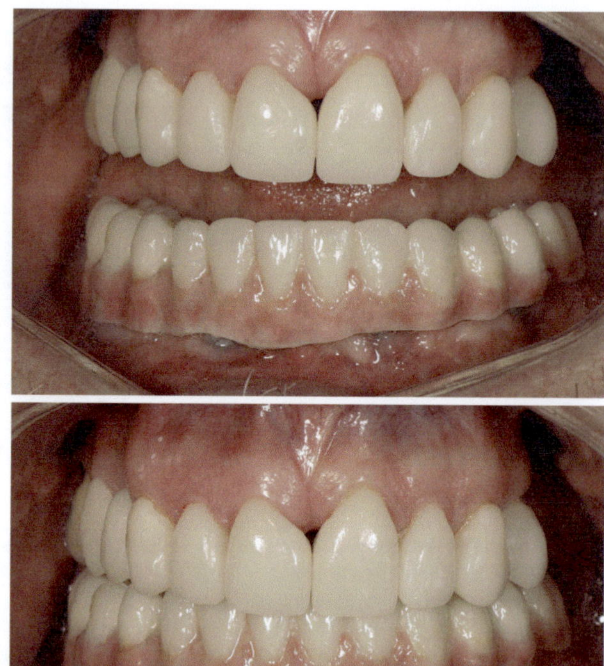

Fig. 4.21 Same patient with final zirconia entire arch mandibular reconstruction

Pearls

- Patients with myofascial pain syndrome from chronic clenching and grinding need to be treated beforehand with Botox, behavioral therapy, and muscle relaxants.
- Model surgery must be done on the casts to determine the adequate amount of alveoloplasty necessary to hide the transition zone.
- Advise patients to keep a liquid diet until the first post-op check.

Pitfalls

- Using original fixtures for the chosen implant system and new drills for the implant osteotomies is necessary to decrease the chance of bone overheating and not a perfect fitting of the prosthetic parts.

- Prosthetic complications will occur because of a conservative vertical reduction and irregular alveoloplasty of the jaw arches. This discrepancy will transition into insufficient restorative space for the strength of the prosthesis. Inadequate anterior-posterior spread of the implants and improper angulation of the implant axis will lead to weak and unaesthetic prosthetics. When planning, always strive for the emergence of axes of the multiunit abutments to come as close as possible to the mid-arch posteriorly and palatally on the anterior teeth of the prosthesis.
- Avoid narcotics and over-sedation in these patients since they will need to be active during lab transition and loading the implants.

Further Reading

Graves S, Mahler BA, Javid B, Armellini D, Jensen OT. Maxillary all-on-four therapy using angled implants: a 16-month clinical study of 1110 implants in 276 jaws. Oral Maxillofac Surg Clin North Am. 2011;23(2):277–87. https://doi.org/10.1016/j.coms.2011.02.002, vi. PMID: 21492801.

Babbush CA. Posttreatment quantification of patient experiences with full-arch implant treatment using a modification of the OHIP-14 questionnaire. J Oral Implantol. 2012;38(3):251–60. https://doi.org/10.1563/AAID-JOI-D-12-00001. Epub 2012 Jan 17. PMID: 22250619.

Sclar AG, Cardenas JD, Von Haussen U. Diagnostically driven planning and execution of an all-on-4 treatment concept. Compend Contin Educ Dent. 2015;36(5):332–8; quiz 340. PMID: 26053636.

Butura CC, Galindo DF, Jensen OT. Mandibular all-on-four therapy using angled implants: a three-year clinical study of 857 implants in 219 jaws. Dent Clin North Am. 2011;55(4):795–811. https://doi.org/10.1016/j.cden.2011.07.015. PMID: 21933733.

Rangert B, Jemt T, Jörneus L. Forces and moments on Branemark implants. Int J Oral Maxillofac Implants. 1989;4(3):241–7. PMID: 2700747.

Maló P, Rangert B, Nobre M. "All-on-Four" immediate-function concept with Brånemark System implants for completely edentulous mandibles: a retrospective clinical study. Clin Implant Dent Relat Res. 2003;5(Suppl 1):2–9. https://doi.org/10.1111/j.1708-8208.2003.tb00010.x. PMID: 12691645.

Chapter 5
The PATZI Protocol in Maxillary Full Arch Rehabilitation

Shouvik Ponnusamy and Juan Gonzalez

Abstract Full-arch implant rehabilitation is achieved with a stable configuration of implants supporting a fixed implant-supported prosthesis. However, vast variability exists in this procedure regarding prosthetic success outcomes. The disconnect between surgical and prosthetic success is a pitfall many young surgeons or surgical residents are prone to. This is primarily due to the disconnect between the dedicated surgical and restorative procedures involved with the treatment. In the traditional "all on four" configuration, the surgeon may deem the surgery to be successful simply by being able to place four maxillary implants with appropriate primary stability and insertion torque for immediate loading. However, this definition of surgical success does not necessarily equate to equivalent prosthesis success or address the restorative nuances required of the final prosthesis design for optimal performance. It is important for the surgeon to analyze such prosthetic outcomes and nuances as a direct result of secondary outcomes of the surgery performed, such as prosthetic arch length, antero-posterior (AP) spread, length of distal extension cantilevers, bucco-palatal screw access hole positions, and restorative material thickness. These prosthetic design outcomes are affected directly by surgical implant platform position and configuration and are critical to long-term prosthetic success.

Oftentimes, due to maxillary sinus pneumatization, lack of alveolar bone height or width, or poor quality of bone for immediate loading of implants may indicate the necessity to place extra-alveolar implants. Where if extra-alveolar fixation were not utilized in such a situation, would significant prosthetic pitfalls occur, such as failing to achieve the successful prosthetic outcomes previously mentioned. The authors use the PATZI protocol when planning and performing full-arch implant rehabilitation as a systematic surgical protocol to help achieve ideal prosthetic results while

S. Ponnusamy
Niva Dental Specialists, Austin, TX, USA

J. Gonzalez (✉)
Private Practice, Austin, TX, USA

D. Amin, H. Marwan (eds.), *Pearls and Pitfalls in Oral and Maxillofacial Surgery*, https://doi.org/10.1007/978-3-031-47307-4_5

utilizing various surgical techniques, prioritizing traditional implant placement over extra-alveolar fixation, and accounting for strategic backup plans for potential future salvage procedures—the purpose of this chapter to discuss the PATZI protocol for planning and performing full-arch implant rehabilitation.

PATZI Protocol

PATZI stands for "Posterior, Anterior, Tilted, Zygomatic implant." The protocol begins with placing pterygoid implants first, establishing the most *Posterior* aspect of the fixed prosthesis, virtually eliminating distal cantilever forces. *Anterior* implants are then placed in the pre-maxilla region. The AP spread is finalized at this point, and a third set of implants are prepared to be placed between the anterior and posterior fixtures. *Tilted* implants are the third section of the protocol, specifically addressing the premolar region. If all implant placement attempts were successful at this point, the protocol would be complete, and a stable configuration of six implants would be achieved without a cantilever and with optimal full prosthetic arch length. However, if attempts along the three sections are unsuccessful, a zygomatic implant is placed to address the deficiency. For example, if a pterygoid implant cannot be placed on one side, and the tilted premolar implant position is so anterior (limited posteriorly due to anterior pneumatization of the maxillary sinuses), that it would only allow prosthetic screw access to extend to the first premolar, then a zygomatic implant would be placed, with the implant platform positioned in the first molar region (Fig. 5.1). By following a systematic, consistent, and prosthetically driven protocol, such as PATZI, the surgeon may achieve prosthetic success in addition to surgical success in full-arch implant rehabilitation.

Practical Tips

- Maxillary sinus pneumatization occurs anteriorly in addition to inferiorly; therefore, a traditional "all on four" configuration may result in posterior prosthetic screw access holes only reaching to the canines or first premolars (shortened dental arch), as opposed to second premolars or molars (ideal arch length).
- A shortened prosthetic dental arch leads to poor patient satisfaction and may only be ameliorated with the incorporation of elongated distal extension prosthetic cantilevers, ultimately resulting in undesirable biomechanical forces, leading to prosthetic complications.
- Extra-alveolar fixation follows the vertical craniofacial skeleton buttresses. Pterygoid implants, zygomatic implants, and trans-nasal implants engage the cortical bone of the pterygomaxillary buttress, zygomaticomaxillary buttress, and lateral nasal wall buttress, respectively.

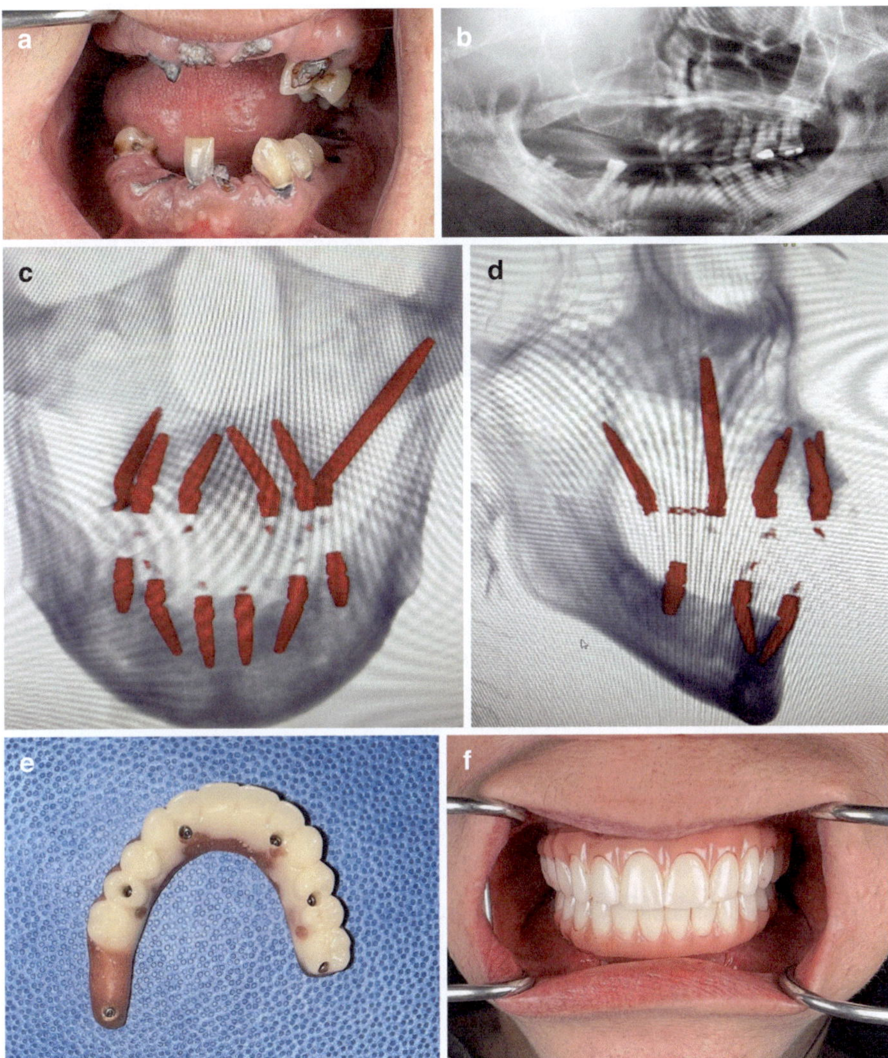

Fig. 5.1 (**a**) Pre-operative retracted intraoral view. (**b**) Pre-operative panoramic X-ray. Extensive periapical radiolucencies of left posterior maxillary teeth, with significant pneumatization of maxillary sinuses bilaterally. (**c**) Post-operative frontal 3D reconstruction view. Note how the left pterygoid implant was unable to be placed. A posteriorly based zygomatic implant was placed, preserving the superior aspect of the zygomatic bone next to the inferolateral aspect of the orbit for a second zygomatic implant, if indicated in the future. (**d**) Post-operative sagittal 3D reconstruction view. The right pterygoid implant is visualized to be angled anteriorly. A significant AP spread is appreciated. (**e**) Occlusal view of the provisional prosthesis. Note how there is no distal prosthetic cantilever present. If the left zygomatic implant was not placed, an unfavorable cantilever would have existed to attain the first molar occlusal, leading to poor biomechanical forces. (**f**) Post-operative intraoral retracted view. Immediate provisional prostheses are in place. With the arch length extending to the first molar or greater, wide and esthetic smiles are attainable in addition to optimal masticatory function

- Extra-alveolar fixation can be utilized to address the lack of alveolar bone stock and provide improved prosthetic outcomes as opposed to those without extra-alveolar fixation.
- When placing a zygomatic implant in the premolar or molar region, it is important to keep the apex of the zygomatic implant at the inferior and posterior aspect of the body of the zygoma bone. This position is intended to preserve the superior anterior bone stock of the zygoma body; should the initial zygomatic implant or traditional anterior implants fail, a second zygomatic implant may be utilized. Thus, avoid placing a zygomatic implant in the center of the zygoma body; always position the zygomatic implant apices with intention and with future planning in mind.
- The authors believe there is no "one" technique to place zygomatic implants. Intra-sinus, extra-sinus, extra-maxillary, and zygoma anatomy-guided approaches have been described. The authors believe that the planned prosthesis determines the zygomatic implant trajectory.
- Especially in thin soft tissue biotype and lack of keratinized tissue, buccal fat or pedicled subepithelial connective tissue grafts should be placed over the body of the zygomatic implant at the time of placement to reduce post-operative peri-zygomatic soft tissue recession defects.
- Pterygoid implants engage the cortical bone of the pterygomaxillary complex, which, although they do have a significant learning curve, have demonstrated high survival rates, help attain high insertion torque values, and dramatically increase AP spread from a prosthetic standpoint.

Pearls

- PATZI protocol stands for "Posterior, Anterior, Tilted, Zygomatic implant."
- Always start with placing the pterygoid implants.
- By following a systematic, consistent, and prosthetically driven protocol, such as PATZI, the surgeon may achieve prosthetic success in addition to surgical success in full-arch implant rehabilitation.
- By placing six implants along the maxillary arch instead of four, if one fails, the prosthesis may remain loaded on five implants while the failed implant is addressed.

Pitfalls

- The disconnect between surgical and prosthetic success is a pitfall many young surgeons or surgical residents are prone to.
- When utilizing osteotomes during pterygoid implant placement, sound, and haptic feedback are the primary indicators of being in the correct anatomical location and trajectory for optimal cortical stability.

Further Reading

Ponnusamy S, Holzclaw D, Gonzalez J. A systematic approach to restoring full arch length with maxillary fixed implant reconstruction: the PATZI protocol. Int J Oral Maxillofac Implants. 2023;38(5):996–1004.

Fueki K, Igarashi Y, Maeda Y, Baba K, Koyano K, Sasaki K, Akagawa Y, Kuboki T, Kasugai S, Garrett NR. Effect of prosthetic restoration on masticatory function in patients with shortened dental arches: a multicentre study. J Oral Rehabil. 2016;43(7):534–42. https://doi.org/10.1111/joor.12387.

Markowitz BL, Manson PN. Panfacial fractures: organization of treatment. Clin Plast Surg. 1989;16(1):105–14.

Ponnusamy S, Miloro M. A novel prosthetically driven workflow using zygomatic implants: the restoratively aimed zygomatic implant routine. J Oral Maxillofac Surg. 2020;78(9):1518–28. https://doi.org/10.1016/j.joms.2020.05.030.

Holtzclaw D, Telles R. Pterygoid fixated arch stabilization technique (PFAST): a retrospective study of pterygoid dental implants used for immediately loaded full arch prosthetics. J Implant Adv Clin Dent. 2018;10:6–17.

Chapter 6
Practical Tips for Alveolar Ridge Augmentation

Victoria A. Mañón and Victor M. Mañón

Abstract Prosthetic rehabilitation of the partially or completely edentulous patient requires adequate height and width of the bony alveolar ridge, particularly when using dental implants. Resorption of alveolar bone after tooth loss occurs in bucco-lingual and apico-coronal dimensions but may be accelerated in patients with periodontal disease, periapical bone loss due to dental infections, and/or trauma. Without adequate bone, treatment options may be limited without completing a ridge augmentation procedure. The purpose of this chapter is to review the indications for alveolar ridge augmentation, the various available techniques, and ridge augmentation materials.

Evaluation of the Defect

Evaluation of the defect to be reconstructed includes a clinical examination of the hard and soft tissues and a radiographic evaluation. This includes evaluating the defect's location, size, and the donor site's characteristics. Defect sizes may range from localized minimal defects to generalized, complex defects. The reconstruction of generalized complex defects can be aided by using computed tomography (CT) and computer-generated three-dimensional (3D) models. This information helps the surgeon determine how much bone grafting material is necessary and, therefore, will determine which material/donor site to use. The site of the defect should also be evaluated for the presence of infection, foreign bodies, root tips, and pathology. Additionally, the quality of the soft tissue, including the amount of keratinized gingiva, mucosal thickness, and the presence of scar tissue, should also be assessed and

V. A. Mañón (✉)
Bernard and Gloria Katz Department of Oral and Maxillofacial Surgery,
University of Texas Health at Houston, Houston, TX, USA
e-mail: victoria.a.manon@uth.tmc.edu

V. M. Mañón
Private Practice, Kingwood, TX, USA

D. Amin, H. Marwan (eds.), *Pearls and Pitfalls in Oral and Maxillofacial Surgery*, https://doi.org/10.1007/978-3-031-47307-4_6

documented. Inadequate soft tissue may require that soft tissue grafting procedures be planned in addition to bone augmentation.

Techniques for Bone Augmentation

There are multiple surgical techniques available for the augmentation of the alveolar ridge. Selection of the most appropriate technique will be determined by the location of the area to be grafted, the size of the defect, treatment goals (achieving alveolar height, width, or both), available materials (donor site availability or other commercial grafts), and operator experience and comfort.

Pearl: The success of these techniques may vary from surgeon to surgeon. Choosing the correct surgical procedure will vary based on the surgeon's skill level and comfort. The technique with the most predictable results should be selected by the respective surgeon.

Onlay Block Grafts

- Cortical and cancellous autogenous bone harvested from an intraoral or extraoral site and placed at the defect site.

  - Intraoral sites: mandible (symphysis, ramus; Fig. 6.1).
  - Extraoral sites: rib, iliac crest, tibia.

- The block can be shaped in various fashions, including saddle or veneer grafts, to address horizontal and vertical defects of the maxilla and mandible.

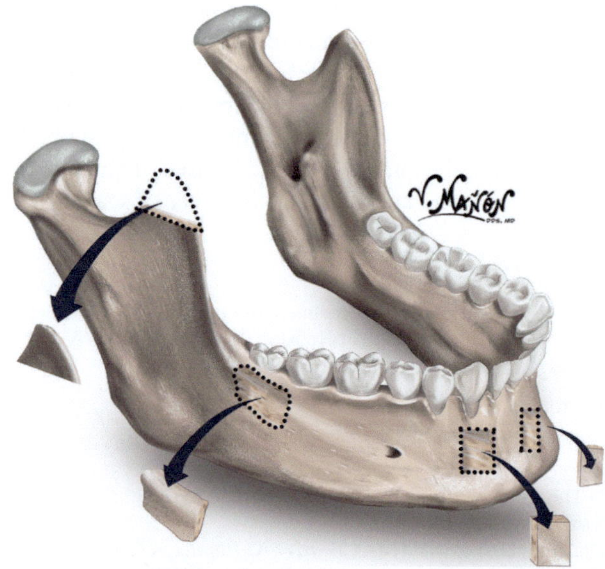

Fig. 6.1 Potential intraoral sites for harvesting onlay block grafts from the mandible include the coronoid, mandibular ramus, body, parasymphysis, and symphysis. Other intraoral sites include the maxillary tuberosity (not shown)

- The block is secured by placing screws through the cortical portion of the graft.
- Major disadvantages include
  - Donor site morbidity.
  - Increase surgical time to harvest.
  - Graft exposure results in an increased risk of infection and total loss of the graft.

Guided Bone Regeneration (GBR)

- Use a particulate graft covered by a membrane that stabilizes the graft material and prevents the ingrowth of non-osteogenic cells.
- Autologous bone, allogeneic bone, xenografts, or alloplasts may be used as the particulate.
- The membrane may be resorbable or non-resorbable.
  - Non-resorbable membranes require primary soft tissue closure over the membrane. Failure to do so may result in wound dehiscence, infections, and loss of the graft. Additionally, a second surgery is required to remove the membrane.
  - Resorbable membranes may lead to tenting, resulting in less space maintenance. While a second surgery is unnecessary, the catalytic process leads to an acidic environment, potentially impacting overall bone formation. Additionally, the rate of resorption, if accelerated, may be less ideal as a physical membrane beyond 1 month of use.
- GBR may be predictably used for the augmentation of horizontal defects.
  - Smaller defects may be successfully grafted with allograft or autograft.
  - Larger defects may require non-resorbable meshes or tenting screws with a staged approach.
- Ample blood supply and angiogenesis are critical for the success of the graft.
  - When the tooth is lost, the blood supply from the periodontium is lost. Blood supply is provided from the surrounding soft tissues and supraperiosteal blood vessels.
  - A round bur may be used to decorticate the bone to stimulate bleeding into the grafted area.

Distraction Osteogenesis (DO)

- Separation of the alveolar ridge from the underlying bone while maintaining attachment to the lingual periosteum, with slow separation of the fragments.
- Osteotomies are created, and a distraction device is placed. Devices can be internal or external.

- A bone that most closely resembles natural bone is regenerated between the fragments.
- It can be used for the distraction of the midface, maxilla, mandible, and cranial vault.
- Osteogenesis can be divided into four phases:

  - Initial placement of the distractor.
  - Latency phase: after placement of the distractor, the device is not activated for 24 h to 5 days, depending on the site to be distracted.
  - Active distraction phase: activation of the device, usually once or twice daily, for days to weeks, involving incremental traction on the bony callus.
  - Consolidation phase: The distractor is left in place for several weeks while the formed immature primary bone mineralizes. The device is removed after the completion of this phase.

- Advantages of the procedure include the generation of natural host bone in a controlled manner, concomitant generation of surrounding soft tissue, and, if initially overcorrected, resistance to relapse.
- Disadvantages of this procedure include potential malpositioning of the distracted segment due to muscle pull or improper placement of the device, risk of infection due to mucosal or soft tissue dehiscence, malocclusion, and scarring.

Osteoperiosteal Split Ridge Procedure

- Splitting of the edentulous mandibular ridge into vestibular and buccal cortical plates and opening the space in between with osteotomes.
- Primarily beneficial for the widening of the alveolar ridge.
- The procedure may occur in single or multiple stages depending on the density of the bone or the span of the bone to be expanded. Unusually dense bone or spans greater than the length of three or more teeth may require multiple stages.
- After completing the split, the site may be allowed to heal for 4–6 months, or an implant may be immediately placed if primary stability is achievable (Fig. 6.2).
- Risks include undesirable ridge fracture through the buccal plate and damage to the mental nerve (anterior mandible).

Elevation of the Maxillary Sinus with Grafting

- Elevation of the maxillary sinus membrane with the placement of grafting material.
- Used primarily in patients with pneumatized sinuses of the posterior maxilla.

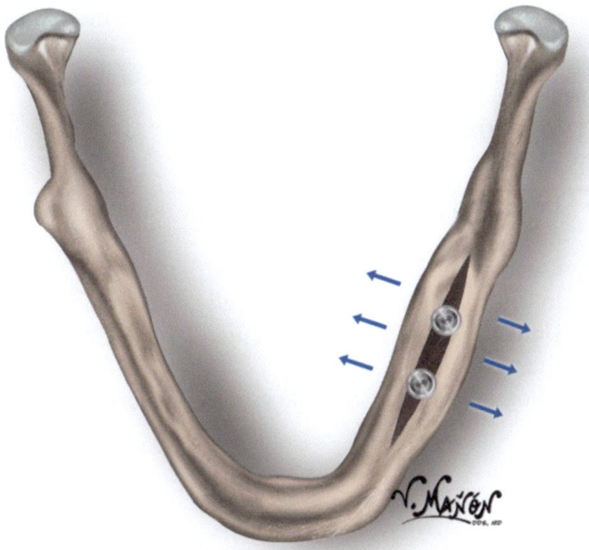

Fig. 6.2 Widening of the edentulous alveolar ridge can be achieved with an osteoperiosteal split ridge procedure. Dental implants may be immediately placed if primary stability is achievable during the split

- Various grafting materials can be placed after the elevation of the sinus membrane in order to generate the formation of bone.
- There are two primary techniques used to elevate the sinus membrane:

  - Direct, lateral window technique.
  - An indirect technique using osteotomes.

LeFort I Osteotomy with Grafting

- Down-fracturing and repositioning the atrophic maxilla in an inferior and anterior position with the placement of grafting material.
- Augmentation of the lateral maxilla may also be completed simultaneously.
- Various grafting materials may be used to fill the resulting space and the floor of the nose.

Bone Grafting Materials

Autografts

- Bone or tissue obtained from the same individual.
- Osteogenic, inductive, and conductive properties
- It is considered the gold standard for grafting materials.

- A major disadvantage includes donor site morbidity.

Allografts

- Bone or tissue obtained from the same species, but a genetically different individual
- Osteoconductive only
- In dentistry, the source is typically cadaveric bone.
- Unlike autografts, there is an increased risk of disease transmission but no donor site morbidity.
- Allografts are a resorbable grafting material.

Xenografts

- Bone obtained from a species other than humans and is used as a calcified matrix.
- Osteoconductive only.
- Bovine bone is commonly used.
- Xenografts resorb at different rates depending on differences in manufacturer processing.

Alloplastic Grafts

- Synthetic grafting material that is not obtained from a human or other animal source.
- Examples include hydroxyapatite and bioglass.
- The characteristics of each material vary with each product.
- Osteoconductive only.

Pearl: Areas grafted with resorbable materials may result in loss of the augmented bone if dental implants are not placed in the region of the graft within the timeframe of the grafting material's duration.

Pitfall: Dental implants placed in bone grafted with non-resorbable materials may fail the implant due to the formation of fibrous attachment instead of osseointegration.

Ceramic-Based Bone Graft Substitutes

- Bone grafts include ceramics, such as calcium sulfate, bioactive glass, or calcium phosphate.
- Various products have varying properties based on the material used and therefore have different applications and clinical behaviors, including the rate of resorption.

Polymer-Based Bone Graft Substitutes

- Polymers may be natural or synthetic and can be further divided into degradable or non-degradable.
- Degradable synthetic and natural polymers can be reabsorbed into the body.

Growth Factors

- Human growth factors or morphogens are responsible for regulating cellular activity for the purpose of generating (production and resorption) bone.
- It may require a carrier medium, such as collagen, for delivery.
- Examples include tumor growth factor-beta (TGF-beta), insulin-like growth factors I and II, platelet-derived growth factor (PDGF), fibroblast growth factor (FGF), and bone morphogenic proteins (BMPs).

Tissue-Engineering Techniques

- Recapitulation of an embryonic process uses a combination of materials, usually particulate bone, stem cells, and growth factors. Various combinations have been described.
- Typically used for larger continuity defects, particularly in cases of benign pathology.
- The graft may be stabilized with a titanium mesh and reconstruction plate.
- Advantages include no donor site morbidity and decreased hospital stay (as compared to free flap surgery).
- Disadvantages include the inability to develop surrounding soft tissue and significant swelling associated with the use of BMP.

Further Reading

Hansson S, Halldin A. Alveolar ridge resorption after tooth extraction: a consequence of a fundamental principle of bone physiology. J Dent Biomech. 2012;3:1758736012456543. https://doi.org/10.1177/1758736012456543. Epub 2012 Aug 16. PMID: 22924065; PMCID: PMC3425398.

Herford AS, Nguyen K. Complex bone augmentation in alveolar ridge defects. Oral Maxillofac Surg Clin North Am. 2015;27(2):227–44. https://doi.org/10.1016/j.coms.2015.01.003. PMID: 25951958.

Tolstunov L, Hamrick JFE, Broumand V, Shilo D, Rachmiel A. Bone augmentation techniques for horizontal and vertical alveolar ridge deficiency in oral implantology. Oral Maxillofac Surg Clin North Am. 2019;31(2):163–91. https://doi.org/10.1016/j.coms.2019.01.005. PMID: 30947846.

Brody-Camp S, Winters R. Craniofacial distraction osteogenesis. In: StatPearls. Treasure Island, FL: StatPearls Publishing; 2022. https://www.ncbi.nlm.nih.gov/books/NBK560915/.

Tolstunov L, Hicke B. Horizontal augmentation through the ridge-split procedure: a predictable surgical modality in implant reconstruction. J Oral Implantol. 2013;39(1):59–68. https://doi.org/10.1563/AAID-JOI-D-12-00112.

Kumar P, Vinitha B, Fathima G. Bone grafts in dentistry. J Pharm Bioallied Sci. 2013;5(Suppl 1):S125–7. https://doi.org/10.4103/0975-7406.113312. PMID: 23946565; PMCID: PMC3722694.

Block MS. The processing of xenografts will result in different clinical responses. J Oral Maxillofac Surg. 2019;77(4):690–7. https://doi.org/10.1016/j.joms.2018.10.004. Epub 2018 Oct 12. PMID: 30414391.

Melville JC, Mañón VA, Blackburn C, Young S. Current methods of maxillofacial tissue engineering. Oral Maxillofac Surg Clin North Am. 2019;31(4):579–91. https://doi.org/10.1016/j.coms.2019.07.003. Epub 2019 Aug 21. PMID: 31445759.

Part II
Anesthesia

Chapter 7
Practical Tips for Managing Pediatric Anesthesia

Sharif Mohamed

Abstract Understanding the physiological and anatomical differences between pediatric and adult patients is crucial in delivering safe anesthesia to pediatric patients. Examples of basic respiratory differences include prominent occiput, an oversized tongue, the larynx being more anteriorly cephalad, alveolar ventilation is much higher in neonates, and type I diaphragmatic muscle fibers are less, so they can get fatigued easier. These differences slowly disappear as the child grows, and the rate of disappearance of these differences differs from one child to another; thus, every pediatric patient's anesthetic plan must be individually tailored and titrated to adapt to every child-specific need.

In Anesthesiology, it is essential to realize the three distinct phases of care: Preoperative, Intraoperative, and postoperative. The Intraoperative phase of care contains three more sub-phases of care: Induction, Maintenance, and emergence. The purpose of this chapter is to discuss how to deliver safe anesthesia to the pediatric patient population along the three different phases of care.

Preoperative Practical Tips

- Sedation: Separation anxiety starts at 9 months. It could be overcome non-pharmacologically by well-selected parental presence during the induction or child-life age-appropriate distraction techniques. Separation anxiety could also be overcome pharmacologically by oral midazolam (0.5 mg/kg with a max of 20 mg, which takes 15 min to start working).
- Upper Respiratory Infections (URIs): Three red flags will need the procedure to be rescheduled in 6+ weeks: Active wheezing, fever, and somnolence. Other signs of URIs put the patient on the moderate risk spectrum, like runny nose,

S. Mohamed (✉)
Department of Pediatric Anesthesia, University of Texas Medical Branch, Galveston, TX, USA
e-mail: shmohame@utmb.edu

D. Amin, H. Marwan (eds.), *Pearls and Pitfalls in Oral and Maxillofacial Surgery*, https://doi.org/10.1007/978-3-031-47307-4_7

coughing, and congestion. In this situation, if the anesthesia provider is comfortable managing complications like laryngospasms, the procedure can proceed; if not, it should be postponed for 2 weeks.

- Family history: In the pediatric population, family history is a unique risk factor for postoperative nausea and vomiting (PONV). So if parents had PONV, the kid is at a higher risk of having PONV, especially if the surgery is more than 30 min and the kid is 3 years old or older. Another essential point to ask is if there is any history of problems with anesthesia running in the family, like fever under anesthesia "Malignant Hyperthermia (MH)" since this will impact the anesthetic plan by avoiding MH triggers like inhalational anesthetics and succinylcholine. The breathing circuit should be washed with high flow or a filter, and vaporizer should be removed.
- History and Physical: Important points to verify in history:

  - Does the kid snore during sleep? If yes, is it every single night? If yes, this kid has an element of sleep apnea, so minimize opioids, use half of what is usually used, and augment analgesia with NSAIDs or IV Acetaminophen.
  - Was the kid born with heart defects, turning blue, or heart murmurs? If yes, then the kid may need further cardiac assessment.
  - Was the kid born in preterm labor? If the anesthetic is happening within the 60 weeks postconceptual age, the baby will need to be admitted on telemetry overnight for risk of apnea of prematurity.
  - Was the kid intubated as a neonate before? If yes, expect an element of subglottic stenosis that may need the breathing tube's downsizing.
  - Is the kid known to have asthma or need breathing treatment? If yes, then auscultate the front and back of the chest to listen to the lung base; if wheezing on the day of surgery, then postpone for 6 weeks and refer to a pediatrician for optimization with inhalers/steroids.

- Syndromic patients: Kids known to have any syndromic congenital anomalies or developmental delays will need a closer assessment of their cardiac function and facial features to assess difficulty with intubation. A short mandible, prominent upper teeth, limited neck extension, and dysmorphic features are signs of difficult intubation. Kids who are bedridden or wheelchair-bound, or any kid less than 1 year old will need to avoid succinylcholine due to the risk of fatal hyperkalemia unless it is an emergency. Kids under 1 year old may have a hidden myopathy that did not show yet since they did not start walking.

Intraoperative Practical Tips

Induction

- Standard monitors include EKG, blood pressure, and pulse oximeter. Temperature measurement is only essential if significant temperature changes are expected (neonates, any use of active warming devices) or surgery is more than 1 h.
- Medications: Standard induction medications plus emergency medications to be used in case of pediatric emergencies, which include: Atropine (20 mic/kg with a minimum of 100 mics), Succinylcholine (2 mg/kg), and Epinephrine (10 mic/kg, another syringe of 1 mic/kg may be needed if severe bronchospasms or pulmonary hypertensive crisis is expected).
- If suspecting a difficulty with airway management, have backup plans like video-assisted laryngoscopy equipment, fiberoptic, and LMA. If expecting difficulty with airway management, keep the patient spontaneously breathing by inhalational induction; after three failed intubation trials, consider waking up the patient and aborting the procedure. Multiple trials can cause airway edema and convert a cannot intubate scenario into a cannot ventilate scenario, a life-threatening scenario that may need a surgical airway. A straight laryngoscope blade is more helpful in kids under 2 years old since the larynx is more anterior and cephalad, and the tongue is bigger compared to the oral cavity size. I always teach to use the straight blade as a curved blade, i.e., go to the Valecula and do not catch the epiglottis. The reason is that not catching the epiglottis is a less traumatic intubation with less risk of laryngeal edema, and it is technically more straightforward. It allows visualization of the epiglottis, which is the standard gold landmark for the airway. It avoids stimulating the vagus. It gives a bigger space for instrumenting and visualizing the glottic opening.
- Inhalational induction: Works quickly in babies due to higher alveolar ventilation wash-in ratio. It is essential to wait for the inhalational anesthetic to equilibrate at the brain level, which needs extra few minutes. The main benefit of inhalational induction is that it maintains the spontaneous breathing effort intact.
- Laryngospasms: If trying to ventilate a patient and, after optimization, still cannot ventilate with no chest rise, then consider this a laryngospasm until proven otherwise. First action is to deliver positive pressure ventilation, starting at 20 cmH_2O but can go up on the APL valve to 70. If this does not help, consider deepening the kid back into deep anesthesia by pushing propofol 1 mg/kg or more. Deepening works if an IV is available during a laryngospasm (laryngospasm during extubation). If deepening does not work or the kid has no IV, consider an IM injection of Succinylcholine 2 mg/kg. After breaking a laryngospasm, consider reintubation and fully awake extubation to avoid another laryngospasm.

Maintenance

- Fluid balance: Give a 20 mL/kg fluid bolus of lactated ringer for short procedures. If the procedure is more than an hour, then maintenance may need to be calculated, and dextrose 10% may be used for maintenance in neonates.
- Temperature: Babies have a bigger body surface area compared to their body mass. This makes them get cold quicker, so a warming blanket may be helpful for longer surgeries. However, due to the same physical principle, they can get overheated too quickly, so the core body temperature needs to be monitored anytime active warming is used.
- Cardiopulmonary reserves: Pediatric patients have limited reserves; thus, they drop their oxygen saturation quickly if ventilation is interrupted. This is because their oxygen demand is higher (higher metabolic rate), and their oxygen supply is lower (lungs collapse easier) when apneic.
- Ventilation: Historically, babies are better ventilated using pressure mode rather than volume mode. Pressure mode compensates for tube leaks when an uncuffed tube is used and avoids the risk of pneumothorax if compliance suddenly changes.
- Medications: Muscle relaxants are rarely needed in most infants because inhalational anesthetics have some muscle-relaxing effect, giving enough muscle relaxation for most surgeries, yet extra muscle relaxation may be needed. Succinylcholine is only used for emergencies, so non-depolarizing muscle relaxants are the most commonly used. To achieve analgesia, you can use opioids (use fewer opioids if the kid has sleep apnea), or NSAIDs (usually avoided in kids less than 6 months old), or IV acetaminophens, or a low dose of ketamine (0.1–0.2 mg/kg), or adding some nitrous to the gas mixture which can provide some intraoperative analgesia but no postoperative analgesia.

Emergence

- Deep vs. awake extubation: Deep extubation avoids coughing and bucking, and it is speedy extubation that saves time when there is production pressure, yet the patient has to be a good candidate (no risk of aspiration, not known to be a difficult airway) and the anesthesia provider has to be comfortable dealing with deep extubation complications (laryngospasm). The checklist for successful deep extubation is a patient who is spontaneously breathing, on 100% oxygen, and does not respond to suctioning. When working alone and not comfortable dealing with laryngospasm, I recommend doing awake extubation.
- If coughing and bucking prevention is a genuine concern, but at the same time, deep extubation is not preferred, then awake extubation could be done with an umbrella coverage of some IV lidocaine (1.5 mg/kg) and/or remifentanil infusion (0.2–0.4 mic/kg/min) which can smoothen the awake extubation and minimize coughing.

Postoperative Practical Tips

- PACU can be bypassed if the patient fulfilling the below criteria:

  - Neuro: awake, aware, alert.
  - Respiratory: Can breathe and cough freely, with more than 92% oxygen saturation when on room air.
  - Cardiac: Blood pressure and heart rate are within 20% of admission numbers.
  - Musculoskeletal: Patient can move four limbs.

- Discharge after PACU should be to Home/Floor/ICU depending on the patient's status, so if pediatric anesthesia is delivered in a location with no pediatric floor or ICU, there has to be an agreement with a nearby facility equipped with a pediatric floor and ICU for emergency admissions.
- Postoperative analgesia could be achieved by long-acting opioids (morphine, hydromorphone), NSAIDs (Ibuprofen, ketorolac), Acetaminophen, and regional analgesia (nerve blocks, infiltration). A postoperative pain management plan must be discussed with any family before discharge to home.

Pearls

- Understanding the physiological and anatomical differences between pediatric and adult patients is essential.
- There are three phases of care: Preoperative, intraoperative, and postoperative.
- Consider rescheduling patients with upper respiratory infections.

Pitfalls

- Consider thorough assessments for kids with syndromic congenital anomalies or developmental delays.
- Avoid hypothermia in babies.
- Avoid muscle relaxants in most infants.

Further Reading

Ellen McCann M, Kain ZN. The management of preoperative anxiety in children: an update. Anesth Analg. 2001;93(1):98–105. https://doi.org/10.1097/00000539-200107000-00022.

Lalwani K. Pediatric anesthesia: a problem-based learning approach. Oxford: Oxford University Press; 2018.

Lerman J, Cote CJ, Steward DJ. Manual of pediatric anesthesia. Berlin: Springer; 2016.

Overview of mechanical ventilation in neonates. UpToDate. n.d. https://www.uptodate.com/contents/overview-of-mechanical-ventilation-in-neonates. Accessed 5 Oct 2022.

Phillips NM, Street M, Kent B, Haesler E, Cadeddu M. Post-anesthetic discharge scoring criteria: key findings from a systematic review. Int J Evid Based Healthcare. 2013;11(4):275–84. https://doi.org/10.1111/1744-1609.12044.

Chapter 8
Managing Difficult Sedations

Vickas Agarwal and Thomas Schlieve

Abstract The ability to perform safe and effective outpatient intravenous sedation makes oral and maxillofacial surgery unique among other dental and medical specialties. The goal of every sedation is to create a safe and comfortable environment for both the patient and the operator so that a procedure can be completed successfully with efficient patient analgesia and amnesia. This chapter aims to provide tips and techniques for managing difficult sedations, specific patients with severe anxiety, those with frequent upper airway obstructions during sedation, and sedations in the elderly population.

Practical Tips

- Regardless of the patient or procedure, standard monitors must be used at all times, with emergency equipment immediately available

  - 3 lead EKG
  - Pulse oximeter
  - Blood pressure and pulse
  - Capnography and end-tidal CO_2
  - Supplemental oxygen delivered via a non-invasive device during sedation
  - Suction
  - Bag valve mask or another method of delivering positive pressure ventilation

V. Agarwal
Oral and Maxillofacial Surgery, Virginia Commonwealth University,
Richmond, Virginia, USA
e-mail: agarwalv@vcu.edu

T. Schlieve (✉)
Oral and Maxillofacial Surgery, UT Southwestern Medical Center, Parkland Memorial
Hospital, Dallas, TX, USA
e-mail: thomas.schlieve@utsouthwestern.edu

D. Amin, H. Marwan (eds.), *Pearls and Pitfalls in Oral and Maxillofacial Surgery*, https://doi.org/10.1007/978-3-031-47307-4_8

- Respiratory adjuncts (oral and nasal airways, endotracheal tubes, laryngoscope, etc.)
  - Stethoscope
  - Intravenous access equipment
  - Emergency drugs

- The key to effective sedation is profound local anesthesia

  - Recommend use of long-acting local anesthetic such as bupivacaine for all nerve blocks.

- Use the appropriate anesthetic at the appropriate time on the appropriate patient for the appropriate procedure.

  - Propofol—rapid onset (less than 1 min), short duration (<10 min), can be given as a bolus or infusion

    Bolus for short-term sedation—for a short procedure or toward the end of a procedure

    Infusion for continuous sedation—reserved for more prolonged procedures

    Decreases blood pressure, heart rate, systemic vascular resistance, and respiratory drive

  - Dexmedetomidine—slower onset (10–15 min), long duration (1–2 h), can be given as bolus or infusion.

    Bolus pre-procedure for long-term anesthesia for an intermediate or long-term procedure

    Decreases blood pressure, heart rate, and systemic vascular resistance with no decrease in respiratory drive

- Pre-emptive management of postoperative nausea and vomiting (PONV)

  - Consider perioperative administration of dexamethasone IV—additionally can reduce post-operative edema
  - Ask about PONV during consultation visit—what has worked for the patient in the past? Consider supplementation with an anti-emetic such as ondansetron.

- *Management of patients with severe anxiety*

  - Allow additional time during a consultation visit to discuss techniques to make the patient feel more comfortable on the day of the procedure.

    Does the patient prefer to know what is happening intraoperatively? If so, talk the patient through the steps of the procedure as they are happening. Allow the patient to select music to play in the room during the procedure and make notes in the patient chart for return visits.

  - Use of nitrous oxide and topical ethyl chloride spray or topical lidocaine before venipuncture—once intravenous access is established, wean off of nitrous oxide to 100% oxygen before the start of the procedure.

- Use of topical oral anesthetic before sedation starts to allow sufficient time prior to injections.
- Pre-medication before the procedure starts with a benzodiazepine such as Midazolam.
- Consider oral sedation with a benzodiazepine such as Triazolam in patients who may not be able to tolerate obtaining intravenous access.

- *Management of patients with frequent upper airway obstructions*

  - Perform thorough pre-anesthetic consultation—be aware of patients with a history of obstructive sleep apnea (OSA), increased body mass index (BMI), retrognathia, etc.
  - Proper positioning of the operative chair

    The patient's upper body should be approximately 45–60° from the floor—avoid laying the patient supine if possible.

    - Functional residual capacity (FRC) is up to 0.5 L lower in the supine patient due to abdominal contents displacing the diaphragm, restricting its expansion, and limiting thoracic expansion.

    Headrest or pillow should be under the occiput of the patient to allow for neck extension unless otherwise contraindicated.

  - Have additional staff available to support the airway and perform jaw thrusts as needed during the procedure.
  - Consider using a laryngeal mask airway (LMA), other supraglottic devices, or a high-flow nasal cannula if available.
  - Limit the use of opioids intra- and post-operatively to reduce the potential for respiratory depression.

- *Management of elderly patients*

  - The primary caregiver (if applicable) should be present at the consultation visits to aid in providing history, medication list, daily schedule, etc.
  - Allow additional time for a consultation visit to obtain a complete and thorough pre-anesthetic evaluation
  - It is imperative to determine if the patient has medical decision-making capacity or has a court-appointed healthcare proxy
  - Determine the patient's level of exercise tolerance

    Inquire about metabolic equivalents (METs).
    Four or more METs (climbing a flight of stairs without rest or becoming short of breath) is considered sufficient.

  - Obtain a medical consultation for patients with uncontrolled or complex endocrine, cardiac or pulmonary conditions, recent cardiac or cerebrovascular events, or those on anticoagulation/antiplatelet medication.

Consider delaying elective treatment in the setting of recent cardiac, pulmonary, or cerebrovascular events.

Consider treatment under local anesthetic in multiple visits or treatment under general anesthesia in the operating room for acute treatment.

- Be aware of physiologic changes that occur with age

  Decreased sensitivity of baroreceptors, stiffening of peripheral vasculature and myocardium, decreased lung compliance, decreased blood flow to peripheral organs, less sensitive cough reflex.

  Any of the above can put an elderly patient at higher risk for hypotension, hypoventilation, end-organ damage, slower metabolism of anesthetic agents, and aspiration.

- Administer anesthetic agents at lower doses, and a slower rate—these patients have an increased response to a smaller dose as compared with younger patients.

  Avoid benzodiazepines and anticholinergic medications when possible, as these agents can potentiate delirium.

- Expect a longer recovery for elderly patients

  Slower metabolism of drugs

  May require additional assistance with transport

Pearls

- The key to effective sedation is profound local anesthesia.
- Use the appropriate anesthetic at the appropriate time on the appropriate patient for the appropriate procedure.

Pitfalls

- Consider pre-medication prior to procedure.
- Perform thorough pre-anesthetic consultation—be aware of patients with a history of obstructive sleep apnea (OSA), increased body mass index (BMI), and/or retrognathia.
- For elderly patients: administer anesthetic agents at lower doses and at a slower rate.

Further Reading

Fonseca RJ. Oral and maxillofacial surgery. 3rd ed. Amsterdam: Elsevier; 2018.

American Association of Oral and Maxillofacial Surgeons (AAOMS). Parameters of care: AAOMS clinical practice guidelines for oral & maxillofacial surgery, sixth edition. J Oral Maxillofac Surg. 2017;75(Suppl 1):e34–49.

Pardo MC, Miller RD. Basics of anesthesia. 7th ed. Amsterdam: Elsevier; 2018.

Fossum K, Love SL, April MD. Topical ethyl chloride to reduce pain associated with venous catheterization: a randomized crossover trial. Am J Emerg Med. 2016;34(5):845–50.

Chapter 9
Non-opioid Analgesic Pain Management

Dina Amin, Victoria A. Mañón, and Franco Pedro

Abstract Liposome bupivacaine injectable suspension (LB, EXPAREL®, Pacira Pharmaceuticals Inc., San Diego, CA) is a long-acting bupivacaine hydrochloride (HCL). LB is loaded in a multivesicular liposome (DepoFoam) which causes a slow and prolonged release of bupivacaine HCL. Several studies have demonstrated that LB infiltration reduces postoperative pain after third molar extraction and/or dental implant surgery. Furthermore, LB injection reduced postoperative pain in abdominal wall augmentation, total knee arthroplasty, augmentation mammaplasty, and/or mastectomy with tissue expander and/or implant reconstruction. The purpose of this chapter is to review the pearls and pitfalls in utilizing Liposome Bupivacaine Injectable Suspension for postoperative pain management.

Practical Tips

Preoperative Consideration

- LB should be used cautiously in patients with hepatic disease.
- LB is contraindicated for patients who are allergic to amide local anesthetics and/or its preservatives.
- LB vial is available in two doses: 133 mg (10 mL) and 266 mg (20 mL).
- For adults, the maximum dose of LB is 266 mg.

D. Amin (✉)
Department of Oral and Maxillofacial Surgery, University of Rochester, Rochester, NY, USA
e-mail: dina_amin@urmc.rochester.edu

V. A. Mañón
Department of Oral and Maxillofacial Surgery, University of Texas Health at Houston, Houston, TX, USA

F. Pedro
Dallas Fort-Worth Oral and Maxillofacial Surgery, Irving, TX, USA

© The Author(s), under exclusive license to Springer Nature Switzerland AG 2024
D. Amin, H. Marwan (eds.), *Pearls and Pitfalls in Oral and Maxillofacial Surgery*, https://doi.org/10.1007/978-3-031-47307-4_9

- Do not use the vial if there is a color variation (LB normal color is white to off-white); there is particulate within the solution, previously frozen vials and/or exposed to high temperatures (>104 °F or 40 °C).
- The recommended dose is based on the surgical site size and the required volume to cover the area.
- For large surgical sites, LB expansion is recommended. Expansion can be done with normal saline, ringer lactate solutions, or bupivacaine HCL.
- LB vial should not be expanded (i.e., diluted) with water or other hypotonic agents.
- To ensure early analgesic onset: (1) expand LB with bupivacaine HCL, or (2) inject bupivacaine HCL immediately before LB injection.
- It is contraindicated to use LB with a non-bupivacaine local anesthetic because the non-bupivacaine local anesthetic will accelerate the release of bupivacaine from the multivesicular liposomes (DepoFoam) and lead to a shorter duration and/or unpredictable analgesia time.
- Before administering LB, make sure that the antiseptic solution is dry. LB should not come into contact with antiseptic solutions such as povidone-iodine.

Intraoperative Consideration

LB Injection Protocol

- Gently shake LB vile to resuspend the liposome particles.
- Use a 25-gauge needle to maintain the structural integrity of LB particles.
- Aspirate before injection to avoid intravascular injection.
- The intravascular injection can result in cardiac and neurological side effects such as convulsions or cardiac arrest.
- Inject LB slowly and deeply (1–2 mL per injection) into soft tissue (Fig. 9.1).
- Use the moving needle technique (injecting while withdrawing the needle).
- Ensure injection sites overlap.
- If non-bupivacaine local anesthetics were used, the surgeon should wait at least 20 min before injecting LB.

  - Non-bupivacaine local anesthetics should not be administered into a surgical site after LB has been injected.
  - When bupivacaine is co-administered with LB, consider maintaining a ratio of 1:2 (LB to bupivacaine).
  - Always remember that the toxic effects of these local anesthetics are additive.

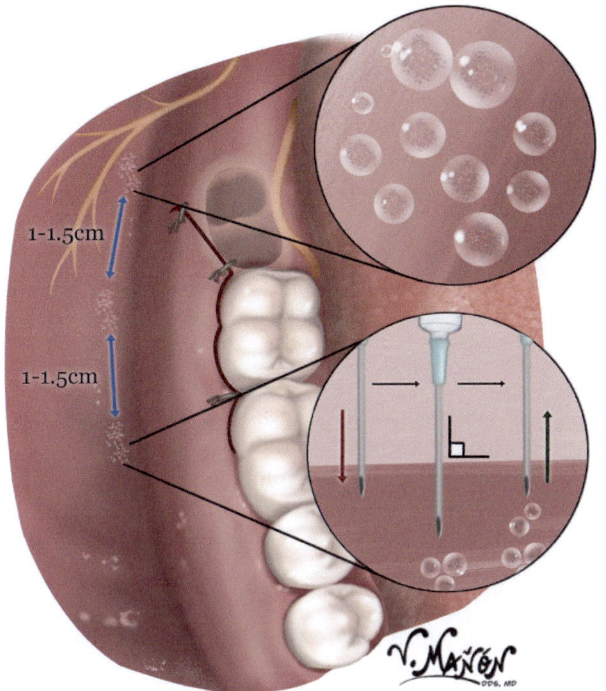

Fig. 9.1 The preferred injection locations after the third molar surgery

Postoperative Consideration

- The duration of action for LB injection is 72 h.
- Systemic plasma levels can persist for 96 h.
- LB injection has been associated with adverse side effects, including:

    - Central nervous system (CNS) reactions

        Symptoms include nausea, vomiting, CNS excitation and/or depression, persistent anesthesia, paresthesia, weakness, and paralysis.
        Excitatory symptoms usually proceed to convulsions. Those symptoms may include restlessness, anxiety, dizziness, tinnitus, blurred vision, pupillary dilation, or tremors.
        Depressive symptoms may include drowsiness that progresses to unconsciousness and respiratory arrest.
        Reported neurological symptoms have been slow, incomplete, or without recovery.

- Cardiovascular system reactions

  LB depresses cardiac conductivity and excitability, which may lead to atrioventricular block, ventricular arrhythmias, and cardiac arrest.
  LB decreases cardiac output and arterial blood pressure by decreasing cardiac contractility via peripheral vasodilation.

- Allergic reactions

  Reported allergic reactions are rare but may be due to hypersensitivity to the anesthetic or other components of the solution.
  Cross-reactivity to other amide-anesthetics has been reported.

- Chondrolysis

  This complication has been primarily seen after non-approved infusion of local anesthetics into the shoulder joint.
  Symptoms include joint pain, stiffness, and limited range of motion.
  There is no effective treatment for chondrolysis; management techniques have included arthroplasty or joint replacement.

- Methemoglobinemia

  Patients at risk for the development of methemoglobinemia include those with glucose-6-phosphate deficiency, congenital or idiopathic methemoglobinemia, infants less than 6 months of age, existing cardiac or pulmonary compromise, or concurrent exposure to oxidizing agents and their metabolites.
  Methemoglobinemia is a complication that has been associated with the use of other local anesthetics.
  Symptoms include cyanotic skin discoloration and/or abnormal coloration of blood. Elevated methemoglobin levels have also been associated with seizures, coma, arrhythmias, and death.
  The offending agent should be discontinued immediately.
  Supportive care is often sufficient and includes supplemental oxygen, hydration, etc. More severe cases may require treatment with methylene blue, hyperbaric oxygen, or blood transfusion.

Pearls

- The recommended dose is based on the surgical site size and the required volume to cover the area.
- For adults, the maximum dose of LB is 266 mg.
- LB injection is technique sensitive; adhering to the recommended protocol will ensure optimum outcomes.

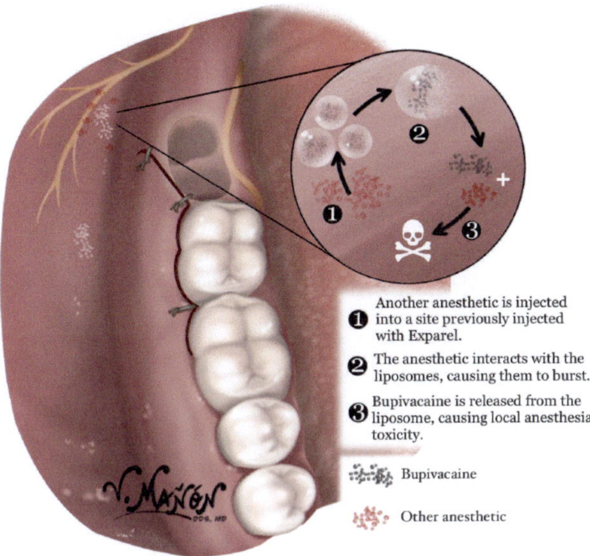

Fig. 9.2 The interaction between the liposomal anesthetic and local anesthetic with bursting liposomes

Pitfalls

- Consider a 25-gauge needle or larger to maintain the structural integrity of LB particles.
- Consider expanding LB with bupivacaine HCL to ensure the early analgesic onset (Fig. 9.2).
- LB injection is technique sensitive; adhering to the recommended protocol will ensure optimum outcomes.
- Before administering LB, make sure that the antiseptic solution is dry.

Further Reading

Lieblich SE, Danesi H. Liposomal bupivacaine use in third molar impaction surgery: INNOVATE study. Anesth Prog. 2017;64(3):127–35. https://doi.org/10.2344/anpr-64-02-03. PMID: 28858553; PMCID: PMC5579813.

Kaye AD, Armstead-Williams C, Hyatali F, et al. Exparel for postoperative pain management: a comprehensive review. Curr Pain Headache Rep. 2020;24(11):73. https://doi.org/10.1007/s11916-020-00905-4.

Ilfeld BM, Viscusi ER, Hadzic A, et al. Safety and side effect profile of liposome bupivacaine (exparel) in peripheral nerve blocks. Reg Anesth Pain Med. 2015;40(5):572–82. https://doi.org/10.1097/AAP.0000000000000283.

Mooney M, Parker T, Bussell A. Does liposomal bupivacaine injection reduce postoperative opioid requirements or improve quality of life measures for maxillary orthognathic surgery?: a prospective randomized, controlled double-blind trial. J Oral Maxillofac Surg. 2018;76(10):e32–3.

EXPAREL (bupivacaine liposome injectable suspension). 2022. https://www.accessdata.fda.gov/drugsatfda_docs/label/2018/022496s9lbl.pdf. Accessed 24 Nov 2022.

Iero PT, Mulherin DR, Jensen O, Berry T, Danesi H, Razook SJ. A prospective, randomized, open-label study comparing an opioid-sparing postsurgical pain management protocol with and without liposomal bupivacaine for full-arch implant surgery. Int J Oral Maxillofac Implants. 2018;33(5):1155–64.

Surdam JW, Licini DJ, Baynes NT, Arce BR. The use of exparel (liposomal bupivacaine) to manage postoperative pain in unilateral total knee arthroplasty patients. J Arthroplasty. 2015;30(2):325–9.

Vyas KS, Rajendran S, Morrison SD, et al. Systematic review of liposomal bupivacaine (exparel) for postoperative analgesia. Plast Reconstr Surg. 2016;138(4):748e–56e.

Part III
Craniomaxillofacial Trauma

Chapter 10
Minimizing Complications in Tracheostomy and Cricothyrotomy

Hisham Marwan ⓘ, Victoria Manon, and Dina Amin ⓘ

Abstract Surgical airway management is an essential skill for oral and maxillofacial surgeons. There are two main surgical airway procedures: tracheostomy and cricothyrotomy. Technique-related complications are preventable. Emergency surgical management of the airway is associated with more complications. Complications include bleeding, tracheal-esophageal communication, a false passage between the trachea and sternum, emphysema, pneumothorax, pneumomediastinum, accidental decannulation, and tracheal stenosis. Preventing complications is easier than managing them. The purpose of this chapter is to explain the surgical technique for tracheostomy and cricothyrotomy and how to avoid intraoperative and postoperative complications.

Practical Tips for Tracheostomy

Preoperative

- Securing the airway before elective tracheostomy is important to prevent complications.
- Patient positioning with a good size shoulder roll to help extend the neck is vital.

H. Marwan
Department of Surgery, The University of Texas Medical Branch, Galveston, TX, USA
e-mail: Himarwan@utmb.edu

V. Manon
University of Texas Oral and Maxillofacial Surgery Resident, McGovern Medical School,
UTHSC School of Dentistry at Houston, Houston, TX, USA

D. Amin (✉)
Department of Oral and Maxillofacial Surgery, University of Rochester, Rochester, NY, USA
e-mail: dina_amin@urmc.rochester.edu

D. Amin, H. Marwan (eds.), *Pearls and Pitfalls in Oral and Maxillofacial
Surgery*, https://doi.org/10.1007/978-3-031-47307-4_10

- For overweight patients and females with big breast tissues, tapping the chest from the shoulder toward the feet will help retract the tissues away—careful padding before taping to prevent pressure ulcers.
- Identifying thyroid hypertrophy is vital to prevent complications. In case of enlarged thyroid tissue, it is advisable to divide the thyroid isthmus (Fig. 10.1).

Intraoperative

- The transverse incision is recommended since the amount of exposure is similar to the vertical incision, and the scar is better concealed.
- The incision should be placed about one finger breadth below the cricoid.
- Avoid any injury to the cricoid to prevent subglottic stenosis.
- Stay in the midline!
- Once the thyroid isthmus is identified, a right angle is used to lift the isthmus from the pretracheal fascia. Judicious use of electrocautery will help control the bleeding.
- For overweight patients, creating a Bjork flap and suturing the edges of the anterior tracheal wall with 2–0 Nylon to the skin edges is recommended. This will help tremendously in accidental dislodgement of the fresh tracheostomy.
- Before entering the airway, ensure the assistant and the scrub nurse check the balloon of the tube, which is lubricated with jelly for easy insertion.

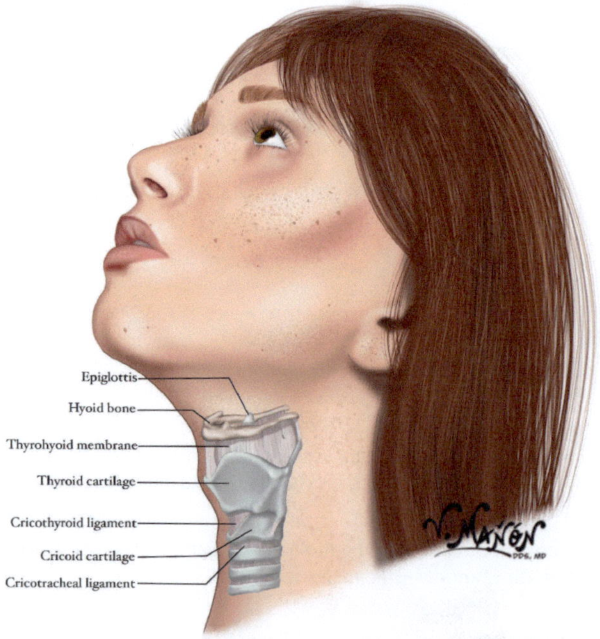

Fig. 10.1 The anatomical landmark for tracheostomy and cricothyrotomy

- At this stage, communication with the anesthesiologist is essential. The anesthesiologist should have direct access to the tube, and they are ready to pull the tube away from the surgical field.
- The anesthesiologist should never completely pull the tube out. The tube needs to be pulled up to create enough space for the tracheostomy tube. In case of failure to place the tracheostomy tube, the anesthesiologist should advance the endotracheal tube back again and ventilate the patient.
- Insertion of the tracheostomy tube should be done under direct vision. No blind attempt should be made.
- In case of a large tumor that displaces the trachea, careful dissection, hemostasis, careful studying of the radiographic images (if available), and sticking the field with a syringe filled with saline and aspirating to find air usually will help identify the trachea.
- The cricoid hook should be engaging the cricoid until the anesthesiologist confirms end-tidal CO_2.
- Suturing the superior edge of the tracheostomy tube plate will help prevent accidental dislodgement.
- Placement of Mepilex under the tracheostomy flange will help prevent pressure ulcers.

Postoperative

- Chest X-ray postoperatively will help determine the distance of the tracheostomy tube from the carina.
- In postoperative bleeding, packing SURGICEL® Absorbable Hemostat (oxidized regenerated cellulose) [New Brunswick, New Jersey] at the surgical bed will help control the oozing from the surgical site. However, the surgeon should manage active and profuse bleeding in the operating room.

Practical Tips for Cricothyroidotomy

Preoperative

- Knowing the cause of the airway obstruction (e.g., foreign body, edema, infection, laryngeal, or thyroid tumor) is helpful. The approach may vary depending on the type of upper airway obstruction.
- Cricothyroidotomy is not advised in laryngeal cancer and trauma patients where laryngotracheal disjunction is suspected.
- In children: The hyoid bone is higher; the surgeon should know the airway differences between adults and children.

Postoperative

- The conversion of cricothyroidotomy to tracheostomy is done once the patient is stable to prevent tracheal stenosis.
- Monitor the patient for subglottic stenosis.

Pearls

- Meticulous surgical technique is key in preventing complications.
- Always check the balloon of the tracheostomy cannula before entering the airway.
- Consider the conversion of cricothyroidotomy to tracheostomy once the patient is stable.

Pitfalls

- It is advisable to use a Bjork flap for overweight patients.
- Failure to insert the tracheostomy cannula under direct vision can result in a false passage.
- Cricothyroidotomy in acute laryngeal disease does not provide adequate ventilation.

Further Reading

Davis K, Campbell RS, Johannigman JA, Valente JF, Branson RD. Changes in respiratory mechanics after tracheostomy. Arch Surg. 1999;134(1):59–62.

Donaldson L, Raper R. Successful emergency management of a bleeding tracheoinnominate fistula. BMJ Case Rep. 2019;12(12).

Porter JM, Ivatury RR. Preferred route of tracheostomy–percutaneous versus open at the bedside: a randomized, prospective study in the surgical intensive care unit. Am Surg. 1999;65(2):142–6.

White AC, Kher S, O'Connor HH. When to change a tracheostomy tube. Respir Care. 2010;55(8):1069–75.

Chapter 11
Practical Tips for Open Reduction and Internal Fixation of Mandibular Subcondylar Fracture

Hisham Marwan ⓘ, Victoria Manon, and Dina Amin ⓘ

Abstract Mandibular subcondylar fractures are fractures below the most inferior point of the sigmoid notch. The reported incidence is 25% to 35%, depending on the study. Unlike most facial fractures, mandibular condyle fractures are due to indirect trauma. Typically, direct forces (i.e., trauma) to symphysis and/or parasymphysis will generate indirect forces. Transmitting the indirect forces (i.e., trauma) often results in mandibular condyle fracture/s. Several classification systems have been proposed. However, the most commonly used classification divides the mandibular condyle into three areas: (1) condylar head, (2) condylar neck, and (3) subcondyle. Condylar head fractures are located at the level of the temporomandibular joint (TMJ) capsule (i.e., intracapsular or diacapitular). Condylar neck fractures extend from the TMJ capsule superiorly to the level of the sigmoid notch inferiorly. Subcondylar fractures are below the sigmoid notch. Appropriate treatment of a mandibular condyle fracture re-establishes pre-injury occlusion, vertical facial height, speech, and mastication. There are various treatment approaches: (1) soft diet, (2) closed reduction (CR) with maxillomandibular fixation (MMF), and/or (3) open reduction and internal fixation (ORIF). The purpose of this chapter is to review pearls and pitfalls for ORIF of mandibular condyle/ subcondylar fractures.

H. Marwan
Department of Surgery, The University of Texas Medical Branch, Galveston, TX, USA
e-mail: Himarwan@utmb.edu

V. Manon
University of Texas Oral and Maxillofacial Surgery Resident, McGovern Medical School, UTHSC School of Dentistry at Houston, Houston, TX, USA

D. Amin (✉)
Department of Oral and Maxillofacial Surgery, University of Rochester, Rochester, NY, USA
e-mail: dina_amin@urmc.rochester.edu

D. Amin, H. Marwan (eds.), *Pearls and Pitfalls in Oral and Maxillofacial Surgery*, https://doi.org/10.1007/978-3-031-47307-4_11

Practical Tips

Preoperative Consideration

- The gold standard for diagnosing mandibular condyle/subcondylar fractures is computed tomography (CT) scans without contrast.
- Always look for concomitant mandibular fractures.
- Identifying fracture/s (1) location (head, neck, or subcondyle), (2) angulation, (3) dislocation, and/or (4) comminution will help to formulate the surgical plan.
- To avoid long-term functional complications such as cross and/or open bite, consider ORIF for fracture/s causes >2 mm shortening of the and/or angulated ≥30° (Fig. 11.1).

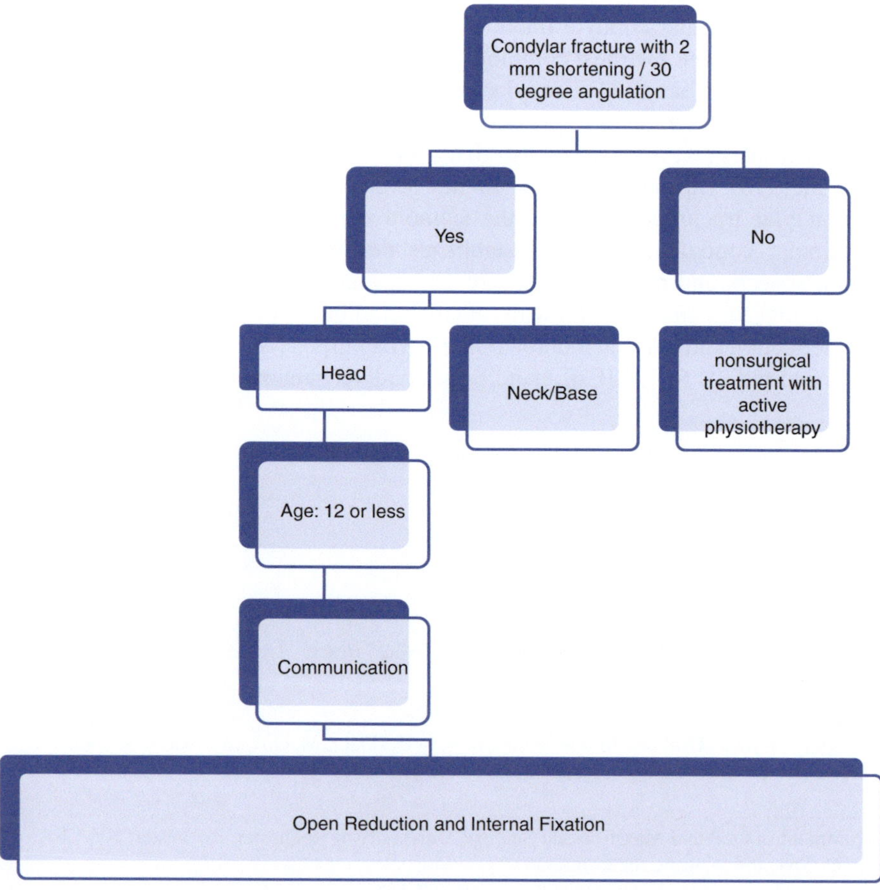

Fig. 11.1 Algorithm for management of mandibular condylar process fracture

Intraoperative Consideration

- The main surgical approaches for mandibular condyle/ subcondylar fractures are (1) preauricular, (2) high submandibular, (3) retromandibular, or (4) endoscopic (Fig. 11.2).
- The pre-auricular approach provides limited exposure to the condylar neck and subcondylar fractures. The pre-auricular approach is advised to treat condylar neck fractures.
- The high submandibular approach provides adequate exposure to condylar neck and subcondylar fractures. However, the risk of the marginal mandibular branch of the facial nerve injury is high because the incision lies immediately on top of the nerve (Fig. 11.3).
- Retromandibular approach has three modifications: (1) transparotid, (2) anteroparotid, and (3) retroparotid approaches.
- Anteroparotid and transparotid approaches have a lower incidence of facial nerve injury than retroparotid.
- The retromandibular approach provides direct and broad access to the condylar neck and subcondylar fractures. To minimize facial nerve injury, consider using a hand-held nerve stimulator to help localize the nerve branches.
- Do not use muscle relaxants while approaching the fracture.
- Once the buccal and marginal mandibular branches are identified, carefully dissect them with a McCabe nerve dissector.
- Once the fracture is exposed, ask the anesthetist to provide a muscle relaxant. Minimizing muscle pull will help with fracture mobilization and reduction.

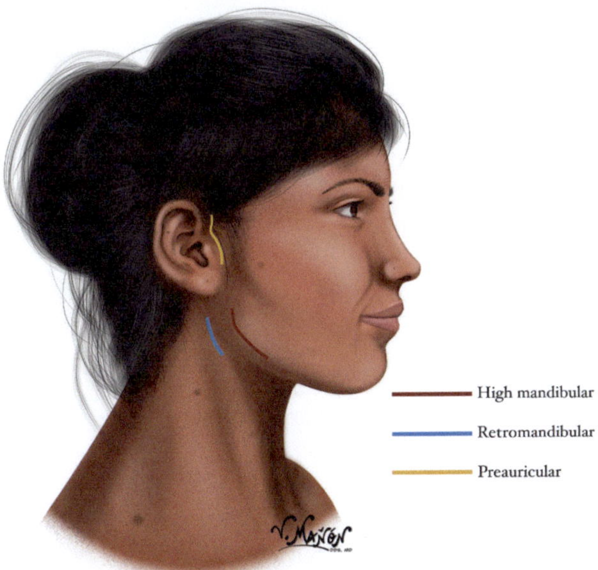

Fig. 11.2 Different surgical approaches for ORIF of mandibular condylar fractures

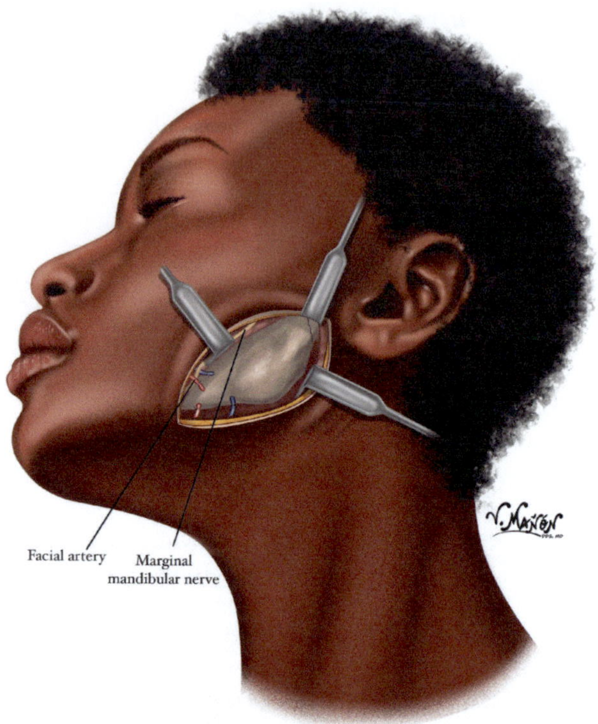

Fig. 11.3 High submandibular approach. Notice the location of the marginal mandibular branch

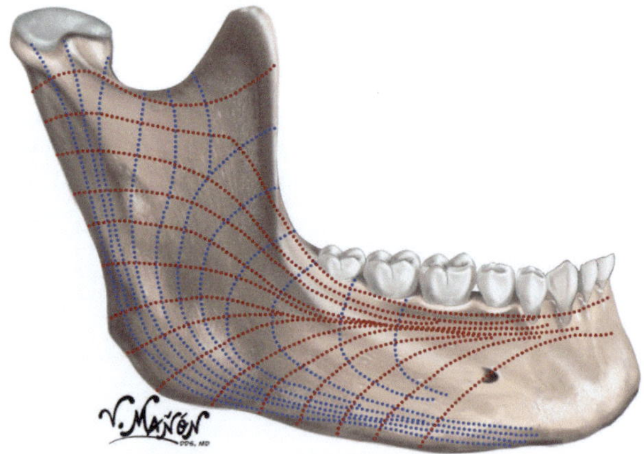

Fig. 11.4 Lines of compression and tension of the condylar process

- Do not use intermaxillary fixation (IMF) because it prevents proper fracture reduction.
- Careful alignment of the fracture segments with good anatomic reduction is important.
- Consider following Myers Lines of Osteosynthesis for more stable fixation (Fig. 11.4).

- Fixation can be done with (1) 2 mini plates following Myers lines of Osteosynthesis, (2) trapezoidal plate (best long-term results), or (3) geometric 3D plate.
- Always pay attention to the assistant during retraction to prevent neuropraxic injury with excessive pressure.
- Careful closure of the parotid-masseteric fascia with watertight closure will prevent the formation of sialocele.
- Consider cosmetic skin suturing technique; up to 8% of patients complain of postoperative scarring.

Postoperative Consideration

- Transient facial nerve paresis is common. It should resolve within 3 to 6 months.
- Sialocele is a rare complication, and it can be managed conservatively with aspiration/pressure, a scopolamine patch, and a Botox injection.

Pearls

- Consider open reduction and internal fixation (ORIF) to prevent long-term functional complications.
- For accurate nerve stimulation results, avoid muscle relaxants while approaching the fracture. In contrast, to help fracture reduction, muscle relaxants are advised.

Pitfalls

- Intra-operative intermaxillary fixation (IMF) is not recommended, as it will hinder accurate fracture reduction.
- Avoid nerve injury due to retraction by paying attention to the retraction technique.

Further Reading

Marwan H, Sawatari Y. What is the most stable fixation technique for mandibular condylar fracture? J Oral Maxillofac Surg. 2019;77(12):2522.e1–2522.e12. https://doi.org/10.1016/j.joms.2019.07.012.

Ellis E, et al. Surgical complications with open treatment of condylar process fractures. J Oral Maxillofac Surg. 2000;58:950–8.

Satishchandran S, Umorin M, Manhan AJ, Abramowicz S, Amin D. Does the treatment approach for mandibular condyle fractures impact self-perceived quality of life? J Oral Maxillofac Surg. 2022;S0278-2391(22):00971–5. https://doi.org/10.1016/j.joms.2022.10.006; Epub ahead of print.

Bagheri SC, Bell RB, Khan HA. Current therapy in oral and maxillofacial surgery. St Louis, MO: Mosby/Elsevier; 2011.

Chapter 12
Pearls and Pitfalls in Endoscopic Open Reduction and Internal Fixation of Mandibular Subcondylar Fracture

Victoria Manon and Hisham Marwan

Abstract Mandibular subcondylar fractures are fractures below the most inferior point of the sigmoid notch. There are various treatment approaches: (1) soft diet, (2) closed reduction (CR) with maxillomandibular fixation (MMF), and/or (3) open reduction and internal fixation (ORIF). Recently, several studies have shown the superiority of the ORIF approach compared to the closed treatment.

On the other hand, the risk of facial nerve injury is high with the open approach; therefore, new minimally invasive procedures are investigated and trialed. One of the most unique and well-studied approaches is the endoscopic approach for the subcondylar fracture. The purpose of this chapter is to review pearls and pitfalls in endoscopic ORIF of mandibular subcondylar fractures.

Practical Tips

Preoperative Consideration

- A careful imaging study is necessary to assess the feasibility of the endoscopic approach.
- Relative contraindications are (1) comminuted fractures, (2) displacement of the proximal segment medially and behind the distal segment, and/ or (3) proximal segment length < 3 cm.
- Remember that this technique has a steep learning curve; case selection is crucial.

V. Manon
University of Texas Oral and Maxillofacial Surgery Resident, McGovern Medical School, UTHSC School of Dentistry at Houston, Houston, TX, USA

H. Marwan (✉)
Department of Surgery, The University of Texas Medical Branch, Galveston, TX, USA
e-mail: Himarwan@utmb.edu

D. Amin, H. Marwan (eds.), *Pearls and Pitfalls in Oral and Maxillofacial Surgery*, https://doi.org/10.1007/978-3-031-47307-4_12

Intraoperative Consideration

- Intermaxillary fixation (IMF) is generally not required for isolated mandibular subcondylar fracture. The author recommends IMF with unstable fracture segments.
- This approach is considered a transoral approach. The incision is similar to the mandibular sagittal split osteotomy incision.
- Careful protection of the Stenson's duct during incision to prevent Stenson's duct stenosis.
- Wide periosteal dissection is required with releasing the Pterygomasseteric sling. This step is critical to help mobilize the fractured segments.
- The dissection should proceed toward the sigmoid notch; then, the sigmoid notch retractor should be placed gently at the notch.
- The first assistant should hold the retractors with the mounted scope, and the primary surgeon should perform the ORIF.
- During fixation, the right-angle drill and screwdriver are easier to use than the transbuccal trocar.
- The optical retractor is a specialized mount to hold the scope and provide retraction simultaneously. The retractor should be placed behind the posterior border of the ramus. Be careful when retracting not to displace the fracture (Fig. 12.1).
- The authors recommend using a 4 mm diameter rigid scope with 0-degree and 30-degree optic lenses.
- The right-angle drill should be set at 15000 rounds per minute (rpm) or less to prevent overheating the bur and possible breakage.
- One of the most challenging steps in this procedure is fixation. Using a Trapezoid plate will simplify fixation and provide adequate stability to the fractured segments (Fig. 12.2).
- Using a long nerve hook to hold the plate while drilling is helpful. Confirm the plate's position before drilling.
- It is critical to place the first screw at the inferior part of the plate, do not tighten the screw to allow plate adjustment if needed. The second screw should be placed at the superior part.

Postoperative Consideration

- The risk of facial nerve injury is extremely low to non-existent.
- Wrapping the head with pressure dressing such as Coban for 24 h will help reduce the amount of swelling postoperatively.
- Always obtain a radiographic image postoperatively to assess the reduction and fixation after the procedure.

Fig. 12.1 The optical retractor is placed at the posterior border of the ramus

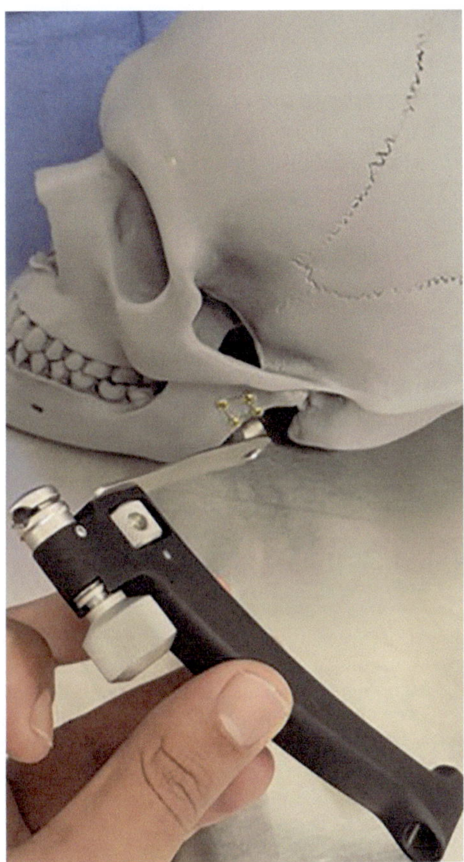

Fig. 12.2 The use of a trapezoid plate for endoscopic fixation for the subcondylar fracture

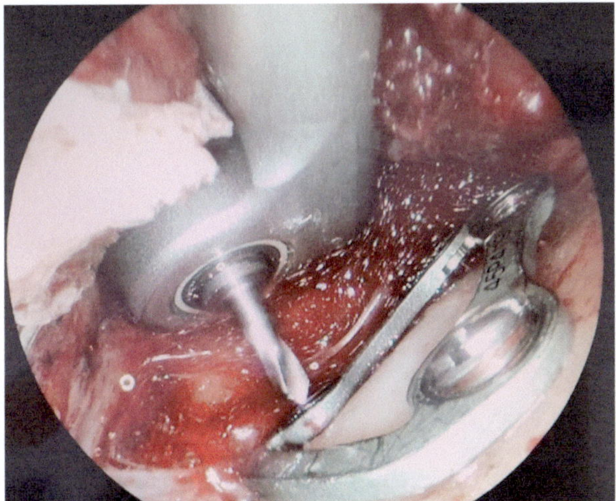

Pearls

- Appropriate use of an endoscope can facilitate fracture visibility.
- Appropriately designed instruments facilitate fracture reduction and fixation.
- Always release the Pterygomasseteric sling.

Pitfalls

- Intra-operative intermaxillary fixation (IMF) is recommended with unstable fracture segments.
- Consider using the right-angle drill and screwdriver for fixation.
- Consider using a trapezoid plate.

Further Reading

Anehosur V, Joshi A, Rajendiran S. Endoscopic-assisted intraoral open reduction internal fixation of mandibular subcondylar fractures: initial experiences from a tertiary-care maxillofacial center in India. Craniomaxillofac Trauma Reconstr. 2018;11(3):183–91. https://doi.org/10.1055/s-0037-1603457; Epub 2017 Jun 12. PMID: 30087747; PMCID: PMC6078704.

Anehosur V, Kulkarni K, Shetty S, Kumar N. Clinical outcomes of endoscopic vs. retromandibular approach for the treatment of condylar fractures-a randomized clinical trial. Oral Surg Oral Med Oral Pathol Oral Radiol. 2019;128(5):479–84. https://doi.org/10.1016/j.oooo.2018.12.007; Epub 2018 Dec 14. PMID: 31227460.

Marwan H, Sawatari Y. What is the most stable fixation technique for mandibular condylar fracture? J Oral Maxillofac Surg. 2019;77(12):2522.e1–2522.e12. https://doi.org/10.1016/j.joms.2019.07.012.

Chapter 13
Pearls and Pitfalls in Orbital Fracture Repair

Darin T. Johnston and David B. Powers

Abstract The position and movement of the globe are affected by the osseous confines of the orbit, multiple supporting ligaments, and the intraorbital fat. Orbital fractures can disrupt these structures leading to diplopia and cosmetic deformities. Therefore, clinical and radiographic findings drive indications for surgical intervention. Orbital fractures can be repaired in acute or subacute phases. However, inadequate reduction of herniated orbital contents or implant malposition may worsen the functional and cosmetic outcomes requiring a revision procedure. A complete understanding of the deep orbit anatomy and intraoperative imaging can prevent these errors. The purpose of this chapter is to review pearls and pitfalls in orbital fracture repair.

Practical Tips

Preoperative Consideration

Radiographic Evaluation

- Use the bone and soft tissue computed tomography scans (CT) windows to identify the location and size of the displaced orbital fractures and extraocular muscle morphology.
- Disruption of the fascioligamentous sling frequently correlates with a rounded or vertically orientated inferior rectus muscle. The Orbital Index is a simple tool

D. T. Johnston
Uniformed Services University, Craniomaxillofacial Trauma/Reconstruction, Oral and Maxillofacial Surgery, David Grant Medical Center, Fairfield, CA, USA

D. B. Powers (✉)
Oral and Maxillofacial Surgery, Division of Plastic, Maxillofacial and Oral Surgery, Duke Craniomaxillofacial Trauma Program, Craniomaxillofacial Trauma and Reconstructive Surgery, Durham, NC, USA
e-mail: david.powers@duke.edu

D. Amin, H. Marwan (eds.), *Pearls and Pitfalls in Oral and Maxillofacial Surgery*, https://doi.org/10.1007/978-3-031-47307-4_13

that relies on these radiographic findings to help predict the risk for post-traumatic enophthalmos (Fig. 13.1).

- Notable findings include intraorbital and intraocular emphysema, blood, and foreign bodies; lens subluxation; and position of the periorbital tissues.
- Neurosurgical consultation is warranted for displaced orbital roof fractures.

Clinical: Initial Consultation

- A thorough clinical examination of the globe's appearance and function is important.
- Dyscoria (abnormal pupil shape) and an easily compressible globe may indicate globe rupture.
- Other pertinent findings that merit ophthalmologic consultation include (1) changes in visual acuity, visual fields, and/ or color perception; (2) asymmetric intraocular pressures; (3) restricted eye movements; (4) eyelid ptosis; (5) binocu-

Fig. 13.1 The orbital index stratifies fractures by size, location, and inferior rectus muscle rounding. Each component is scored from 0 to 2; the composite score is the sum of its component values. A score of 4 or more predicts that the patient is more likely to develop enophthalmos without repair. *CT* computed tomography. (Reproduced from De Ruiter)

THE ORBITAL INDEX

1. SIZE§ (score 0-2)
   - ☐ <1cm² = **0 points**
   - ☐ 1-2cm² = **1 point**
   - ☐ >2cm² = **2 points**

2. LOCATION† (score 0-2)
   - ☐ Anterolateral = **0 points**
   - ☐ Anterolateral = **1 point**
   - ☐ Posterolateral = **1 point**
   - ☐ Posterolateral = **2 points**

3. ROUNDING OF THE INFERIOR RECTUS MUSCLE¥ (score 0-2)
   - ☐ Inferior rectus muscle height-to-width ratio <1 = **0 points**
   - ☐ Inferior rectus muscle height-to-width ratio ~1 = **1 point**
   - ☐ Inferior rectus muscle height-to-width ratio >1 = **2 points**

§Approximated as the product of the largest defect size measured on sagittal CT multiplied by that on coronal CT.

†One point assigned if the fracture involves the posterior floor and one point assigned if the fracture involves the medial floor

¥Assessed on coronal CT. Score 0 if wider than tall, score 1 if round, and score 2 if tallerthan wide.

lar and monocular diplopia; (6) hyphema, (7) dyscoria, (8) anisocoria, (9) abnormal pupillary light reflex, and/ or (10) trigeminal paresthesia.

- Entrapment of extraocular muscles or periorbital tissue within the fracture may lead to muscular necrosis, regardless of displacement. These patients are frequently pediatric and present with restricted eye movements, nausea, vomiting, and symptoms of trigeminocardiac reflex, including bradycardia, hypotension, or apnea. Emergent surgical intervention is indicated.

Clinical: Follow-Up Exam

- When non-operative management is employed, the initial follow-up exam should be performed at 2 weeks. Restricted extraocular movements, globe malposition, binocular diplopia, and an Orbital Index Score predictive of developing enophthalmos indicate early repair.
- A second follow-up exam should be performed in 1–3 months.
- Subacute and late repair, when indicated, can be performed with similar outcomes as early repair.

Ophthalmologic Consultation

- Ophthalmologic consultation should be considered for all patients with positive findings outlined above before surgical intervention.
- Persistent diplopia associated with ophthalmoplegia or hypoglobus may be improved with Fresnel prisms or strabismus surgery.

Intraoperative Consideration

- Include both eyes in the surgical field for comparison of globe position and projection.
- Before incision, determine the range and laxity of eye movements with forced duction.
- Alert the anesthesia provider that a trigeminocardiac reflex may occur during globe retraction and reduction of the orbital contents.

Transconjunctival Approach

- The second (inferior) vascular arcade is a reliable landmark for the curvilinear incision.

- Care is taken to avoid perforating the skin or tarsal plate. The inferior orbital rim should be continuously palpated to guide a combination of sharp and blunt dissection directly to the inferior orbital rim.
- The incision can be extended medially or laterally with a transcaruncular extension or lateral canthotomy. A low threshold for medial or lateral extensions helps minimize the force required for adequate retraction of the eyelid.
- Retraction of the eyelid should be gentle to prevent iatrogenic injury.
- The periosteum must be closed over any surgical implant to prevent scar contracture of the anterior and posterior lamellae. This can be accomplished with interrupted 5–0 or 6–0 Vicryl sutures. The conjunctiva can be closed with several interrupted 6–0 fast-absorbing gut sutures, with some small openings to facilitate the evacuation of a potential post-operative hematoma. If Frost sutures are maintained postoperatively, it is unnecessary to close the conjunctiva.

Transcutaneous

- The subciliary approach can provide adequate access for isolated orbital floor fractures. It is challenging to access the medial orbital wall.
- Following incision and hemostasis with electrocautery, the orbicularis oculi are identified and undermined several millimeters caudally with curved scissors. A submuscular pocket is then developed lateral to medial with blunt scissors several millimeters below the inferior tarsal margin. The stepped musculocutaneous flap is completed by incising the narrow muscular bridge inferior to the tarsal plate. The periosteum is then excised anterior to the arcus marginalis, and the dissection proceeds as described below.
- Access to the lateral orbital rim is obtained by extending the skin incision laterally up to 2 cm lateral to the lateral canthus. Initially, the lateral orbital rim is approached in a supraperiosteal plane, followed by a periosteal incision over the lateral rim superior to the lateral canthal attachments. If additional exposure is needed, the canthal limbs can be fully elevated.
- The incidence of iatrogenic lid pathology is minimized in two ways. First, maintain a cuff of preseptal orbicularis oculi attached to the tarsal plate. Second, approximate, with limited sutures, the periorbita without including the adjacent orbicularis oculi muscle. The subtarsal approach is also acceptable.

Transantral and Endoscopic Transnasal

- The transantral approach can be augmented with endoscopy. Minimal globe manipulation is required making this approach optimal for patients with globe injuries who require an acute surgical intervention for orbital floor fractures. A thin, flexible implant, such as porous polyethylene, can be placed.
- The endoscopic transnasal approach allows for a minimally invasive reduction of medial orbital wall fractures and the release of an entrapped medial rectus muscle.

Orbital Dissection and Reduction of Orbital Contents

- Meticulous elevation of the periosteum overlying the anterior part of the inferior orbital rim will provide a distinct band of periosteum that is easily identified during wound closure.
- The inferior oblique will not be visualized if the dissection is maintained in the subperiosteal plane. Its origin will remain adherent to periorbita and does not require reinsertion.
- The surgeon should be intimately familiar with the landmarks of the deep orbit. These are reliable features to guide a safe and complete dissection of the orbit and are not likely to be disrupted following facial trauma:
  - Infraorbital nerve: the bundle runs parallel to the medial orbital wall and aids in establishing the correct depth of dissection in acute or delayed repairs. Following the nerve posteriorly will traverse the inferior orbital fissure.
  - The inferior orbital fissure: There are no critical structures within the fissure. The zygomatic nerve is posterior, and the infraorbital neurovascular bundle is inferior. The contents can be cauterized and incised to facilitate the reduction of orbital contents.
  - Sphenotemporal buttress: Rising superiorly and posteriorly from the fissure is the orbital plate of the greater wing of the sphenoid. The middle portion buttresses the temporal bone and is rarely fractured or displaced.
  - Palatine plate: Medial to the inferior orbital fissure/sphenotemporal buttress and superior to the infraorbital nerve is the orbital plate of the palatine bone. This stable process is rarely displaced and is the posteromedial extent of orbital dissection. An implant should rest on this stable ledge.
- Displaced fragments of the orbital floor and walls are either removed or maintained external to the orbital implant.
- A nerve hook helps reduce orbital contents. The dissection and reduction processes are complete once stable ledges are established lateral, posterior, and medial to the orbit defect. A stable superior margin should be established in cases of medial or lateral wall defects.
- When dissecting the medial orbital wall, the anterior and posterior ethmoidal arteries should be anticipated and prophylactically cauterized if encountered. Minimal pressure is applied to the medial orbital wall during dissection to prevent the fracture from worsening.
- When late repairs or revisions are performed, dissection of periorbita from the infraorbital neurovascular bundle can be tedious. Bipolar electrocautery and blunt dissection with cotton-tip applicators are invaluable. Sometimes it may be necessary to divide small portions of herniated orbital contents to establish circumferential exposure of the defect.
- Inadequate posterior dissection and reduction of orbital contents will prevent correct implant placement. An error in this situation is to undersize the implant or entrap non-reduced periorbital contents leading to postoperative globe malposition or restricted movements.

- Results of a forced duction test are compared to the pre-procedure findings to confirm that the implant does not restrict periorbital tissues.

Titanium Implants

- Contour intraoperatively to replicate orbital topography.
- It can be secured to the orbital rim and cantilevered posteriorly in rare cases when inadequate stable osseous ledges remain.
- Anatomic and patient-specific implants facilitate the reconstruction of multiwall or significant defects.

Porous Polyethylene

- They are contoured intraoperatively to approximate orbital contours.
- It is easier to visualize on CT imaging if it also contains titanium.
- If exposed or infected must be removed due to bacterial impregnation of material and the inability of antibiotics to eradicate causative organisms.

Intraoperative Imaging and Navigation

- Intraoperative CT adds minimal time to a procedure and can detect implants that are incorrectly contoured, sized, or positioned. The intraoperative revision rate for orbital implants is 31%, the highest of any facial trauma subunit. If CT is unavailable intraoperative plain film imaging (anterior-posterior and lateral skull) can detect gross errors in implant contour and position.
- Intraoperative navigation can guide intraorbital dissection and implant placement in complicated primary repairs and all secondary reconstructions. The current best practice is to confirm navigation with intraoperative CT.

Postoperative Consideration

- Immediately confirm normal pupil size and reactivity, compressible globe, and intact visual acuity in the postoperative setting. Diplopia and extraocular muscle exams are not reliable immediately postoperative.
- Antibacterial eye drops or ointment is prescribed for patients with conjunctival incisions.
- Postoperative diplopia may take 9–12 months to resolve completely.

Pearls

- Orbital Index is a simple tool that helps to predict the risk for post-traumatic enophthalmos.
- Ophthalmologic consultation should be considered for patients with changes in visual acuity, visual fields, and/ or color perception; asymmetric intraocular pressures; restricted eye movements; eyelid ptosis; binocular and monocular diplopia; hyphema, dyscoria, anisocoria, abnormal pupillary light reflex, and/ or trigeminal paresthesia.
- Intraoperative CT adds minimal time to a procedure and can detect implants that are incorrectly contoured, sized, or positioned. The intraoperative revision rate for orbital implants is 31%, the highest of any facial trauma subunit.
- Postoperative diplopia may take 9–12 months to resolve completely.

Pitfalls

- The subciliary approach can provide adequate access for isolated orbital floor fractures. It is challenging to access the medial orbital wall.
- Consider medial and/ or lateral extensions when performing a transconjunctival approach.
- Cauterize the anterior and posterior ethmoidal arteries if encountered during medial wall dissection.
- Minimal pressure is applied to the medial orbital wall during dissection to prevent the fracture from worsening.

Further Reading

Manson PN, Clifford CM, Su CT, Iliff NT, Morgan R. Mechanisms of global support and post-traumatic enophthalmos: I. The anatomy of the ligament sling and its relation to intramuscular cone orbital fat. Plast Reconstr Surg. 1986;77(2):193–202.

De Ruiter BJ, Kotha VS, Lalezar FD, Swanson MA, Kumar AR, Barmettler A, Prendes MA, Davidson EH. Orbital index: a novel comprehensive quantitative tool for prediction of delayed enophthalmos in orbital floor fracture management. Plast Reconstr Surg. 2022;150(3):625e–9e.

Evans BT, Webb AA. Post-traumatic orbital reconstruction: anatomical landmarks and the concept of the deep orbit. Br J Oral Maxillofac Surg. 2007;45(3):183–9.

Liu EH, Najarali Z, Farrokhyar F, Banfield L, McRae M. Resolution of diplopia in late repair of enophthalmos following facial trauma. J Craniofac Surg. 2018;29(4):1006–11.

Cuddy K, Khatib B, Bell RB, Cheng A, Patel A, Amundson M, Dierks EJ. Use of intraoperative computed tomography in craniomaxillofacial trauma surgery. J Oral Maxillofac Surg. 2018;76(5):1016–25.

Yu DY, Chen CH, Tsay PK, Leow AM, Pan CH, Chen CT. Surgical timing and fracture type on the outcome of diplopia after orbital fracture repair. Ann Plast Surg. 2016;76(Suppl 1):S91–5.

Chapter 14
Practical Tips for Surgical Management of Naso-Orbitoethmoid Fractures

Nathan Dombrowski, Suzanne Barnes, and George Kushner

Abstract Naso-orbitoethmoid (NOE) fractures occur in an area of the face rich in anatomy, functional subunits, and esthetic concerns. This makes repairing these fractures relatively difficult regarding surgical access and technique. Most NOE fractures occur with other midfacial or frontal sinus fractures. An intricate understanding of the underlying anatomy can provide invaluable insight into when these fractures require surgical repair. Over the years, different classifications have been proposed, but the one generally accepted is the Markowitz and Manson classification, published in 1991. This classification system includes the following: Type I fractures, defined as a single-segment central fragment without injury to the medial canthal tendon (MCT); Type II fractures, defined as comminution of the central fragment without fractures involving the bony segment where the MCT inserts; and Type III fractures, defined as comminution of the central fragment with fractures involving the bony segment where the MCT inserts or detachment of the MCT. Not surprisingly, the surgery becomes increasingly more difficult with the progression from Type I to Type III fractures. Careful consideration of the Markowitz Classification system reveals indications for surgery, which include weakness or violation of the MCT, violation of nasolacrimal drainage or the nasofrontal outflow tract (NFOT), loss of the nasal buttress, and comminution to the medial orbital wall. The purpose of this chapter is to review pearls and pitfalls for surgical management of naso-orbitoethmoid fractures.

N. Dombrowski
Oral and Maxillofacial Surgery, University of Louisville School of Dentistry, Louisville, KY, USA

S. Barnes · G. Kushner (✉)
Department of Oral and Maxillofacial Surgery, University of Louisville School of Dentistry, Louisville, KY, USA
e-mail: george.kushner@louisville.edu

D. Amin, H. Marwan (eds.), *Pearls and Pitfalls in Oral and Maxillofacial Surgery*, https://doi.org/10.1007/978-3-031-47307-4_14

Practical Tips

Preoperative Consideration

- Adequate computed tomography (CT) imaging is required to evaluate the involvement of the nasolacrimal apparatus, nasofrontal outflow tract (NFOT), degree of comminution, and type of fracture. Axial, coronal, and sagittal views and 3D reconstruction of the scans should be thoroughly examined to determine the extent of injuries.
- Be sure to note any telecanthus. A bowstring test is typically done to evaluate the MCT.
- Perform an excellent nasal examination, including bimanual and speculum examination, to note the integrity of the septum.
- Consider ophthalmological evaluation to rule out globe injury in the case of orbital fracture.
- Considering the types of exposure necessary to treat the fracture is paramount to success. These include but are not limited to coronal, existing lacerations, gull-wing, open sky, maxillary vestibular, transconjunctival, subciliary, and transcaruncular approaches.
- A preoperative discussion with the patient regarding esthetics can help determine the appropriate incisions.
- If severely comminuted, a coronal approach may be best to recover the full extent of the bony fragments. Additionally, calvarial bone grafts can be harvested as needed.
- Type I fractures can sometimes be exposed solely through a maxillary vestibular incision.
- Type II and III fractures usually require a larger exposure, with coronal being the preference in most cases.
- When accessing through a coronal approach, using a Mayfield headrest and placing the patient in reverse Trendelenburg can help position the patient.
- With panfacial fractures, NOE fractures tend to be treated last after adequate reduction and fixation of facial buttresses have been accomplished to restore proper facial height and width.

Intraoperative Consideration

- Keep dissection in a subperiosteal plane to avoid iatrogenic injury during the procedure. This area tends to be rich in anatomy.
- Identification of the MCT should be a priority. The decision on how to proceed with fixation usually emanates from assessing if the MCT is attached to a bony fragment that is amenable to fixation or whether the MCT needs reattachment via transnasal wiring or a canthal barb.

- Next, assess the medial orbital rim for the degree of comminution and available bony stock for fixation. Plate fixation is typically dictated by fracture and comminution patterns.
- Low-profile plates are preferred in this area due to easy palpability.
- Plates should be fixated to stable segments first; then, attention should be turned to fixating the more comminuted segments with screws or wire if needed.
- Reconstruction of the medial orbital wall should be done to restore proper orbital volume.
- Screw holes placed along the orbital rim can aid in the fixation of the medial orbital wall.
- Using an incision through the caruncle with Iris scissors can help with the passage of the canthal barb and minimize iatrogenic injury.
- Make sure the wire has a dense piece of MCT to attach, or the wire may pull through.
- Resuspension of the MCT should be in a posterior and superior direction.
- The canthal barb can either be passed directly through bone or suspended and fixated to an ipsilateral plate if severe comminution of the medial orbital wall exists. Just like a pulley, the wire can be pulled through the most posterior hole of the plate and then contoured back up the medial wall of the orbit to be secured to a centrally placed screw in the frontal bone.
- A 2.0-mm-long drill bit can be utilized to make a hole through the nasal cavity in a superior and posterior direction if the barb is passed directly through the bone. It is prudent to use a malleable retractor on the opposing side to protect the orbit.
- Take note of the frontoethmoidal suture on the medial wall of the orbit! This can be used to identify the level of the cribriform plate, which one should stay inferior to while drilling.
- Transnasal wiring can be done with an awl, spinal, or a suture. Either way, the wire or suture can be secured with two separate screws on the orbital rim.
- The intercanthal distance can usually be approximated to inter alar distance.
- It is appropriate to aim for a minimal overcorrection of the intercanthal distance.
- As stated, grafting may be required before canthopexy if severe comminution exists.
- It should be noted that if bilateral canthopexies are performed, they should be secured as separate units. This is because if loosening or failure were to occur on one side, the other would also loosen and/or fail.
- Reducing the nasal septum can help reestablish nasal projection and a proper nasal airway. This can be done using the Asch forceps. Be sure to seat the beaks fully posteriorly until they are completely over the septum and not crushing the tissue of the columella.
- A suture through the anterior nasal spine (ANS) can assist with a severely displaced septum as a means of fixation.
- Intraoperative CT can be used to assess for restoration of premorbid orbital volume and the projection of the NOE complex.
- Doyle splints can be placed to secure the septum. Consider placing external nasal splints to assist in soft tissue healing around the nasal bone fracture. This can be done with Xeroform gauze, thermoplastic splints or plaster splints.

- Reconstruction of the nasal bone can be done at this point and is usually accomplished with calvarial dorsal strut grafts, which can be secured to the frontal bone with a straight plate or Y-plate.
- Overcorrecting nasal projection usually has a better outcome than underprojection regarding the perception of intercanthal width.
- Layered closure is preferred. Failure to resuspend the flap near the frontozygomatic suture has been shown to produce an aged face.

Postoperative Consideration

- Complications can include cosmetic or functional deficits. Cosmetically, these include telecanthus, saddle nose deformity, and poorly placed surgical incisions resulting in scars.
- Enophthalmos can result if orbital reconstruction does not restore proper orbital volume.
- Nasolacrimal injury is a common complication with epiphora as a result. This can be treated with dacryocystorhinostomy for up to 4–6 weeks from the injury.
- Cerebrospinal fluid (CSF) leaks can occur if the cribriform plate is violated. However, usually these resolve with observation in 2–10 days.
- If there is a persistent CSF leak, a neurosurgeon should be consulted to provide lumbar drainage or extracranial versus intracranial procedures.
- Saline solution nasal spray can help treat symptoms of rhinosinusitis. This is due to irrigation and clearance of the nasolacrimal duct, the frontonasal duct, and the Ostia of the maxillary sinus.
- Mucolytics such as guaifenesin can be helpful in the postoperative period to aid in the clearance of mucus. They effectively thin the mucus, allowing for more straightforward clearance when the mucociliary apparatus may be hypofunctional due to edema.
- Decongestants may also be considered. They typically act via alpha adrenergic-mediated vasoconstriction. These agents should be used for up to 3 days due to tachyphylaxis.
- Lastly, intravenous (IV) antibiotics with sinus flora coverage are indicated for up to 24 h after the surgery. There is no benefit to further antibiotic therapy.

Pearls

- With panfacial fractures, NOE fractures tend to be treated last after adequate reduction and fixation of facial buttresses have been accomplished to restore proper facial height and width.
- Intravenous (IV) antibiotics with sinus flora coverage are indicated for up to 24 h after the surgery.
- The frontoethmoidal suture on the medial wall of the orbit can be used to identify the level of the cribriform plate.

Pitfalls

- The selected surgical approach is paramount to success.
- Resuspension of the medial canthal tendon (MCT) should be in a posterior and superior direction.
- Overcorrecting nasal projection usually has a better outcome.

Further Reading

Markowitz BL, Manson PN, Sargent L, et al. Management of the medial canthal tendon in nasoethmoid orbital fractures: the importance of the central fragment in classification and treatment. Plastic Reconstruc Surg. 1991;87:843.

Miloro M, Ghali GE, Larsen PE, Waite PD. Peterson's principles of oral and maxillofacial surgery—third edition: Volume One. Shelton, CT: People's Medical Publishing House; 2012.

Kademani D, Tiwana P. Atlas of oral and maxillofacial surgery. St. Louis, MO: Elsevier; 2016.

Dorafshar A, Rodriguez E, Manson P. Facial trauma surgery: from primary repair to reconstruction. St. Louis, MO: Elsevier; 2020.

Chapter 15
Pearls and Pitfalls for Surgical Management of Panfacial Fractures

Yoh Sawatari

Abstract Panfacial fracture are facial fractures simultaneously involving the upper, middle, and lower thirds of the face. Fractures of the frontal sinus, maxilla, zygomatic complex, nasoethmoid-orbital (NEO), and mandible are the most common. Management of panfacial fracture requires an understanding of the interrelationship between the horizontal and vertical buttresses of the face. Panfacial fractures result in loss of anterior projection and increased horizontal and decreased vertical dimensions of the face. Panfacial fracture complexity is based on the number of fractures, the degree of fracture comminution and displacement, and the stability of fractured segments. A systematic approach to evaluation, planning, and execution is necessary to achieve the most optimal results. Inadequate early treatment leads to secondary deformities that are challenging to treat. The purpose of this chapter is to review pearls and pitfalls for surgical management of panfacial fractures.

Practical Tips

Preoperative Consideration

Airway

- This can be secured with tracheostomy or submental intubation to allow for full facial exposure and placement of intermaxillary fixation (IMF).

Y. Sawatari (✉)
Oral and Maxillofacial Surgery, University of Miami, Miami, FL, USA
e-mail: ysawatari@med.miami.edu

Radiographic Evaluation

1. Careful evaluation of the maxillofacial computed tomography (CT) scan, including axial, coronal, sagittal views, and 3D reconstruction.

   (a) Identify fractures.

       - Orbit.
       - Frontal: A careful assessment of the anterior and posterior table fractures. Displaced posterior table fracture will result in a dural tear and CSF leak. A combined neurosurgical approach is indicated in these cases.
       - Orbito zygomatico maxillary complex (including sagittal fracture at the root of the arch).
       - Naso-orbitoethmoidal.
       - Lefort I, II, III.
       - Mandible.

         - Condylar process.
         - Body.
         - Angle.
         - Symphysis/parasymphysis.

   (b) Identify the degree of comminution.
   (c) Identify the degree of displacement.

       - The more severely comminuted and/or displaced the fracture, the more complex the reduction.
       - For severely comminuted fractures, consider primary bone grafting to provide stability and support.

   (d) Identify stable bony reference points.

Clinical Evaluation

1. Identify clinical injury.
2. Identify functional deficits.

   (a) Malocclusion.
   (b) Entrapment.
   (c) Nerve deficits.

3. Identify facial deformity.

   (a) Asymmetry.
   (b) Enophthalmos and dystopia.
   (c) Loss of anterior facial projection.
   (d) Increased transverse facial dimension.

Plan

1. Confirm the necessity of surgical intervention.
2. Confirm which fractures require surgical intervention.
3. Choose the access type to expose stable bony references and unstable fracture segments.
4. Determine the sequence of reduction and fixation (Fig. 15.1).

   (a) Generally, bring unstable bone to be stable.
   (b) Peripheral to center.
   (c) Varies depending on levels of comminution and reliability of peripheral reference.
   (d) Sequence (Bring unstable to stable): The reconstruction sequence depends on the clinical findings and the fracture pattern. However, these are generally the sequence recommended.

   - Dentate mandible.
   - Non-dentate mandible.
   - Intermaxillary fixation.
   - Frontal bone.
   - Zygomaticofrontal junction.
   - Zygomaticosphenoid confirmation.
   - Zygomaticotemporal junction.
   - Nasofrontal junction.

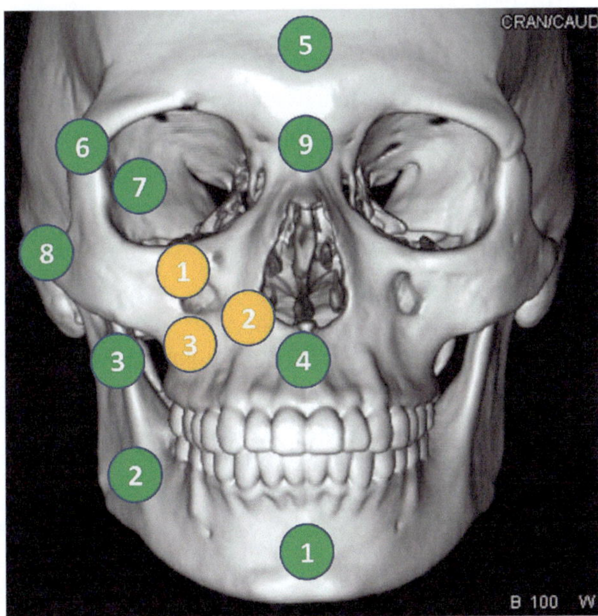

Fig. 15.1 The author's preferred sequence of reduction and fixation for panfacial fracture

(e) Sequence (Converge facial components):

- Orbital rim.
- Piriform rim.
- Zygomaticomaxillary buttress.

Intraoperative Consideration (Execution)

1. Expose all stable references and fracture segments per the plan.
2. Reduce and fixate per the determined sequence of repair.
3. Do intraoperative CT scan after the mandible ORIF. This will ensure the mandible is well reduced before establishing the maxillo-mandibular complex.
4. Carefully re-attach the medial canthal tendon in type II and III NOE fracture cases. This is very important from an esthetic perspective.
5. The zygomatic arch (ZT suture) alignment is a key landmark for successful zygomaticomaxillary complex reconstruction. The correct alignment of the ZT suture will ensure adequate AP projection of the face and minimize the medio-lateral rotation.
6. Consider bone grafting for comminuted fracture segments. The calvarial bone graft is readily available with a coronal approach.
7. Intraoperative analysis (intraoperative CT and navigation), assess for restoration of:

    (a) preoperative projection and symmetry
    (b) restoration of orbital volume

8. Postoperative analysis.

    (a) Restoration of functional deficits.
    (b) Restoration of preinjury facial contour.

Postoperative Consideration

- Keep the head elevated for the first 2 days to help reduce the edema.
- A postoperative antibiotic is recommended for 3 days after the surgery.
- Frequent visual checks, including visual acuity and motility, are recommended.
- Sinus precaution and monitoring the signs of CSF leak is important, particularly in panfacial fractures with dural involvement.

Complications

1. Failure in assessment.

   (a) Clinical.
   (b) Radiographic.

2. Underestimation of the problem (fractures that can have a significant effect on outcome leading to increased transverse dimension and decreased anterior projection).

   (a) Symphysis of mandible flare.
   (b) Oblique fractures of the mandible.
   (c) Condylar complex fractures.

     - The combination of these fractures will increase facial width. Therefore, careful exposure of the lingual surface of the mandible to ensure accurate reduction is vital for successful results.

   (d) Palatal split.
   (e) Sagittal fracture of the root of the zygomatic arch.
   (f) Zygomaticosphenoid junction.
   (g) Orbit.

3. Failure of the plan:

   (a) This includes failure to plan and perform a bone grafting procedure for severely comminuted fractures.

4. Failure of execution.

Pearls

- Extra-oral approach to the mandible is recommended for Parasyymphysis fracture with condylar fractures and oblique mandibular fractures. Extraoral access provides better visualization and allows for accurate reduction and prevention of increased posterior mandibular width
- ORIF of the condylar/subcondylar fracture is essential to prevent loss of the posterior facial height.

- The ZT and ZS are excellent landmarks for the adequacy of midface reconstruction.
- Intraoperative CT scans are beneficial in identifying any misalignment or improper reduction. If you start with the mandible first approach, obtaining an intraoperative scan after mandibular ORIF is important.

Pitfalls

- The reconstruction of panfacial fracture may be delayed because other life-threatening injuries which must be addressed first. Delaying surgical intervention will make the reconstruction more difficult.
- Bone grafting may be indicated for comminuted panfacial fractures.

Further Reading

Kim J, Choi JH, Chung YK, Kim SW. Panfacial bone fracture and medial to lateral approach. Arch Craniofac Surg. 2016;17(4):181–5. https://doi.org/10.7181/acfs.2016.17.4.181; Epub 2016 Dec 23. PMID: 28913280; PMCID: PMC5556833.

Chapter 16
Pearls and Pitfalls for the Reconstruction of Gunshot Injuries to the Face

Janet Sung and Baber Khatib

Abstract Gunshot wounds to the face frequently present complex challenges to the reconstructive surgeon as they can cause significant bone and soft tissue defects and have high rates of tissue necrosis, ischemia, and infection. High-velocity (>1200 ft. per second, e.g., rifles) ballistic injuries produce debilitating soft tissue avulsions, hard tissue defects, sequential necrosis, and tissue loss over several days. Patients who have attempted suicide or been shot at close range with a shotgun can have similar injuries. Low-velocity bullets can result in the comminution of bone but do not typically cause such avulsive defects and rarely result in significant sequential necrosis and tissue loss. Initial management of gunshot injuries to the face is in accordance with Advanced Trauma Life Support (ATLS). After patients are stabilized, they are taken for debridement and damage control, often on the same day as arrival. This involves wound washout, examination under anesthesia, surgical hemostasis, conservative debridement of clearly nonviable tissues, wound closure, and/or packing. Occasionally, some bony fixation may be applied if it can be done easily and quickly. When tissue viability is questionable, it should be left to heal with ensuing necrotic areas debrided every 48 h with short trips to the operating room (OR). Immediately after injury, while patients are marginally stable and in a profound inflammatory state, extended and lengthy procedures should be avoided. Once the patient is stable and the injuries are no longer evolving, one can plan and approach the reconstruction. The purpose of this chapter is to review pearls and pitfalls for the reconstruction of gunshot injuries to the face.

J. Sung
Head and Neck Surgical Associates/Legacy Emanuel Trauma Center, Portland, OR, USA

B. Khatib (✉)
Head and Neck Surgical Associates, Legacy Emanuel Trauma Center, Portland, OR, USA

© The Author(s), under exclusive license to Springer Nature Switzerland AG 2024
D. Amin, H. Marwan (eds.), *Pearls and Pitfalls in Oral and Maxillofacial Surgery*, https://doi.org/10.1007/978-3-031-47307-4_16

Practical Tips

Preoperative Consideration

- Utilize virtual surgical planning, custom surgical guides and plates, intraoperative navigation, and intraoperative imaging for predictable results.
- Repeated plate bending decreases fatigue resistance and increases the risk of plate fracture. Consider custom plate fabrication.
- If accurate occlusal relationships are critical for virtual planning, take impressions. Computed tomography (CT) scans cannot capture occlusal anatomy accurately.
- With orbital and mandibular reconstruction, the uninjured side can be mirrored to the injured side to approximate the pre-traumatic form, which can then be used to prebend plates or design custom plates. If both sides are fractured, the least comminuted side is virtually corrected and then mirror imaged to the contralateral side.

Intraoperative Consideration

- Stage your reconstruction.

  - Midface and orbital reconstruction because of their importance in establishing proper facial width.
  - Oromandibular reconstruction.
  - Palatomaxillary reconstruction.
  - Internal orbital reconstruction.
  - Soft tissue reconstruction—lip, nose, etc.
  - Dental rehabilitation.

- GSW to the mandible:

  - Treat open or closed?

    Open reduction and internal fixation (ORIF), when possible, is associated with a lower complication rate.

    If extensive comminution and open treatment would result in the removal of many displaced fragments, consider closed treatment via maxillomandibular fixation or external fixation to allow for bony healing while maintaining the spatial relationship of the mandibular fragments.

    If there is significant soft tissue disruption, especially in GSWs of the floor of the mouth, consider closed treatment. If lingual musculature and mucosa have completely detached from the mandible, open treatment will detach buccal mucosa and musculature and thus the remaining blood supply.

  - Bony defects:

    If the size is <6 cm with adequate soft tissue, consider single-stage reconstruction with bone graft.

If inadequate soft tissue or bony defect >6 cm, consider reconstruction with a vascularized bone flap.

– Figures 16.1 and 16.2 present two cases with extensive facial injury related to GSW.

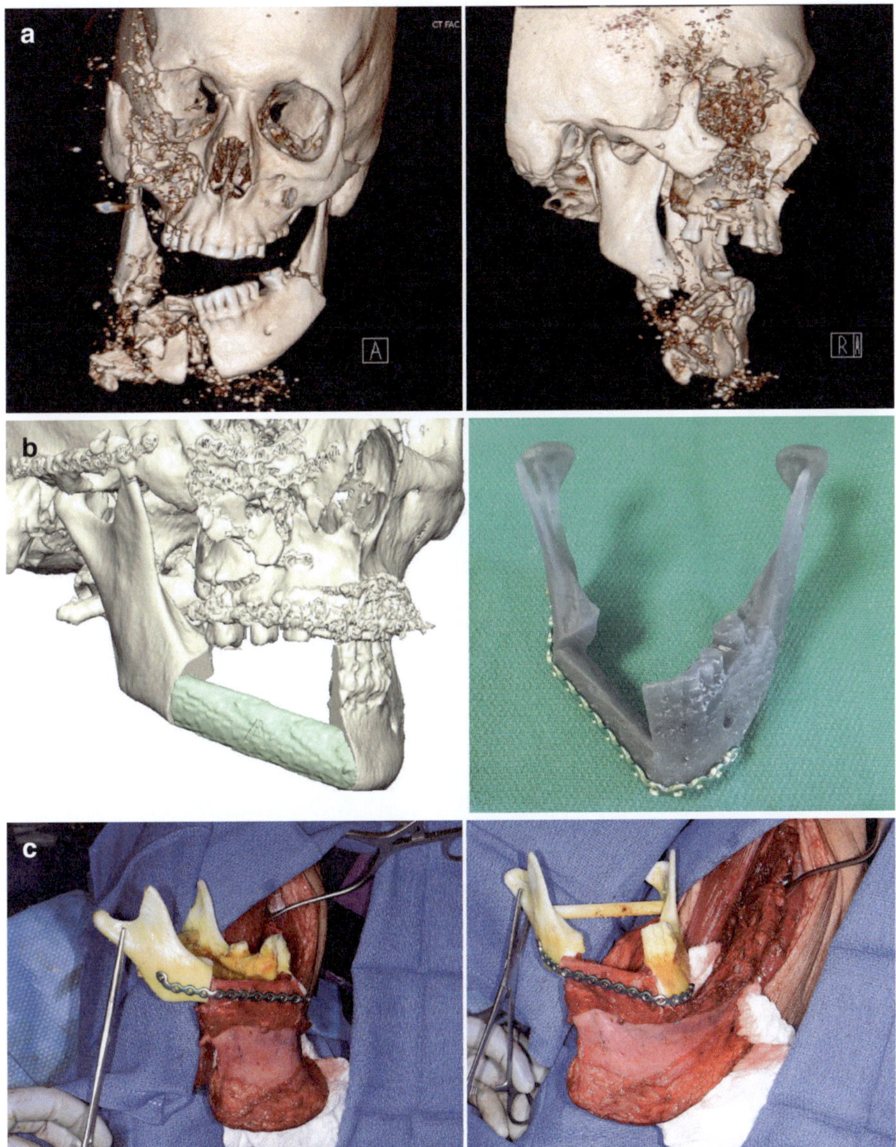

Fig. 16.1 (**a**) Gunshot wound to the face, initial CT 3D reconstruction after presenting to Legacy Emanuel Hospital. (**b**) Virtual surgical planning for mandible reconstruction with a fibula osteocutaneous tissue transfer. The 3D model is printed in-house to allow a prebent plate to be fabricated before the OR. (**c**) Intraoperative shaping of the fibula on "resected model" showing excellent adaptation of the plate to the fibula and model. (**d**) Post-operative imaging

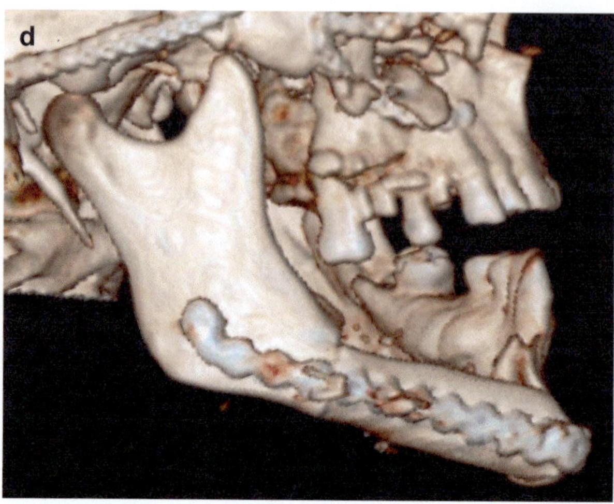

Fig. 16.1 (continued)

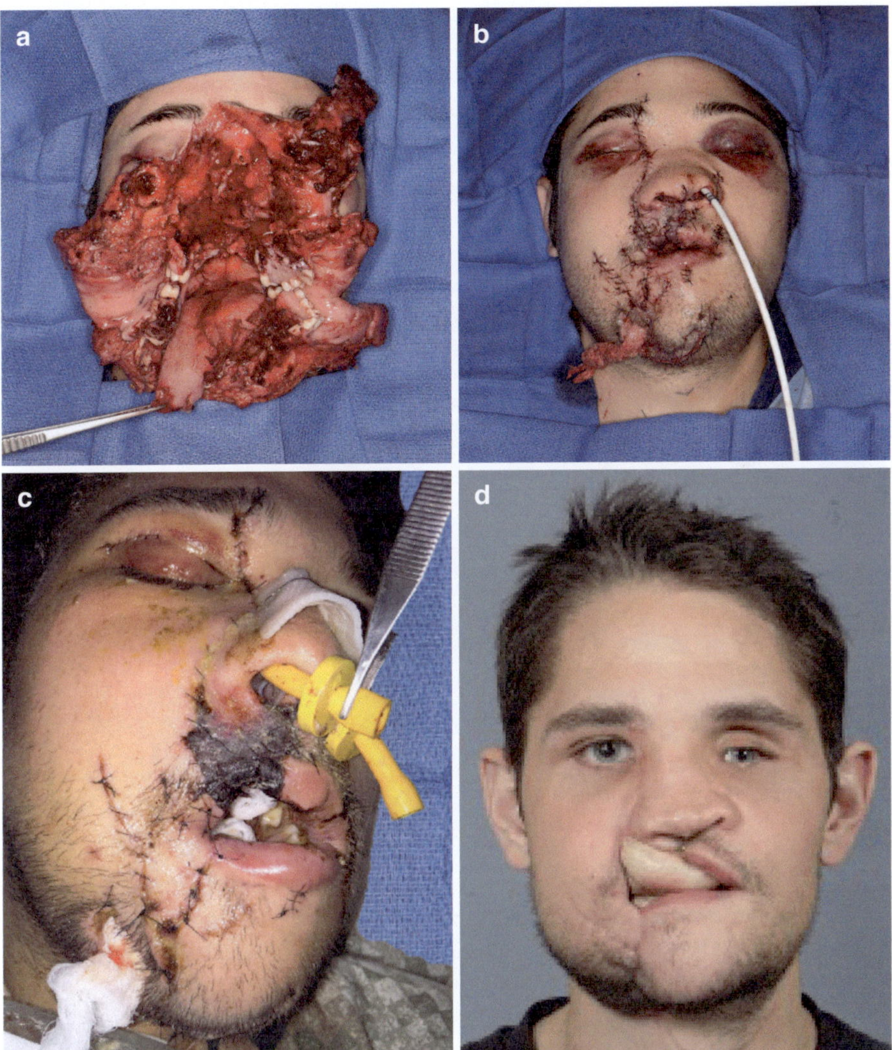

Fig. 16.2 (**a**) Initial washout and minimal selective debridement of a self-inflicted gunshot wound after presenting to Legacy Emanuel Hospital. (**b**) Initial repair with particular attention to key anatomic landmarks. Note early venous congestion of the upper lip. (**c**) Soft tissue necrosis of right upper lip, philtrum. (**d**) Delayed repair, osteocutaneous fibula-free flaps for maxilla and mandible. (**e**) Soft tissue revision delayed Abbe flap and fibula flap debulking

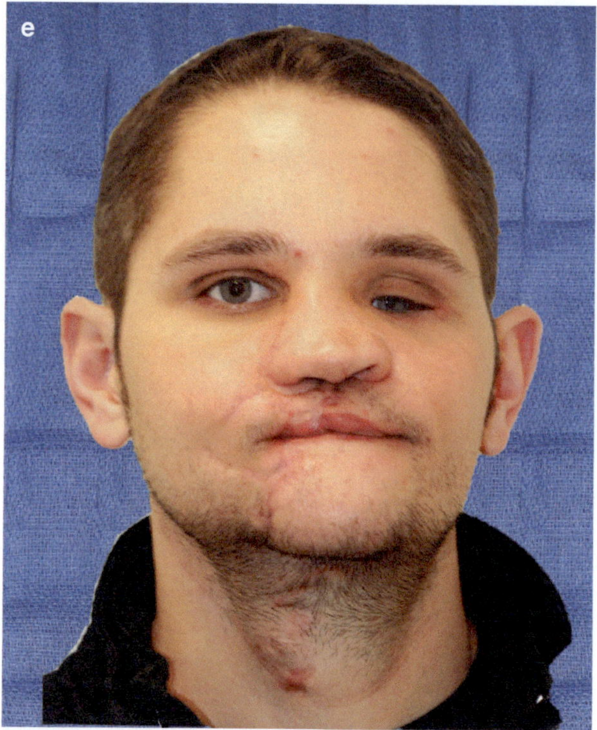

Fig. 16.2 (continued)

Pearls

- The amount of soft tissue loss and the damage to surrounding tissues depends mainly on the type of weapon used (high velocity vs. low velocity).
- When tissue viability is questionable, it should be left to heal with ensuing necrotic areas debrided every 48 h with short trips to the operating room.
- Attempt to stage the reconstruction.
- Always obtain impression or optical scans for the occlusion to reestablish the maxillo-mandibular relationship.

Pitfalls

- Bending the plate to span the defect will result in plate weakness and future breakage; using VSP and a custom-made plate will prevent this problem.
- Avoid ORIF in comminuted segments, as it will increase the chances of devascularization.

Further Reading

Powers DB, Delo RI. Characteristics of ballistic and blast injuries. Atlas Oral Maxillofac Surg Clin North Am. 2013;21(1):15–24.

Ostrander BT, et al. Contemporary management of mandibular fracture nonunion—a retrospective review and treatment algorithm. J Oral Maxillofac Surg. 2018;76(7):479–1493.

Ellis E 3rd, Muniz O, Anand K. Treatment considerations for comminuted mandibular fractures. J Oral Maxillofac Surg. 2003;61(8):861–70.

Kaufman Y, Cole P, Hollier LH Jr. Facial gunshot wounds: trends in management. Craniomaxillofac Trauma Reconstr. 2009;2(2):85–90.

Khatib B, Gelesko S, Amundson M, Cheng A, Patel A, Bui T, Dierks EJ, Bell RB. Updates in management of craniomaxillofacial gunshot wounds and reconstruction of the mandible. Facial Plast Surg Clin North Am. 2017;25(4):563–76.

Chapter 17
Pearls and Pitfalls in the Management of Post-Traumatic Facial Deformities

Hisham Marwan ⓘ

Abstract Management of post-traumatic facial deformity is very challenging. The goal of the reconstruction is similar to the primary repair; restore function and pre-injury form. The ideal management starts with a comprehensive preoperative assessment and collection of data, followed by formulating a treatment plan that addresses the patient's complaints. There are several differences between primary repair and secondary revision of facial fracture, including lack of mobility of segments affected due to malunion (bony or fibrous), loss of stable reference points with subsequent reduction in the accuracy at the fracture junction. These differences necessitate a more elaborate exposure and Osteotomies of the facial skeleton to mobilize the segments. The purpose of this chapter is to review pearls and pitfalls in managing post-traumatic facial deformities.

Practical Tips

Preoperative and Intraoperative Consideration

- Identify the reason for the deformity. Is it because of the delay in the primary repair or failure to appropriately managed the initial injury? Sometimes, the patient may elect not to have surgery after the initial trauma.
- The patient and the surgeon should accept that the results might be less than ideal. Counseling the patient is important.
- Obtain the preinjury computed tomography (CT) scans, if possible. It will provide valuable information for planning.
- Plan to use all the available technology CT scan, virtual surgical planning "VSP," navigation, intraoral scanner, etc. to help you plan and execute the procedure as accurately as possible.

H. Marwan (✉)
Department of Surgery, The University of Texas Medical Branch, Galveston, TX, USA
e-mail: Himarwan@utmb.edu

D. Amin, H. Marwan (eds.), *Pearls and Pitfalls in Oral and Maxillofacial Surgery*, https://doi.org/10.1007/978-3-031-47307-4_17

- For post-traumatic enophthalmos, diplopia, and dystopia, consider ophthalmological evaluation since some of the ophthalmological symptoms (blurry vision and diplopia) might worsen after surgery.
- Carefully identify the cause of the orbital deformity, internal orbital wall, periorbital wall, or a combination. Understanding the difference will help in planning and correcting the deformity.
- For zygomatic post-traumatic deformity, using VSP is the key to optimum results. The mirror imaging technique allows the reconstruction of the unilateral defect of the zygoma and the orbit as accurately as possible.
- For zygomatic post-traumatic deformity reconstruction, custom guides and plates will help replicate the plan. However, using the corrected stereolithographic model to bend the readily available midface plates is a cheaper and faster alternative.
- For cases with malocclusion, dental impressions, and dental casts, clarify the compensatory movements of the dentition and how to plan to fix it.
- Malocclusion management is driven by the re-establishment of the occlusion, not as much by the alignment of bone or symmetry.
- If the origin of the malocclusion is the mandible, consider orthodontic and prosthetic evaluation for mild occlusal discrepancies. If the mandible fracture is not fully healed (fibrous union, non-union), it may separate segments at the fracture line. Finally, if the mandible fracture is fully healed, it depends on the location:

  - If the fracture is anterior to the mental foramen, an osteotomy can be performed at the fracture site.
  - If the fracture is posterior to the mental foramen and in the dentate area, consider nerve lateralization and osteotomy.
  - If the fracture is posterior to dentition (mandibular condylar or subcondylar) with normal functional condyle, consider sagittal split osteotomy, vertical ramus osteotomy, or inverted L osteotomy.
  - If the fracture is posterior to dentition (mandibular condylar or subcondylar) with an ankylosed condyle, consider total joint replacement.
  - If the fracture is posterior to dentition (mandibular condylar or subcondylar) with unstable pseudoarthrosis (rare), consider repositioning the condyle into the fossa with ramus osteotomy to correct the occlusion.

- If the origin of the malocclusion is the maxilla, Consider orthodontic and prosthetic evaluation for mild occlusal discrepancies. If the maxilla fracture is not fully healed (fibrous union, non-union), it may separate segments at the fracture line. Finally, if the maxilla fracture is fully healed, a Lefort 1 osteotomy would help to mobilize the segment.
- If the deformity is severe and cannot be corrected with osteotomy, consider camouflaging technique with fat grafting and alloplastic materials.

Postoperative Consideration

- Correcting post-traumatic deformity requires broader and multiple exposures and longer recovery.
- The use of an occlusal splint and intermaxillary fixation with wires or elastics is recommended to minimize the relapse in case of post-traumatic malocclusion.

Pearls

1. The goal of management of post-traumatic deformity is similar to the primary injury; restore the function and esthetic.
2. Identifying the reason for the poor initial result is the key to understanding the deformity and how to solve it.
3. The use of all available technological aids will help achieve excellent results (VSP, Intraoperative scans, and navigation).

Pitfalls

1. Malunion will require osteotomy and subsequent bone grafting.
2. Extensive soft tissue exposure during surgical approach might result in soft tissue changes and poor cosmesis.
3. Malocclusion-related post-traumatic deformity will require a period of IMF to help stabilize the maxilla and mandible and prevent future relapse.

Further Reading

Zhang SL, Gui H, Lin Y, Shen G, Xu B. Navigation-guided correction of midfacial post-traumatic deformities (Shanghai experience with 40 cases). J Oral Maxillofac Surg. 2012;70(6):1426–33; ISSN 0278–2391.

Gong X, He Y, An J, Yang Y, Huang X, Liu M, Zhao Y, Zhang Y. Application of a Computer-Assisted Navigation System (CANS) in the delayed treatment of zygomatic fractures: a randomized controlled trial. J Oral Maxillofac Surg. 2017;75(7):1450–63; ISSN 0278–2391.

Part IV
Head and Neck Pathology

Chapter 18
Pearls and Pitfalls in the Diagnosis and Management of Vascular Lesions

Anastasiya Quimby

Abstract Vascular lesions in the head and neck comprise a wide array of abnormalities present at birth or in childhood. Management of vascular lesions differs depending on the specific type. Although some vascular lesions have distinct clinical presentations that make the diagnosis straightforward, others may pose diagnostic and management challenges owing to the complex anatomy of the region. Commonly, their superficial component extends to deeper tissue, involves vital organs, and/or extends intracranially. While most vascular lesions are sporadic solitary entities, syndromic associations exist and thus must be ruled out in certain cases. Correct diagnosis is key to the appropriate management of vascular lesions. Numerous classifications and terms have been used to classify vascular lesions, making the task of diagnosis even more difficult. The International Society for the Studies of Vascular Anomalies (ISSVA) proposed the classification of vascular lesions. This system is used to classify and guide vascular lesions management. The purpose of this chapter is to review pearls and pitfalls in the diagnosis and management of vascular lesions.

Practical Tips

- Vascular lesions are classified into malformations and tumors (Fig. 18.1).
- Vascular malformations.

  - They are congenital lesions present at birth and continue to grow as the rest of the body grows.
  - Defined as defects in vascular morphogenesis with no neoplastic potential.
  - Classified into simple and combined.
  - Simple malformations are further classified according to the vessels involved: (1) capillary, (2) venous, (3) arteriovenous malformations (AVM), (4) arterio-

A. Quimby (✉)
Department of Surgery, Good Samaritan Hospital, AQ Surgery: Head and Neck
Microvascular Surgery Institute, West Palm Beach, FL, USA

© The Author(s), under exclusive license to Springer Nature
Switzerland AG 2024
D. Amin, H. Marwan (eds.), *Pearls and Pitfalls in Oral and Maxillofacial
Surgery*, https://doi.org/10.1007/978-3-031-47307-4_18

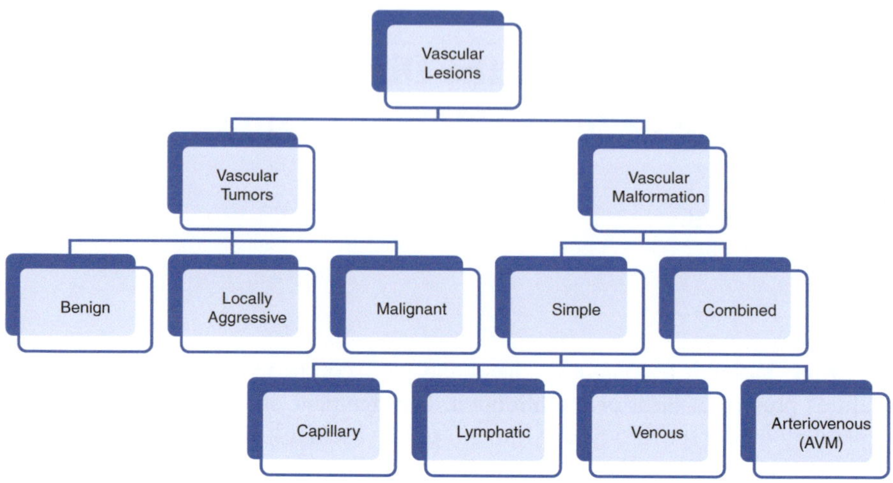

Fig. 18.1 International Society for the Study of Vascular Anomalies (ISSVA) classification of vascular anomalies

venous fistulas (AVF), and (5) lymphatic malformations (historically named lymphangiomas, although they're not true tumors).
- Lymphatic malformations are classified into macrocystic and microcystic lymphatic malformations.
- Combined malformations may be composed of any of the simple ones.
- Vascular malformations can be classified as (1) low-flow (venous) or (2) high-flow (arteriovenous) lesions. This classification has surgical management implications.

- Vascular tumors.

  - They are not present at birth. However, depending on the type, they may present in early childhood (hemangioma) or adulthood (angiosarcoma).
  - The lesions increase in size disproportionately to the rest of the body.
  - They demonstrate endothelial mitoses and have independent growth potential.
  - Classified into (1) benign, (2) locally aggressive, and (3) malignant.
  - Benign vascular tumors are the most common; it includes two subtypes of hemangioma: congenital and infantile.
  - Infantile hemangioma (IH) expresses GLUT-1, unlike other vascular lesions, presents at birth or shortly after, grows rapidly, and involutes by age 1. Large IH is associated with hemangiomas of visceral organs, and PHACE and LUMBAR syndromes must be ruled out.
  - Congenital hemangioma (CH) is present at birth at its maximum size; it doesn't demonstrate growth and does not express GLUT-1. It is divided into three types: rapidly involuting (RICH), partially involuting (PICH), and non-involuting (NICH).

- The most common locally aggressive vascular tumor is Kaposi sarcoma.
- The most common malignant vascular tumor is Angiosarcoma.

Preoperative Consideration

- Diagnosis of vascular lesions is based on history, clinical exam, and radiographic evaluation.

  - History:

    One of the most important history questions to ask patients is whether the lesion in question was present at birth. Vascular malformations are present at birth, and vascular tumors may present in infancy (Infantile or congenital hemangioma) or adulthood (Kaposi's sarcoma, angiosarcoma, hemangiopericytoma).

    The rate of growth and age of the patient can help narrow the diagnosis. A rapidly growing vascular lesion in an infant is likely to be an infantile hemangioma, which is expected to cease growth by 12 months of age. A vascular lesion that appears after birth and remains stable in size may or may not involute (RICH vs. PICH vs. NICH). A rapidly growing lesion in adulthood most certainly signifies aggressive or malignant behavior. Slowly enlarging diffuse masses increase clinical suspicion for lymphatic and arteriovenous malformations.

    Did the lesion rapidly increase in size after infection, hormonal changes, or trauma? Vascular malformations that were previously stable may be provoked into an exuberant growth phase.

    Does it spontaneously bleed? Angiosarcomas are known to have episodes of bleeding.

    What other symptoms does the patient have? Pain, sensory or motor deficits, tinnitus, headaches, hoarseness, respiratory difficulty, and hemoptysis may be suggestive of the involvement of deeper structures.

    Family history of vascular malformations? If present, should warrant genetic evaluation for possible syndromic association (PHACE, LUMBAR).

  - Clinical Evaluation:

    Low-flow malformations clinically present as compressible lesions that can grow to extensive size. Capillary and venous malformation will present positive on diascopy. Venous malformations demonstrate a change in lesion volume with changing body positioning. Lymphatic malformations clinically are soft tissue masses that may present with pain and swelling due to intralesional hemorrhage. These lesions can grow to extensive size traversing tissue planes, causing elephantiasis.

High-flow lesions clinically present as soft compressible pulsatile masses with audible bruit and a purple hue if close to the skin or mucosal surface. Due to their capacity to hold large blood volumes, these lesions have been described to cause a steal phenomenon. Catastrophic bleeding may occur if the blood volume becomes excessive, causing the development of aneurysms.

Steal phenomenon is defined as blood flow shunting from adjacent structures to the focus of vascular malformation. Cerebral AVMs may present with symptoms of transient ischemic attacks due to the "steal" of blood flow by the AVM.

Lymphatic malformations clinically are soft tissue masses that may present with pain and swelling due to intralesional hemorrhage. These lesions can grow to extensive size traversing tissue planes, causing elephantiasis. Radiographic evaluation:

- Ultrasound and flow Doppler is recommended for superficial and easily accessible lesions.
- For head and neck lesions, Gadolinium-enhanced magnetic resonance imaging (MRI) is recommended.

High-flow lesions present as hypo- or isointense on T1 and hyperintense on T2. Flow voids are characteristic of high-flow vascular lesions.
Low-flow lesions vary in presentation depending on the type.

Venous malformations (VM) present as hypo- or isointense on T1 and hyperintense vascular channels on T2 and may include phleboliths, which are pathognomonic for VM.
Lymphatic malformations are classified into macrocystic (channels >2 cm squared) and microcystic (channels <2 cm squared). These lesions present with no flow and may or may not demonstrate cystic cavity enhancement on T2, depending on the degree of hemorrhage. Lymphatic malformations demonstrate cystic septae enhancement, unlike the rest of the vascular lesions.

- Computed tomography scans (CT) are usually avoided due to poor soft tissue resolution and ionizing radiation, as the majority of vascular lesion patients are pediatric. CT scans are helpful when intrabony lesion is present, and the degree of bony destruction needs to be assessed.
- Always remember that the lesion may extend deep into underlying organs, carry a risk of airway obstruction, or have an intracranial extension. Obtaining appropriate imaging is essential.
- More than five cutaneous IH warrants imaging evaluation of visceral organs.
- CT angiography with 3D reconstruction or MRA are recommended to evaluate AVM (high-flow lesions).

- Arteriogram is another means of demonstrating the extent of high-flow lesions. Given the availability and low risk of obtaining cross-sectional imaging such as MRI, the role of arteriograms has remained the same in the initial evaluation of AVMs.

Intraoperative Consideration

- Do not perform in-office biopsies if a vascular lesion is suspected.
- IH management.

  - Observation is recommended, as they are expected to involute within the first year of life.
  - Consider Propranolol as a systemic agent in cases with orbital or airway involvement.
  - Consider surgical intervention for managing excess tissue and/or scar after the lesion has been involuted.

- Low-flow vascular malformations managements.

  - Consider neodymium-doped yttrium aluminum garnet (Nd: YAG) laser or intralesional sclerotherapy.
  - The recommended sclerosing agents are sodium tetradecyl sulfate (STS), ethanol, doxycycline, or bleomycin.

- Lymphatic malformations managements.

  - They can be managed with surgery and/or intralesional sclerotherapy.
  - For macrocystic lymphatic malformation.

    Consider fine needle aspiration. The advantages of fine needle aspiration are (1) it decreases the volume of intralesional fluid and (2) it allows for histopathologic confirmation of the diagnosis.
    Doxycycline is a sclerosing agent of choice.

  - For microcystic lymphatic malformation.

    Bleomycin is the sclerosing agent of choice.

- High-flow vascular malformations managements.

  - A multidisciplinary team is highly recommended for the management of high-flow vascular lesions.
  - Surgical interventions are reserved for symptomatic patients with high-flow lesions or those who have not responded to non-surgical therapy.
  - Patients should be typed and screened, and blood banks are advised to have blood products ready.

- Preoperative embolization of the feeding vessels is carried out 24–48 h before surgery. This will avoid the development of collateral flow. However, post-embolization bleeding may occur.
- Radiation exposure during embolization can be up to 6 Gy per treatment. Patients may undergo 10 or more treatments. Alopecia is a common complication.
- External carotid ligation has also been shown to be an effective method of limiting flow to the lesions.
- If the overlying mucosa or skin has obvious vasculature, excision of the mucosa and/ or skin is recommended because it will recur and expand.
- If bone resection is planned, one must be prepared for significant bleeding. Bone wax and Gelfoam powder can be used to stop bleeding.
- Reconstruction is usually necessary with large AVMs; therefore, a microvascular surgeon should be available.

Postoperative Consideration

- Removal of lesions involving the aerodigestive tract warrants post-operative admission to the ICU for airway monitoring or ventilation maintenance if the patient was left intubated.
- With the removal of large vascular lesions, post-op bleeding has the potential to be catastrophic; thus, adequate venous access and the ability to activate mass transfusion protocol are essential.
- Vascular malformations are likely to recur; therefore, routine follow-up must be established for the patient.

Pearls

- Diagnosis of vascular lesions is based on history, clinical exam, and imaging.
- Understanding clinical presentations and course is important for management.
- For high-flow vascular malformation, complete excision, with or without preoperative embolization, provides the highest rate of successful treatment.

Pitfalls

- For high-flow vascular malformation, ligation or embolization of major feeder vessels alone is not recommended.
- Embolization with alcohol to superficial areas can result in significant tissue necrosis.

Further Reading

Bertino F, Trofimova AV, Gilyard SN, Hawkins CM. Vascular anomalies of the head and neck: diagnosis and treatment. Pediatr Radiol. 2021;51(7):1162–84. https://doi.org/10.1007/s00247-021-04968-2; Epub 2021 Apr 16.

Nair SC. Vascular anomalies of the head and neck region. J Maxillofac Oral Surg. 2018;17(1):1–12. https://doi.org/10.1007/s12663-017-1063-2; Epub 2018 Jan 5. PMID: 29382987; PMCID: PMC5772031.

Oomen KPQ, Wreesmann VB. Current classification of vascular anomalies of the head and neck. J Oral Pathol Med. 2022;51(10):830–6. https://doi.org/10.1111/jop.13353; Epub 2022 Oct 20.

Puttgen KB, Pearl M, Tekes A, Mitchell SE. Update on pediatric extracranial vascular anomalies of the head and neck. Childs Nerv Syst. 2010;26(10):1417–33. https://doi.org/10.1007/s00381-010-1202-2; Epub 2010 Aug 10.

Colletti G, Valassina D, Bertossi D, Melchiorre F, Vercellio G, Brusati R. Contemporary management of vascular malformations. J Oral Maxillofac Surg. 2014;72(3):510–28. https://doi.org/10.1016/j.joms.2013.08.008; Epub 2013 Oct 16.

Chapter 19
Pearls and Pitfalls in the Management of Ameloblastoma

Caitlyn McGue, Kolina Mah-Ginn, Victoria A. Mañón, Allen C. Cheng, and Chi T. Viet

Abstract Ameloblastomas are benign tumors of the maxilla and mandible originating from odontogenic epithelium involved with tooth formation. They preferentially occur in the mandible (75%) and are most commonly found in the third molar area of either jaw. Clinically, they present as asymptomatic expansions of the jaw bones. Radiographically they appear as well-defined, expansile uni- or multilocular radiolucencies. Diagnosis is typically made with an incisional biopsy. Although benign, they can be locally aggressive and invade and resorb bone and soft tissue. However, they are unable to undergo true perineural invasion. Very rarely, ameloblastomas may undergo malignant transformation into either ameloblastic carcinoma (invasive) or malignant ameloblastoma (metastatic).

The two most common histopathologic patterns are follicular and plexiform, both of which demonstrate columnar cells with nuclei polarized away from the basement membrane.

Because enucleation and curettage have a 70–85% recurrence rate and microscopic disease has been found to extend up to 8 mm beyond radiographic disease, ameloblastomas are treated by bone resection with 1.0–1.5 cm margins. When adequately resected, cure rates are 98%.

The molecular biology of ameloblastoma is an area of active research. V600E BRAF mutations have been identified as a common mutation in mandibular ameloblastomas. The clinical significance of this finding is still being investigated, but it is intriguing because approved targeted therapies for this mutation are already on the market. Case reports of using BRAF/MEK inhibitors to treat ameloblastomas, ameloblastic carcinomas, and malignant ameloblastomas have reported promising

C. McGue · K. Mah-Ginn · C. T. Viet (✉)
Department of Oral and Maxillofacial Surgery, Loma Linda University, Loma Linda, CA, USA

V. A. Mañón
Department of Oral and Maxillofacial Surgery, University of Texas Health Science Center at Houston, Houston, TX, USA

A. C. Cheng
Legacy Good Samaritan Cancer Center and Head and Neck Surgical Associates, Portland, OR, USA

D. Amin, H. Marwan (eds.), *Pearls and Pitfalls in Oral and Maxillofacial Surgery*, https://doi.org/10.1007/978-3-031-47307-4_19

preliminary results. The purpose of this chapter is to review pearls and pitfalls in the surgical management of ameloblastoma.

Practical Tips for the Treatment of Ameloblastoma

Resection

- Resect with 1.0 to 1.5 cm bony margins, one uninvolved anatomical barrier margin, and frozen sections documenting tumor-free margins (when necessary).
- Bony resection should leave adequate bone (about one-half of a tooth socket) between the resection edge and the adjacent tooth for structural support (Fig. 19.1).
- If there is evidence that the tumor has perforated through the cortical bone, a supra-periosteal dissection should be performed in this area as an additional anatomic margin.

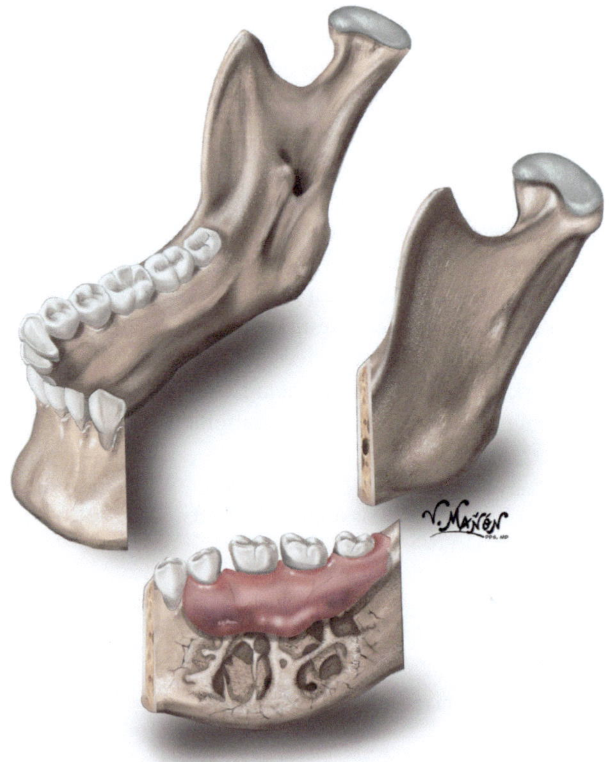

Fig. 19.1 Segmental mandibulectomy of ameloblastoma with 1.0 to 1.5 cm bony margins and one uninvolved anatomical barrier margin

- Examine the freshly resected specimen for areas of unexpected tumor perforation through bone. Correlate these areas with a location in the wound so frozen sections can be taken, if indicated.
- Take a specimen radiograph to assess the tumor's relationship to the bony margins.
- If the inferior alveolar neurovascular bundle is at least 1 cm from the tumor, or it can be isolated and displaced from the resection without dissecting through the tumor, it can be preserved. The tumor should not be entered or exposed to preserve the nerve. Nerve grafting can be considered if the inferior alveolar nerve is resected.
- A marginal mandibulectomy can be considered if the tumor is small enough that a clear margin will still leave adequate support at the inferior border of the mandible. The resection should be curvilinear rather than at right-angles to minimize the risk of a pathologic fracture (Fig. 19.2).

Reconstruction

- For a segmental mandibulectomy, immediate reconstruction is advised.
- The 2.0 mm or thicker titanium fixation plate should be used. Placement of 2–4 bicortical screws in each segment is ideal; 2–3 screws placed on a proximal segment consisting only of the condylar neck and condyle may suffice.

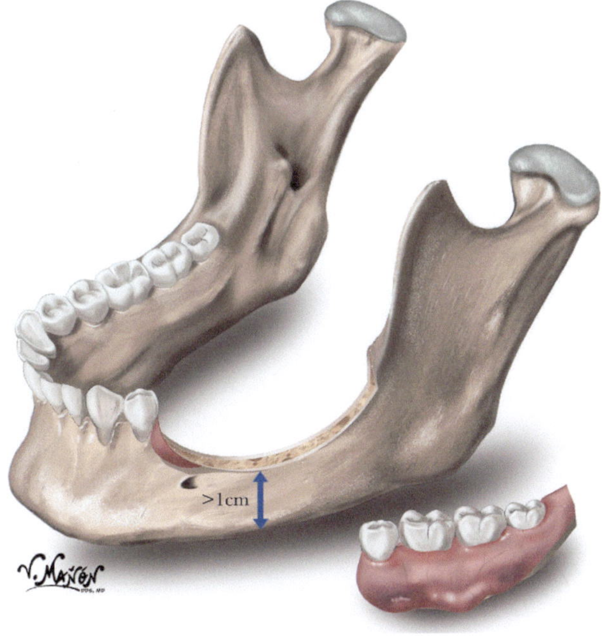

Fig. 19.2 Marginal mandibulectomy of ameloblastoma. Note the distance of the tumor from the inferior border of the mandible and the angulation of the peripheral cuts

- If immediate bone grafting is not feasible, it can be performed approximately 3–4 months after the transoral incision has healed.
- Microvascular free tissue transfer (with or without immediate implant and dental prosthesis placement) and non-vascularized bone grafting with tissue engineering are the two more commonly used reconstruction methods.
- Studies have shown the success of composite tissue-engineered grafts, a combination of allogeneic bone, recombinant BMP-2, and bone marrow aspirate concentrate, even for defects greater than 6 cm (Fig. 19.3).
- If a tissue-engineered graft is used, adequate vascular supply must be available from tissues surrounding the defect site, and tension-free primary closure must be obtained due to vulnerability to microorganism contamination.
- With a proper patient selection, it is possible to perform simultaneous resection and reconstruction, or "jaw-in-a-day," where dental implants and a dental prosthesis are placed concurrently with the primary reconstruction of the jaw (Fig. 19.4).
- Computer-aided surgery simulation improves the accuracy of resection, bony reconstruction, and implant placement and reduces intraoperative time.

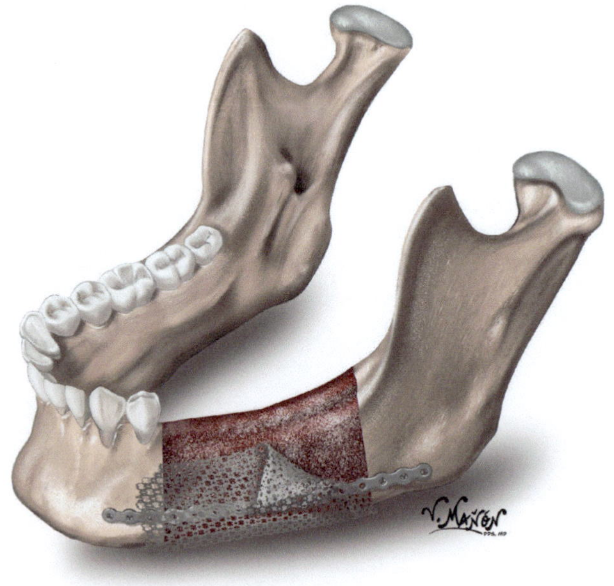

Fig. 19.3 Mandibular reconstruction with composite tissue-engineered grafts

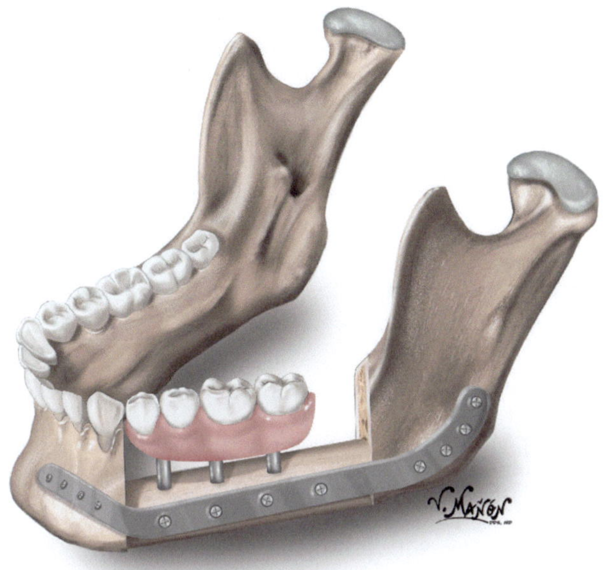

Fig. 19.4 Jaw-in-a-day procedure for mandibular reconstruction

Pearls

- Proper resection with 1–1.5 cm margins has a 98% cure rate.
- If the inferior alveolar nerve bundle is at least 1 cm from the tumor, or if it can be isolated and displaced without disrupting the tumor, it can be preserved. Otherwise, consider nerve grafting.
- Computer-aided surgery should be used when feasible as it improves accuracy and minimizes surgical time.
- Reconstruction can be accomplished with vascularized free flaps or non-vascularized bone grafting with tissue engineering.

Pitfalls

- Enucleation and curettage are not recommended for invasive ameloblastoma because of the high risk of recurrence and the potential for tumor seeding. Margins are usually 1–2 cm beyond the radiographic margin, and if not readily addressed, rapid expansion can result in airway obstruction or restriction of feeding, depending on location.

- Due to the high infection rate, immediate reconstruction should not be performed if there is communication into the oral cavity.
- While a great option with proper patient selection, "jaw-in-a-day" requires significant planning prior to the operation, which must be considered for fast-growing tumors. Another concern is low adherence to computer-assisted surgical planning when changes arise intraoperatively.

Further Reading

Müller H, Slootweg PJ. The growth characteristics of multilocular ameloblastomas. A histological investigation with some inferences with regard to operative procedures. J Maxillofac Surg. 1985;13(5):224–30.

Reichart PA, Philipsen HP, Sonner S. Ameloblastoma: biological profile of 3677 cases. Eur J Cancer B Oral Oncol. 1995;31B(2):86–99.

Marx R, Diane S. Odontogenic tumors. In: Huffman L, editor. Oral and maxillofacial pathology: a rationale for diagnosis and treatment. Vol 1. Hanover Park, IL: Quintessential Publishing Company, Inc; 2012. p. 680–757.

Kunmongkolwut S, Chaisuparat R. Analysis of BRAF V600E expression and disease-free survival in patients with ameloblastoma. Int J Oral Maxillofac Surg. 2022;51(8):1034–42.

Lu Y, Zhang X, Li X. Molecular biology exploration and targeted therapy strategy of ameloblastoma. Arch Oral Biol. 2022;140:105454.

Levine JP, Bae JS, Soares M, et al. Jaw in a day: total maxillofacial reconstruction using digital technology. Plast Reconstr Surg. 2013;131(6):1386–91.

Melville JC, Tran HQ, Bhatti AK, Manon V, Young S, Wong ME. Is reconstruction of large mandibular defects using bioengineering materials effective? J Oral Maxillofac Surg. 2020;78(4):661. e661–29.

Chapter 20
How to Avoid Odontogenic Keratocyst (OKC) Recurrence

Tiffany Han and Waleed Zaid

Abstract Odontogenic keratocyst (OKC) represents 3–11% of odontogenic cysts. It is well documented that these lesions are aggressive and have a high recurrence rate, which is reported to be between 5 and 62%. There are currently three accepted surgical treatments for OKC (marsupialization or decompression, enucleation, and en-bloc resection) as well as several adjunctive therapies (peripheral ostectomy, application of Carnoy's solution, modified Carnoy's solution, liquid nitrogen, and 5% fluorouracil (5-FU)) that might be utilized in combination with the surgical modalities. The purpose of this chapter is to review the most commonly used methods to help in minimizing OKC recurrence.

Practical Tips

Marsupialization

- The decision to marsupialize a cyst should be made during the incisional biopsy.
- Conventionally, the OKC is opened to create a pouch where the cyst lining can be sutured to the mucosa. A prosthetic device such as acrylic resin or a nasopharyngeal airway is often secured to keep the pouch open. Patients are instructed to irrigate the cavity daily for hygiene and to maintain patency.
- Marsupialization alone as a surgical modality in the management of OKC has a 32.3% recurrence rate.
- Combining residual cyst enucleation after marsupialization or decompression reduces the recurrence rate to 14.6%.

T. Han · W. Zaid (✉)
Louisiana State University Health Sciences Center New Orleans, New Orleans, LA, USA
e-mail: wzaid@lsuhsc.edu

D. Amin, H. Marwan (eds.), *Pearls and Pitfalls in Oral and Maxillofacial Surgery*, https://doi.org/10.1007/978-3-031-47307-4_20

Enucleation

- Ensuring the cyst is removed entirely from the bony cavity is critical. However, doing so can be challenging as the cyst lining is friable and only typically composed of 6–8 cells thick.
- Enucleation alone as a surgical modality in the management of OKC has a recurrence rate of 23.1%.
- Combining enucleation with various adjuvant therapy has helped reduce the recurrence rate to 11.5–17.4%.
- Sometimes enucleation might be associated with risks, especially if the cyst is approaching the inferior border of the mandible, which places the patient at risk of a pathological fracture or neurosensory injury of the inferior alveolar nerve.
- It is helpful to document the vitality of all the teeth with roots located within the cyst before enucleation.

En Bloc Resection

- En bloc resection results in a low recurrence rate of 0–8.4% but increases patient morbidity.
- This treatment modality is typically reserved for cases with multiple recurrences or under challenging locations where other surgical modalities are hard to implement (e.g., coronoid process) and, finally, in rare cases, those that have undergone malignant transformation or have led to a pathological fracture.

Peripheral Ostectomy

- This procedure aims to mechanically remove cyst wall remnants or satellite cysts using rotary instruments, usually about 2–3 mm.
- In conjunction with enucleation, this reduces recurrence from 23.1% to 17.5%.
- It may not be feasible to perform peripheral ostectomy depending on the location of the OKC (proximity to teeth or neurovascular bundle, lingual cortex).

Carnoy's Solution and Modified Carnoy's Solution

- The application of Carnoy's solution (absolute alcohol, glacial acetic acid, chloroform, and ferric chloride) aims to fix remnant epithelial lining or satellite cysts.

- Recommended application time for Carnoy's solution is between 3 and 5 min with an expected 1.5 mm bony penetration without penetration into the neurovascular bundle. However, sensory disturbance after 3 min has been reported.
- As an adjuvant therapy along with enucleation, Carnoy's solution has been shown to reduce recurrence to 11.5%.
- The use of modified Carnoy's solution has not shown to be as effective at reducing surgical recurrence, with an estimated recurrence of up to 35–50%.

Liquid Nitrogen

- Cryosurgery promotes 1–3 mm penetration necrosis of epithelial remnants or satellite cysts.
- This procedure involves the application of liquid nitrogen for 1 min followed by a 5-min slow thaw. It is recommended to repeat this procedure for 2 to 3 rounds after enucleation with peripheral ostectomy.
- The estimated recurrence rate with cryotherapy as adjunctive therapy along with enucleation is approximately 14.5–29.2%.

5-Fluorouracil (FU)

- After the cyst's enucleation, 5-FU is coated on a ribbon gauze and placed into a cystic cavity. It is then removed 24 h postoperatively. More recently, the authors have been applying 5-FU to a sheet of non-compressed Gelfoam and packing it in the cavity. This eliminates the need for a second procedure to remove the ribbon gauze after 24 h.
- The recurrence rate using 5-FU is low. Although few studies are available, no recurrences were documented, with a follow-up period of 22 months.

Reconstruction

- Timing dental rehabilitation is essential. Consider postponing reconstructive efforts until after the excision of the cyst or after a period of decompression.
- Although there have been case reports that show success with grafting and immediate implant placement after enucleation, OKC has been shown to recur in grafted sites and can be stressful and costly for patients when dealing with recurrence and graft failure.
- Without bone grafting, a period of 9–12 months delay is recommended after surgical intervention before implant placement.

Pearls

- Complete removal of the cystic lining may be difficult as the lining tends to be thin and friable—adjunctive techniques (peripheral ostectomy, chemical cautery) aid in reducing the recurrence rate.
- Establishing wide access to better visualize the cyst during removal can be helpful in the complete removal of the cystic lining to prevent a recurrence.
- Inferior alveolar nerve can be preserved as odontogenic keratocysts do not invade the epineurium.

Pitfalls

- Failure of initial conservative measures or delayed diagnosis of odontogenic keratocysts can make further surgical intervention considerably more difficult.
- Failure to recognize recurrence on follow-up imaging can lead to devastating outcomes. Recurrence will typically be apparent within 18 months, but a 7–10-year follow-up is recommended. Post-surgical radiolucency should become smaller and radio-opaque over time. An enlarging radiolucency is a sign of recurrence.
- Multiple odontogenic keratocysts should raise suspicion for nevoid basal cell carcinoma syndrome. It is prudent for clinicians to identify these individuals to establish a diagnosis and to make necessary referrals to other healthcare specialties. Close follow-up with these patients is necessary as they are likely to require multiple surgeries.

Further Reading

Neville BW, et al. Oral and maxillofacial pathology. Fourth. 2016.

Pogrel MA. Decompression and marsupialization as a treatment for the odontogenic keratocyst. Oral Maxil Surg Clin. 2003;15:415–27.

Al-Moraissi EA, Dahan AA, Alwadeai MS, Oginni FO, Al-Jamali JM, Alkhutari AS, et al. What surgical treatment has the lowest recurrence rate following the management of keratocystic odontogenic tumor?: A large systematic review and meta-analysis. J Cranio-Maxillo-Facial Surg Off Publ Eur Assoc Cranio-Maxillo-Facial Surg. 2017;45:1.

Voorsmit R. The incredible keratocyst [thesis]. Nijmegen: University of Nijmegen; 1984.

Cassoni A, et al. Keratocystic odontogenic tumor surgical management: retrospective analysis on 77 patients. Eur J Inflamm. 2013;12:209–15.

Frerich B, Cornelius CP, Wietholter H. Critical time of exposure of the rabbit inferior alveolar nerve to Carnoy's solution. J Oral Maxillofac Surg. 1994;52:599–606.

Tay ZW, Sue WL, Leeson RMA. Chemical adjuncts and cryotherapy in the management of odontogenic keratocysts: a systematic review. Adv Oral Maxillofac Surg. 2021;3:100116.

Dashow JE, McHugh JB, Braun TM, Edwards SP, Helman JI, Ward BB. Significantly decreased recurrence rates in keratocystic odontogenic tumor with simple enucleation and curettage using Carnoy's versus modified Carnoy's solution. J Oral Maxillofac Surg. 2015;73:2132–5.

Pogrel MA. The use of liquid nitrogen cryotherapy in the management of locally aggressive bone lesions. J Oral Maxillofac Surg. 1993;51:269–73.

Ledderhof NJ, Caminiti MF, Bradley G, Lam DK. Topical 5-fluorouracil is a novel targeted therapy for the keratocystic odontogenic tumor. J Oral Maxillofac Surg. 2017;75:514–24.

Caminiti MF, et al. 5-Fluorouracil is associated with a decreased recurrence risk in odontogenic keratocyst management: a retrospective cohort study. J Oral Maxillofac Surg. 2021;79(4):814–21.

Isler SC, et al. Immediate implants after enucleation of an odontogenic keratocyst: an early return to function. J Oral Implant. 2012;38:1.

Chapter 21
Preoperative Workup of Oral Cavity Cancer

Victoria A. Mañón, Dina Amin ⓘ, and Hisham Marwan ⓘ

Abstract In 2020, there were 377,713 new cases of oral cavity and lip squamous cell carcinoma in the United States. Oral cancer is the 16th most common cancer in the United States, with ~11,230 deaths per year. In 2022, the 5-year relative survival rate is ~68%; early identification and management of head and neck pathology are imperative for improving survival outcomes. Oral and maxillofacial surgeons are uniquely positioned, in collaboration with other dental colleagues, to identify and manage oral cancer. The purpose of this chapter is to review the preoperative workup for oral cavity cancer.

Identification, Examination, and Preliminary Diagnostic Methods

Head and neck examinations should be routinely performed on all new and existing patients in order to detect any existing or developing lesions within the oral cavity. When an oral cavity lesion is first identified, the first step in diagnosis and management is obtaining and complete medical history, history of the lesion, physical examination, obtaining indicated radiographs, and relevant laboratory testing when indicated.

V. A. Mañón
McGovern Medical School, University of Texas Oral & Maxillofacial Surgery, UTHSC School of Dentistry at Houston, Houston, TX, USA

D. Amin
Department of Oral and Maxillofacial Surgery, University of Rochester, Rochester, NY, USA
e-mail: dina_amin@urmc.rochester.edu

H. Marwan (✉)
Department of Surgery, The University of Texas Medical Branch, Galveston, TX, USA
e-mail: himarwan@utmb.edu

- Obtain or update the patient's medical history:

  - Does the patient have any existing medical conditions requiring a change in surgical management?
  - Is the identified lesion possibly an oral manifestation of an existing or undiagnosed medical condition?

- Obtain a history of the lesion:

  - How long has the lesion been present?
  - Has the lesion changed in size or dimensions?
  - Has the lesion changed in character or features?
  - Are there any symptoms associated with the lesion (i.e., pain, numbness, dysphagia, tender lymph nodes)?
  - What anatomic structures are involved?
  - Are there any associated systemic symptoms?
  - Is the lesion associated with any events (i.e., trauma, history of travel, exposure to toxins)?

- Complete a clinical examination, including information regarding:

  - Anatomic location of the lesion.
  - A detailed description of the physical characteristics of the lesion.
  - Number of lesions (if applicable) and their locations.
  - Size (measured), shape, and growth presentation of the lesion.
  - Color of the lesion.
  - Borders/demarcation (sharp versus ill-defined).
  - Mobility (freely mobile versus fixed).
  - Palpation.
  - Presence of pulsation.
  - Examination of regional lymph nodes.

- Radiographic examination:

  - Bony lesions should be further examined with panoramic imaging, cone beam computed tomography (CBCT), or magnetic resonance imaging (MRI), as indicated.
  - Soft tissue lesions adjacent to the bone may reveal bony or dental reactions or an intraosseous origin of the lesion.

- Nasopharyngoscopic examination: a complete examination of the head and neck is impossible without a careful assessment of the inaccessible areas such as the nasopharynx, the base of the tongue, the vallecula, and the vocal cords.
- After the diagnostic information is obtained, the practitioner should be able to develop a differential diagnosis and treatment plan. A biopsy should be completed as soon as possible if the lesion has multiple suspicious or malignant features (Table 21.1).

Table 21.1 List of historical and clinical features that should raise suspicion for malignancy

Features of lesions suspicious for malignancy
Bleeding
longer duration (>2 weeks)
Erythroplakia
Fixation to adjacent structures (non-mobile)
Rapid growth rate
Indurated on palpation
Ulceration
Increased pain in the region
Non-healing tissue after surgery
History of oral cancer
Bony or dental erosion on imaging

Biopsy: Indications and Techniques

- Indications for biopsy include:

  - Any lesion that presents with the previously reviewed suspicious, malignant (or premalignant) characteristics (Table 21.1).
  - Persistent pathologic conditions that can't be clinically diagnosed.
  - Observed lesions that do not respond as predicted to clinical management (i.e., failure to heal in 10–14 days after removing traumatic source).

- Biopsy techniques typically used for the oral cavity include:

  - Cytology-based procedures.
  - Incisional.
  - Excisional.
  - Aspiration is mainly used for the diagnosis of cervical lymph node.

- Tissue specimens can be further evaluated using viral detection techniques for HPV (In-situ hybridization, p16 immunohistochemical surrogate marker, PCR).

Diagnostic Confirmation and Staging of Oral Cancer

- Once oral cancer has been confirmed with histopathologic diagnosis, the tumor should be staged to determine treatment and prognosis (Table 21.2).

  - Primary tumor (T).
  - Regional lymph nodes (N).

      Clinical nodes (cN).
      Pathologic nodes (pN).

  - Distant metastasis (M).

Table 21.2 Primary tumor (T)

T category	T criteria
TX	Primary tumor cannot be assessed
Tis	Carcinoma in situ
T1	Tumor ≤2 cm with depth of invasion (DOI) ≤5 mm
T2	Tumor ≤2 cm, with DOI* >5 mm and ≤ 10 mm; or tumor >2 cm and ≤ 4 cm, with DOI* ≤10 mm
T3	Tumor >2 cm and ≤ 4 cm with DOI* >10 mm; or Tumor >4 cm with DOI* ≤10 mm
T4	Moderately advanced or very advanced local disease
T4a	Moderately advanced local disease. Tumor >4 cm with DOI* >10 mm; or Tumor invades adjacent structures only (e.g., through cortical bone of the mandible or maxilla, or involves the maxillary sinus or skin of the face) NOTE: Superficial erosion of bone/tooth socket (alone) by a gingival primary is not sufficient to classify a tumor as T4
T4b	Very advanced local disease Tumor invades masticator space, pterygoid plates, or skull base and/or encases the internal carotid artery

- The most significant prognostic factors are tumor size, depth of invasion, nodal status, and distant metastasis.
- Histologic factors associated with poor prognosis include a non-cohesive pattern of invasion (small islands, narrow strands), tumor budding (single cells, clusters of <5 cells at invasive front), perineural and lymphovascular invasion, and bone invasion.
- Approximately 90% of cancers in the oral cavity and oropharynx are squamous cell carcinoma.
- MRI, PET, or CT scans may be used to detect regional node metastasis and other pathologic features of the primary tumor.

  - MRI is superior for detecting extranodal extension, perineural spread, skull base erosion, and intracranial extension.
  - PET is superior for detecting regional node metastasis, distant metastasis to other organs, and second primary tumors.
  - Imaging alone should not replace the need for neck dissection in attempts to detect nodal metastasis.

- Once the tumor has been staged, the need for surgical resection with or without neck dissection and adjuvant treatment can be selected and discussed with the patient.

Tables 21.2, 21.3, 21.4, 21.5, 21.6. TNM staging of oral cavity cancer, adapted from the American Joint Committee on Cancer, Union for International Cancer Control, eighth edition.

Table 21.3 Clinical node (cN)

cN category	cN criteria
NX	Regional lymph nodes cannot be assessed
N0	No regional lymph node metastasis
N1	Metastasis in a single ipsilateral lymph node, 3 cm or smaller in greatest dimension extranodal extension (ENE)(−)
N2	Metastasis in a single ipsilateral node larger than 3 cm but not larger than 6 cm in greatest dimension and ENE(−); or Metastases in multiple ipsilateral lymph nodes, none larger than 6 cm in greatest dimension and ENE(−); or In bilateral or contralateral lymph nodes, none larger than 6 cm in greatest dimension, and ENE(−)
N2a	Metastasis in a single ipsilateral node larger than 3 cm but not larger than 6 cm in greatest dimension, and ENE(−)
N2b	Metastases in multiple ipsilateral nodes, none larger than 6 cm in greatest dimension, and ENE(−)
N2c	Metastases in bilateral or contralateral lymph nodes, none larger than 6 cm in greatest dimension, and ENE(−)
N3	Metastasis in a lymph node larger than 6 cm in greatest dimension and ENE(−); or Metastasis in any node(s) and clinically overt ENE(+)
N3a	Metastasis in a lymph node larger than 6 cm in greatest dimension and ENE(−)
N3b	Metastasis in any node(s) and clinically overt ENE(+)

Table 21.4 Pathological node (pN)

pN category	pN criteria
NX	Regional lymph nodes cannot be assessed
N0	No regional lymph node metastasis
N1	Metastasis in a single ipsilateral lymph node, 3 cm or smaller in greatest dimension extranodal extension (ENE)(−)
N2	Metastasis in a single ipsilateral lymph node, 3 cm or smaller in greatest dimension and ENE(+); or Larger than 3 cm but not larger than 6 cm in greatest dimension and ENE(−); or Metastases in multiple ipsilateral lymph nodes, none larger than 6 cm in greatest dimension and ENE(−); or In bilateral or contralateral lymph node(s), none larger than 6 cm in greatest dimension, ENE(−)
N2a	Metastasis in single ipsilateral node 3 cm or smaller in greatest dimension and ENE(+); or A single ipsilateral node larger than 3 cm but not larger than 6 cm in greatest dimension and ENE(−)
N2b	Metastases in multiple ipsilateral nodes, none larger than 6 cm in greatest dimension and ENE(−)
N2c	Metastases in bilateral or contralateral lymph node(s), none larger than 6 cm in greatest dimension and ENE(−)

(continued)

Table 21.4 Continud

pN category	pN criteria
N3	Metastasis in a lymph node larger than 6 cm in greatest dimension and ENE(−); or Metastasis in a single ipsilateral node larger than 3 cm in greatest dimension and ENE(+); or Multiple ipsilateral, contralateral, or bilateral nodes any with ENE(+); or A single contralateral node of any size and ENE(+)
N3a	Metastasis in a lymph node larger than 6 cm in greatest dimension and ENE(−)
N3b	Metastasis in a single ipsilateral node larger than 3 cm in greatest dimension and ENE(+); or Multiple ipsilateral, contralateral, or bilateral nodes any with ENE(+); or A single contralateral node of any size and ENE(+)

Table 21.5 Distant metastasis (M)

M category	M criteria
M0	No distant metastasis
M1	Distant metastasis

Table 21.6 Prognostic stage groups

When T is…	And N is…	And M is…	Stage group is…
Tis	N0	M0	0
T1	N0	M0	I
T2	N0	M0	II
T3	N0	M0	III
T1, T2, T3	N1	M0	III
T4a	N0, N1	M0	IVA
T1, T2, T3, T4a	N2	M0	IVA
Any T	N3	M0	IVB
T4b	Any N	M0	IVB
Any T	Any N	M1	IVC

Prognosis and Survival Statistics of Oral Cancer

- 5-year relative survival rate

  - Stage I: 76–81%.
  - Stage II: 58–66%.
  - Stage III: 41–59%.
  - Stage IV: 9–32%.

- 65–70% of lesions at the time of identification are stage III or IV.

Further Reading

Sung H, et al. Global cancer statistics 2020: GLOBOCAN estimates of incidence and mortality worldwide for 36 cancers in 185 countries. CA Cancer J Clin. 2021;71(3):209–49. https://doi.org/10.3322/caac.21660. Epub 2021 Feb 4.

Hupp JR, Tucker MR, Ellis E. Principles of differential diagnosis and biopsy. In: Contemporary oral and maxillofacial surgery. 6th ed. St. Louis: Mosby; 2014.

Poon CS, Stenson KM. Overview of the diagnosis and staging of head and neck cancer. Waltham: UpToDate; 2022. https://www.uptodate.com/contents/overview-of-the-diagnosis-and-staging-of-head-and-neck-cancer. Accessed 26 Nov 2022.

Müller S. Update from the 4th edition of the World Health Organization of head and neck tumours: tumours of the oral cavity and mobile tongue. Head Neck Pathol. 2017;11(1):33–40. https://doi.org/10.1007/s12105-017-0792-3. Epub 2017 Feb 28. PMID: 28247230; PMCID: PMC5340733.

Lydiatt WM. At al. Head and neck cancers-major changes in the American joint committee on cancer eighth edition cancer staging manual. CA Cancer J Clin. 2017;67(2):122–37. https://doi.org/10.3322/caac.21389. Epub2017 Jan 27.

Chapter 22
Intraoperative Decisions for Oral Squamous Cell Carcinoma Management

Jeremy Figueroa-Ortiz and Justine Moe

Abstract In the United States, approximately 50,000 people are diagnosed with oral squamous cell carcinoma (OSCC) a year. Surgery remains the primary treatment method for these tumors with radiation with or without chemotherapy used in the adjuvant setting. In this chapter, we focus on the principles of ablative and reconstructive surgery in the management of OSCC. The surgical treatment of OSCC should be tailored to the patient's specific needs to provide personalized surgical care and optimize patient outcomes.

Practical Tips

Preoperative Consideration

- Treatment principles for OSCC follow the National Comprehensive Cancer Network (NCCN) guidelines.
- Treatment considerations should be discussed through multidisciplinary conferences inclusive of several teams, including surgery, medical oncology, radiation oncology, radiology, pathology, dentistry, nutrition, speech and language pathology, social work, anesthesia, and nursing.
- Treatment at high-volume centers with surgical teams equipped in microvascular surgery and intensive care, nursing, and anesthesia teams skilled in managing head and neck cancer patients is associated with improved perioperative and survival outcomes.

J. Figueroa-Ortiz · J. Moe (✉)
Department of Oral and Maxillofacial Surgery, University of Michigan, Ann Arbor, MI, USA
e-mail: jxfo@med.umich.edu; jusmoe@umich.edu

Pre-operative Assessment

- Before the surgical intervention, the patient's premorbid health status, function, lifestyle, and care goals should be considered to optimize outcomes.
- Patient comorbidities overwhelmingly impact planning, complications, morbidity, and mortality. This should be taken into consideration prior to surgical planning. The frailty index can be used to measure the health status of older individuals and serve as a proxy measure of aging and vulnerability to adverse outcomes.
- Poor nutrition (hypoalbuminemia), chronic alcohol use, and smoking can significantly compromise wound healing and contribute to higher infection rates and overall increased complication rates. Failure to remove carcinogenic sources (alcohol, tobacco products) can contribute to recurrence.
- Preoperative speech, swallowing function, and performance status should be considered and objectively measured using validated scales (e.g., functional intraoral Glasgow scale [FIGS]; ECOG performance status).

Intraoperative Consideration

Ablation

- The objective of surgical ablation in OSCC is the resection of the primary tumor to negative margins and the treatment of clinically overt or occult cervical metastases. Ablative interventions should occur only in the context of a previously secured airway, including a tracheostomy when indicated. The management of cervical metastases, including neck dissection and sentinel lymph node biopsy, is discussed in subsequent chapters.
- The standard of care in ablative surgery is the removal of malignancy with negative margins while preserving adequate native tissue for form and function. While the definition of a negative margin remains a point of debate, margins greater than 5 mm and up to 10 mm are widely accepted as adequate. Negative margins should be obtained at all involved component tissues, including mucosa, skin, deep soft tissue, nerve, and bone.
- Despite this controversy, strong data support negative pathologic margins of ≥ 7.0 mm to be associated with better local disease control, with most surgeons finding pathologic margins ≥ 5.0 mm to be adequate.
- The sacrifice of vital structures may be indicated for tumor-free margins as negative margins are predictive of enhanced disease-free survival at 5 years. For example, this may include lingual nerve resection for a retromolar trigone malignancy. Reconstruction of vital structures may be considered on a case-by-case basis.

- Two approaches can be taken when assessing margin status:
  - Specimen-driven margins refer to the assessment of margins from the excised specimen. They allow for comprehensive mucosal margins (e.g., shave margins) or the distance from the tumor to the margin (e.g., radial margins) to be assessed but require close communication between the surgeon and pathologist.
  - Patient (defect)-driven margins refer to margins taken from select locations within the tumor bed, allowing the ablative surgeon to select the margins of interest.
- For soft tissue, specimen-driven analysis has been found to have a sensitivity of 47.6% and a specificity of 96.7%, while defect driven was 47.6% and 84.4%, respectively.
- A close or positive margin may occur due to tumor size, the extent of invasion, and/or aggressive tumor biology and decreases overall prognosis. In these cases, re-resection to negative margins is preferred. However, margin revision is not associated with improved survival, further emphasizing the importance of adequate initial resection. Alternatively, adjuvant radiation for close margins and chemoradiation in the setting of a positive margin is considered to reduce the risk of recurrence.
- Site-specific considerations for tumor ablation are given in Table 22.1. Most OSCC tumors can be resected through a transoral approach. However, alternative approaches are considered for extensive tumors invading adjacent structures and are discussed in Table 22.1.

Reconstruction

- Reconstruction goals include wound coverage and restoration to premorbid form and function.
- Historically, the principles of reconstruction followed the concept of the "reconstructive ladder," which described utilizing the simplest reconstructive intervention to enhance outcomes before employing more complex techniques. The idea of the reconstructive "elevator" or "toolbox" has since been adopted based on utilizing one or a combination of reconstructive techniques of the appropriate complexity to reconstruct form and function (Table 22.2).
- The selection of a reconstructive method should consider recipient site factors (e.g., defect dimensions, location, missing tissue components, quality of surrounding tissue), donor site factors (e.g., dimensions, tissue components, tissue match, donor site morbidities, the arc of rotation and reach for locoregional flaps; pedicle length and geometry for free flaps), patient considerations, and functional goals.
- Osseous reconstruction usually necessitates a free flap. Corticocancellous bone grafts are typically not used due to extensive soft tissue defects often necessitated with oncologic resection or due to the anticipated need for adjuvant radiation.

Table 22.1 Site-specific considerations for ablative and reconstructive surgery

Site	Ablative considerations	Reconstructive considerations
Mandible	<u>Anatomical considerations:</u> • Extent of bony resection should be assessed on presurgical radiologic workup (e.g., panorex, computed tomography) • Mandibular involvement should be suspected with gingival OSCC regardless of imaging or gross clinical assessment <u>Alternative approaches:</u> • Intraoral approach is indicated for most mandibular tumors; however, it may be used in combination with a transfacial approach for an extensive tumor invading skin, with a lip-split approach for posterior tumors, or with a transcervical approach in the setting of concurrent neck dissection <u>Technical considerations:</u> • Marginal mandibulectomy is indicated for OSCC of the alveolar gingiva with no or early mandibular involvement on clinical or radiographic evaluation. • Segmental mandibulectomy is indicated for extensive invasion, condylar involvement, edentulous patients, if anticipated <10 mm remaining following marginal resection. • A supraperiosteal dissection should be completed until at least 1 cm away from the tumor, at which location the periosteum can be incised and subperiosteal dissection can be completed on disease-free bone. • The osteotomy should be planned through dental extraction sites rather than between teeth • If a 1 cm bone margin is not possible while preserving 10 mm of mandibular height at the inferior border, a segmental mandibulectomy rather than a marginal mandibulectomy should be performed • When performing a marginal mandibulectomy, curvilinear osteotomies reduce the risk of fracture • Intraoperative margin evaluation, including bony margins from the native remaining mandible, can be performed with high sensitivity and specificity (up to 89% and 100%, respectively). If the perineural invasion is suspected, intraoperative nerve margins along the proximal inferior alveolar nerve and distal mental nerve should be assessed • In cases of angle-to-angle mandibulectomy, maintenance of the bilateral coronoid processes, when possible, can reduce the risk of lip incompetency and open bite following surgery	• Reconstructive goals: Maintain mandibular form and integrity for mastication and facial profile • Marginal mandibulectomy with a small alveolar soft tissue defect can be reconstructed with primary closure or local flaps (e.g., facial artery myomucosal flap, nasolabial flap) • Marginal mandibulectomy and large soft tissue defects may require regional or free flap reconstruction for soft tissue (ex. supraclavicular flap, radial forearm free flap) • Prophylactic plating may be indicated to prevent fracture if <10 mm mandibular height remaining • Osseous reconstruction of segmental mandibulectomy defects usually requires free flaps, with the fibula free flap serving as a mainstay in this reconstruction, with favorable outcomes. The fibula free flap provides adequate tissue for dental implant placement and enough length for condylar reconstruction • Alternatively, the scapula-free flap can be considered. Osseous free flaps restore mandibular continuity, volume, and stability • Pectoralis major myocutaneous flap can be used for soft tissue reconstruction only for poor free flap candidates

Maxilla	Anatomic considerations: • Gingival involvement necessitates resection of underlying bony tissue • Extent of invasion into the maxilla, maxillary sinus, nasal cavity, and skull base should be established preoperatively • Common sources of bleeding during maxillectomy include pterygoid plexus (venous), posterior superior alveolar artery, and greater palatine artery Alternative approaches: • Brown Classification I/II can be approached transorally • Midfacial degloving incision (sublabial and rhinoplasty incisions) improves access to the bilateral anterior maxilla and paranasal sinuses without the need for facial incisions • The Weber–Ferguson approach allows wide access to the entire maxilla and orbital floor, which is useful for lateral extending tumors • A lip split mandibulotomy improves access to tumors of the posterior maxilla with extension into the pterygoid plates or infratemporal fossa Technical considerations: • Strategies to improve hemostasis include local anesthetic with epinephrine prior to incision and development of mean arterial pressure goals with the anesthesia team, and intraoperative use of topical vasoconstrictor agents • The periosteum should be incised, and the osteotomies should be performed at least 1 cm from the tumor. Tumor extent of the maxillary sinus and nasal cavity should be assessed preoperatively to plan the location of osteotomies • Osteotomies can be completed with a reciprocating saw and finalized with osteotomes with care to avoid disruption of the nasal endotracheal tube • Intraoperative navigation technology can be used to assist in tumor mapping and guide the resection	• Discussion regarding dental rehabilitation should be completed preoperatively. Candidacy for dental/zygomaticus implants may lead to consideration for osseous reconstruction and/or implant placement at the time of resection • The primary reconstructive goal is to separate the oral and sinonasal compartments from one another • An ablative defect without an oro-nasal/antral communication can heal by secondary intention. A postoperative stent may be considered • Obturator reconstruction allows for immediate dental rehabilitation and can redistribute forces to the facial skeleton to prevent undesirable trauma • Zygomatic implants can improve obturator retention and stability • Maxillary defects with large soft tissue defects, extension into the soft palate, retromolar trigone, or buccal mucosa may require reconstruction with soft tissue regional or free flap • Osseous free flaps (including fibula or scapula flaps) may be indicated for maxillary defects with orbital floor or zygoma defects, bilateral anterior maxillary defects, or in cases in which dental implant placement within the flap is desired
Retromolar trigone (RMT)	Anatomical considerations: • OSCC involving the RMT can extend to involve the posterior maxilla, mandible, buccal mucosa, and anterior tonsillar pillar • The lingual nerve is in close proximity to the RMT and may require resection Technical considerations: • Careful dissection to preserve the lingual and inferior alveolar nerves should be performed when possible • Maxillectomy and mandibulectomy may be required as part of the oncologic resection	• Small defects of the RMT may be amenable to local flap reconstruction (e.g., facial artery myomucosal flap [FAMM], buccal advancement flap, palatal flap) • Large defects of the RMT may require soft tissue free flap reconstruction (e.g., radial forearm free flap) • Postoperative therapy to increase mandibular range of motion is indicated to reduce the risk of trismus

(continued)

Table 22.1 Contined

Site	Ablative considerations	Reconstructive considerations
Tongue	<u>Anatomic considerations:</u> • Extensive tongue tumors can involve the floor of the mouth, mylohyoid muscle, lingual mandible, base of the tongue, and suprahyoid muscles • Perineural invasion can involve the lingual and hypoglossal nerves <u>Alternative approaches:</u> • The transoral approach is suitable for most T1/T2 tongue tumors • A lip split mandibulotomy is useful for large posterior tongue tumors • A pull-through submental approach is useful for total or subtotal glossectomies <u>Technical considerations:</u> • Manual palpation can aid in the assessment of tumor depth • Clear margins can be achieved with 1.5–2 cm surgical margins; to preserve function, 1–1.5 cm are typically used	• The reconstructive goal is to restore tongue mobility and bulk for speech, eating, and swallowing • Small tongue defects can heal by secondary intention or can be reconstructed with a split-thickness skin graft or tissue engineering techniques, including acellular dermal matrix • Moderate tongue defects ($\geq$2/3 native tongue present) can be reconstructed with local flaps (e.g., FAMM, submental) or can heal by secondary intention • Lateral tongue defects tend to be amenable to primarily closure • The radial forearm free flap is thin and pliable and can be used to reconstruct the mucosal lining of large tongue defects • Total or subtotal glossectomy defects necessitate reconstruction of tongue volume. Options include the anterolateral thigh flap, the rectus abdominus flap, and the pectoralis major myocutaneous flap. Overall, these defects require volume replacement via fasciocutaneous or myocutaneous free flap
Floor of mouth (FOM)	<u>Anatomic considerations:</u> • The lingual nerve and submandibular duct travel along the floor of mouth and may require resection as part of the ablative surgery <u>Alternative approaches:</u> • The transoral approach is feasible for most tumors isolated to the floor of mouth. <u>Technical considerations:</u> • For ablative defects, including the mandibular gingiva, this margin should be performed early with a division of the periosteum to allow for ease of access for the remainder of the floor of mouth resection • The lingual nerve should be preserved when possible • For ablative defects, including the submandibular duct, the duct should be identified proximally prior to transection to facilitate sialodochoplasty and stenting if needed	• The mucosa of the floor of mouth is relatively displaceable and redundant • Small floor of mouth defects may be reconstructed with floor of mouth advancement and primary closure, split-thickness skin graft, or tissue engineering techniques, including acellular dermal matrix • Resection of the submandibular duct without neck dissection (and subsequent removal of the submandibular gland) necessitates completing a sialodochoplasty with stenting to create a neo-ostium

| Buccal mucosa | Anatomic considerations:
• To achieve negative margins, full-thickness resection of the buccal mucosa, cheek, and overlying skin may be indicated
• The proximity of and possible resection of Stenson's duct with the ablative procedure should be considered
• Full-thickness resection of the cheek will include distal branches of the facial nerve
Alternative approaches:
• The transoral approach may be combined with the transfacial approach for planned full-thickness resection of the cheek
Technical considerations:
• If the planned resection includes Stenson's duct, the proximal duct should be identified
• If cheek skin is within 1 cm of the deep tumor margin, it should be excised along with intraoral tissue | • The reconstructive goal is to ensure healing or replacement of the mucosal lining to prevent postoperative trismus
• Small defects with intact buccinator muscle can heal by secondary intention or can be reconstructed with a split-thickness skin graft or tissue engineering techniques, including acellular dermal matrix
• Large defects with resected buccinator muscle can be reconstructed with local flaps (ex. buccal fat advancement flap) or locoregional or free flaps (ex., submental flap, radial forearm free flap)
• Full-thickness defects, including the skin of the cheek, may require locoregional or free flap reconstruction (ex., radial forearm free flap, anterolateral thigh free flap)
• For resection of a short segment of the distal Stenson's duct, sialodochoplasty with stenting should be considered
• For resection of a longer segment of Stenson's duct, sialodochoplasty may not be feasible; a transoral drain extending to the parotid space should be placed and maintained until the onset of adjuvant radiotherapy |

Table 22.2 The reconstructive toolbox

Reconstructive method	Technique	Example
Primary intention	Closure occurs with direct approximation of skin edges	Direct re-approximation of the mucosal edges of an intraoral ablative defect
Secondary intention	Allowing granulation tissue to fill in wound defect	Ablative defect of the tongue is left open to heal over the course of weeks
Skin graft	Skin from donor site transferred to wound to facilitate healing	Split thickness skin graft from the thigh to reconstruct a floor of mouth defect
Local flap	Transferring adjacent tissue in one part of the body to cover an adjacent defect	Mucosal advancement flap to reconstruct a lip vermilion defect
Regional flap	Donor tissue located at a distance away from the primary defect is transferred with an intact vascular pedicle	Pectoralis major myocutaneous flap to reconstruct a buccal mucosal defect
Free flap	Donor tissue disconnected from its original blood supply from the original location is transferred to the defect in another region of the body	Osteocutaneous fibula free flap to reconstruct a mandibular segmental defect
Tissue engineering	Biomedical engineering of cells, materials, and factors to replace different tissue types	Acellular dermal matrix to reconstruct a mucosal defect

Pearls

1. Optimize preoperative planning: Study imaging and surgical plan and communicate with teams involved with patient care to optimize outcomes and patient disposition.
2. Anticipate intraoperative factors (frozen specimens, invasion of vital structures, etc.) that would change surgical treatment and have a plan.
3. Optimize post-operative nutrition and integrate this with the surgical plan. Consider tube placement in the operating room or coordinate as necessary (Nasogastric tube, Gastrostomy tube, etc.).

Pitfalls

1. Anticipate the possibility of continued post-operative intubation or tracheostomy.
2. Anticipate the location of the endotracheal tube to avoid accidental injury, especially in a maxillectomy—communication with the anesthesia team is critical.

3. Many head and neck cancer patients have aberrant anatomy; an understanding of both normal and the patient's baseline allows for an easier operation and enhanced outcomes.
4. Understanding patient goals and when non-operative palliation is indicated.

Further Reading

U.S. Department of Health and Human Services. Oral cancer 5-year survival rates by race, gender, and stage of diagnosis. Bethesda, MD: National Institute of Dental and Craniofacial Research; 2018.

NCCN guidelines. NCCN. 2022. https://www.nccn.org/guidelines/nccn-guidelines.

Schwam ZG, Judson BL. Improved prognosis for patients with oral cavity squamous cell carcinoma: analysis of the National Cancer Database 1998–2006. Oral Oncol. 2016;52:45.

Piccirillo JF. Importance of comorbidity in head and neck cancer. Laryngoscope. 2000;110:593.

Dequanter D, Lothaire P. Serum albumin concentration and surgical site identify surgical risk for major post-operative complications in advanced head and neck patients. B-ENT. 2011;7:181–3.

Kim DD, Ord RA. Complications in the treatment of head and neck cancer. Oral Maxillofac Surg Clin North Am. 2003;15:213–27.

Zanoni DK, Migliacci JC, Xu B, Katabi N, Montero PH, Ganly I, Shah JP, Wong RJ, Ghossein RA, Patel SG. A proposal to redefine close surgical margins in squamous cell carcinoma of the oral tongue. JAMA Otolaryngol Head Neck Surg. 2017;143:555.

Colevas AD, Yom SS, Pfister DG, Spencer S, Adelstein D, Adkins D, Brizel DM, Burtness B, Busse PM, Caudell JJ, Cmelak AJ, Eisele DW, Fenton M, Foote RL, Gilbert J, Gillison ML, Haddad RI, Hicks WL, Hitchcock YJ, Jimeno A, Leizman D, Maghami E, Mell LK, Mittal BB, Pinto HA, Ridge JA, Rocco J, Rodriguez CP, Shah JP, Weber RS, Witek M, Worden F, Zhen W, Burns JL, Darlow SD. NCCN guidelines insights: head and neck cancers, version 1.2018. J Natl Compr Cancer Netw. 2018;16:479.

Loree TRSE. SIgnificance of positive margins in Oral cavity squamous carcinoma. Am J Surg. 1990;160:410–4.

Nason RW, Binahmed A, Pathak KA, Abdoh AA, Sandor GK. What is the adequate margin of surgical resection in oral cancer? Oral Surg Oral Med Oral Pathol Oral Radiol Endod. 2009;107(5):625–9.

Liao CT, Chang JT, Wang HM, Ng SH, Hsueh C, Lee LY, et al. Analysis of risk factors of predictive local tumor control in oral cavity cancer. Ann Surg Oncol. 2008;15(3):915–22.

Wenig BM. Intraoperative consultation (IOC) in mucosal lesions of the upper aerodigestive tract. Head Neck Pathol. 2008;2(2):131–44.

Kurita H, Nakanishi Y, Nishizawa R, Xiao T, Kamata T, Koike T, Kobayashi H. Impact of different surgical margin conditions on local recurrence of oral squamous cell carcinoma. Oral Oncol. 2010;46:814.

Anderson CR, Sisson K, Moncrieff M. A meta-analysis of margin size and local recurrence in oral squamous cell carcinoma. Oral Oncol. 2015;51:464.

Barroso EM, Aaboubout Y, van der Sar LC, Mast H, Sewnaik A, Hardillo JA, Ten Hove I, Nunes Soares MR, Ottevanger L, Bakker Schut TC, Puppels GJ, Koljenović S. Performance of intra-operative assessment of resection margins in Oral cancer surgery: a review of literature. Front Oncol. 2021;11:628297. https://doi.org/10.3389/fonc.2021.628297.

Kovacs AF. Relevance of positive margins in case of adjuvant therapy of oral cancer. Int J Oral Maxillofac Surg. 2004;33:447–53.

Alicandri-Ciufelli M, Bonali M, Piccinini A, et al. Surgical margins in head and neck squamous cell carcinoma: what is 'close'? Eur Arch Otorhinolaryngol. 2013;270:2603–9.

Moe J, Baker A, Ward B. Surgical factors affecting outcomes in Oral squamous cell carcinoma. In: Kademani D, editor. Improving outcomes in oral cancer. Cham: Springer; 2020.

Hirsch DL, Dierks EJ. Use of a transbuccal technique for marginal mandibulectomy: a novel approach. J Oral Maxillofac Surg. 2007;65(9):1849–51.

Kademani D, Tiwana PS. Atlas of oral et maxillofacial surgery. Amsterdam: Elsevier; 2016.

Wax MK, Bascom DA, Myers LL. Marginal mandibulectomy versus segmental mandibulectomy: indications and controversies. Arch Otolaryngol Head Neck Surg. 2002;128:600–3.

Michael M, Ghali GE, Peter L, Peter W. Peterson's principles of oral and maxillofacial surgery. Shelton: People's Medical Publishing House; 2022.

Murakami K, Sugiura T, Yamamoto K, Kawakami M, Kang YB, Tsutsumi S, Kirita T. Biomechanical analysis of the strength of the mandible after marginal resection. J Oral Maxillofac Surg. 2011;69(6):1798–806. https://doi.org/10.1016/j.joms.2010.07.052. Epub 2011 Jan 26. PMID: 21272980.

Hinni ML, Ferlito A, Brandwein-Gensler MS, Takes RP, Silver CE, Westra WH, Seethala RR, Rodrigo JP, Corry J, Bradford CR, Hunt JL, Strojan P, Devaney KO, Gnepp DR, Hartl DM, Kowalski LP, Rinaldo A, Barnes L. Surgical margins in head and neck cancer: a contemporary review. Head Neck. 2013;35:1362.

Hirsch DL, Dierks EJ. Use of a transbuccal technique for marginal mandibulectomy: a novel approach. J Oral Maxillofac Surg. 2007;65:1849–51.

Brown JS, Rogers SN, McNally DN, Boyle M. A modified classification for the maxillectomy defect. Head Neck. 2000;22(1):17–26. https://doi.org/10.1002/(sici)1097-0347(200001)22:1 <17::aid-hed4>3.0.co;2-2. PMID: 10585601.

Maniglia AJ. Indications and techniques of midfacial degloving: a 15-year experience. Arch Otolaryngol Head Neck Surg. 1986;112:750.

Hanasono MM, Silva AK, Yu P, Skoracki RJ. A comprehensive algorithm for oncologic maxillary reconstruction. Plast Reconstr Surg. 2013;131(1):47–60.

Rogers SN, Lowe D, McNally D, Brown JS, Vaughan ED. Health-related quality of life after maxillectomy: a comparison between prosthetic obturation and free flap. J Oral Maxillofac Surg. 2003;61(2):174–81.

Squaquara R, Kim Evans KF, Spanio di Spilimbergo S, Mardini S. Intraoral reconstruction using local and regional flaps. Semin Plast Surg. 2010;24(2):198–211.

Mathes SJ, Nahai F. Clinical applications for muscle and musculocutaneous flaps. St. Louis, MO: C.V. Mosby; 1982.

Gottlieb LJ, Krieger LM. From the reconstructive ladder to the reconstructive elevator. Plast Reconstr Surg. 1994;93:1503–4.

Chapter 23
Practical Tips in Neck Management: Elective and Therapeutic Neck Dissection

Andrew Beech and Brent Ward

Abstract

- Oral cavity squamous cell carcinoma (OCSCC) is the most common anatomic subsite within the head and neck and represents the 16th most common global malignancy.
- Cervical lymph node involvement is the single most influential prognostic factor, with a survival reduction of 50%.
- Lymphatic metastases are present in 30–40% of patients at diagnosis, and appropriate treatment is essential for disease control.

  - This translates into approximately 70% of patients presenting without occult neck disease with whom an END does not provide a therapeutic benefit and could result in unnecessary morbidity.

- The clinical exam has a sensitivity of 75.76%, a specificity of 66.12%, and a negative predictive value of 66.67% when evaluating for metastatic cervical lymphadenopathy. Staging imaging with CT or MRI has allowed for improved sensitivity for assessment of lymph node size or morphologic atypia, but are not able to evaluate for micrometastasis, as may be present in early-stage (T1–2) oral cavity cancers.
- Failure to perform END in a patient with a cN0 neck who is harboring micrometastasis (pN1) results in nodal relapse, with these patients presenting with a more advanced nodal stage and higher incidence of extracapsular spread with decreased OS and DFS.

A. Beech
Oral and Maxillofacial Surgery, Jefferson Health, Philadelphia, PA, USA

B. Ward (✉)
Oral and Maxillofacial Surgery, Department of Surgery, School of Dentistry,, Michigan Medicine, University of Michigan, Ann Arbor, MI, USA
e-mail: bward@med.umich.edu

D. Amin, H. Marwan (eds.), *Pearls and Pitfalls in Oral and Maxillofacial Surgery*, https://doi.org/10.1007/978-3-031-47307-4_23

- Beyond the primary purpose of END or therapeutic neck dissection, which is to remove metastatic nodal disease, the pathologic staging of pN+ necks guides adjuvant therapy recommendations.
- Considerable controversy remains regarding the appropriate management of the neck in cT1N0 oral cavity cancer.

Elective Neck Dissection

- An END is performed when there is no clinical or radiologic evidence of metastatic cervical lymphadenopathy. The indications for an elective neck dissection have been a topic of controversy.

  - Neck dissections are not without morbidity. Seventy percent of patients who undergo a neck dissection complain of chronic shoulder pain, and 33% have chronic neck discomfort.

- Numerous studies have tried to identify tumor-specific factors which carry an increased risk of nodal metastasis and help to answer the question regarding the management of earlier invasive oral cavity cancer.
- Tumor size has long been known to contribute to cervical metastasis, hence its central role in tumor staging. NCCN recommends an END for cT3-4 N0 OCSCC regardless of the depth of invasion (DOI) or findings on sentinel lymph node biopsy due to the high risk for nodal metastasis.
- Depth of Invasion.

  - The depth of invasion (DOI) of the primary tumor is a promising pathological predictive factor for nodal metastases.
  - DOI correlates with tumor aggressiveness and serves as an independent predictor of nodal metastasis, disease-specific survival (DSS), and overall survival in OCSCC.
  - Subsite location of oral cavity primary tumors has been shown to have different propensities for occult disease in the neck, particularly tongue and floor of mouth primaries representing high-risk sites.
  - Brockhoff and colleagues, in 2017, analyzed 286 patients with OSCC. They analyzed site-specific locations in the oral cavity and the association of DOI with nodal metastasis. Using the Weiss et al. decision analysis cut off of 20% for occult metastasis and DOI, the recommended cut-off for elective neck dissection for oral tongue was 2 mm, the floor of the mouth was 2 mm to 3 mm, retromolar trigone was 3 mm to 4 mm, and alveolus/hard palate was 3 mm to 4 mm. In a multi-institutional follow-up of 283 cT1N0 patients, DOI recommendations were further validated.
  - Spiro et al. found tumors with DOI of less than 2 mm had a rate of cervical metastasis of 7.5% and recommended close observation in these circumstances.
  - Byers and colleagues prospectively evaluated 91 patients with SCC of the oral tongue, who all received a partial glossectomy and neck dissection. Fifty per-

cent of the patients with T2 tumors had pathologic nodal disease. In patients with T1 disease and > 4 mm DOI, there was a greater than 20% of occult metastasis. Thus, their recommendation was END for T2–T4 patients and T1 patients with >4 mm DOI.

  – Moe et al. performed a prospective, blinded study of 30 cT1N0 specimens comparing DOI measured at the time of frozen section analysis of the main specimen and the DOI as determined on permanent assessment. They found these values had a statistically significant correlation and supported the use of intraoperative DOI on frozen section analysis when deciding whether to perform an elective neck dissection for patients with cT1N0 disease.

- Critics of DOI argue that there is heterogeneity between centers in measuring tumor depth. Ebrahimi et al. did not find this translated into clinically relevant differences in the prognostic impact of DOI or tumor thickness.
- D'Cruz et al. in 2015 published their results on the survival benefit of END in patients with a T1–T2, N0 OSCC. A critical evaluation of the study shows more than 85% of patients had primary disease of the tongue, a known higher-risk site for nodal metastasis. In addition, 85% of the patients in the study had a DOI greater than 3 mm, which, as described above, has been shown to cross the 20% risk in many studies, indicating the need for dissection. T2 tumors were lumped in with the T1 tumor group, which created statistical significance in the analysis. When T1 tumors were evaluated alone, they were not found to have a statistically significant decrease in DFS and OS. This study failed to validate neck dissection in all patients, as a neck dissection would have been performed at most institutions for oral tongue primary tumors with T2 stage or DOI of greater than 3. As a result, this fails to answer the question regarding the management of superficial invasive cT1N0 oral cavity tumors.
- The "National randomized trial evaluating elective neck dissection for early stage oral cancer (SEND study) with meta-analysis and concurrent real-world cohort" evaluated END in their randomized prospective study. They also pooled T1 and T2 tumors in their data. A median DOI was 4.5 mm and 5 mm in the resection only and resection with END groups, respectively. At most institutions, a DOI greater than 3-4 mm would have warranted an END, and thus the study design fails to answer the question regarding the management of the neck in patients with superficially invasive cT1N0 disease.
- The extent of neck dissection.

  – The lymph node drainage pathways have been previously well described in the series by Shah et al. In patients undergoing END, found the disease in 3% of level IV and 0.5% in level V specimens.
  – Numerous studies, including the prospective trial by the Brazilian Head and Neck group, found no statistically significant difference in recurrence rate between MRND and Selective Neck Dissection (SND).
  – SND involving levels I-III or I-IV is appropriate for N0 disease.

- Sentinel lymph node biopsy's role in managing T1–2N0 OCSCC disease is discussed in detail elsewhere in this text but not ascribed to by the authors in most clinical scenarios.

Therapeutic Neck Dissection

- A therapeutic neck dissection is performed when there is clinical evidence of cervical lymph node involvement, either with cervical lymphadenopathy on physical exam, on staging imaging (CT or PET), or positive biopsy (FNA or SLNBx).
- The addition of radiation therapy and realization of the morbidity associated with the radical neck dissection has followed a trend toward more focused lymph node removal and preservation of the CN XI, SCM, and IJ vein with the MRND.
- Andersen et al. compared MRND versus RND and did not find a statistically significant increase in recurrence with the preservation of the spinal accessory nerve.
- SND followed by adjuvant radiation is adequate in the setting of N1 and N2 disease in works by Byers et al. and Medina et al., although there is a lack of prospective randomized evidence comparing SND versus MRND in the N+ neck.

Pearls

- Cervical lymph node metastasis in oral cavity cancer is the single most important prognostic factor.
- Elective neck dissection (END) is performed when there is no clinical or radiologic evidence of metastatic cervical lymphadenopathy, but tumor-specific factors suggest an increased risk of lymph node involvement of greater than 20%.
- Proposed decision-making strategies include: watch and wait, sentinel node biopsy, END guided by the depth of invasion (DOI), and END in all oral cavity cancer.
- The authors generally recommend END for cT2–4 tumors or cT1 tumors with DOI greater than 2–4 mm depending on the anatomic subsite (Table 23.1).

Table 23.1 Validation of the DOI for T1 oral SCC based on the different subsites. Reprinted with permission from Elsevier, Journal of Oral and Maxillofacial Surgery Lic# 551371493895

Summary comparing our study and prior recommendations		
	Brockhoff et al.	Current Study
Tongue	2 mm	2 mm[a]
Floor of mouth	2–3 mm	3 mm
Retromolar trigone	3–4 mm	No data
Alveolus/hard palate	3–4 mm	See below
Upper gingiva		3 mm
Lower gingiva		4 mm
Hard palate		No neck dissection

[a]Risk of 18%

Feng et al. Elective Neck Dissection in T1N0 OSCC. J Oral Maxillofac Surg 2020

Pitfalls

- Failure to perform END in cN0 patients harboring micrometastasis, who develop the regional cervical disease, is associated with decreased OS and DFS.
- Careful assessment of study design and population is necessary when evaluating the application and generalizability of previous END studies as it relates to the management of cT1N0 disease.

Further Reading

Pentenero M, Gandolfo S, Carrozzo M. Importance of tumor thickness and depth of invasion in nodal involvement and prognosis of oral squamous cell carcinoma: a review of the literature. Head Neck. 2005;27:1080–91.

Byers RM, El-Naggar AK, Lee YY, et al. Can we detect or predict the presence of occult nodal metastases in patients with squamous carcinoma of the oral tongue? Head Neck. 1998;20:138–44.

Brockhoff HC 2nd, Kim RY, Braun TM, Skouteris C, Helman JI, Ward BB. Correlating the depth of invasion at specific anatomic locations with the risk for regional metastatic disease to lymph nodes in the neck for oral squamous cell carcinoma. Head Neck. 2017;39:974–9.

Feng Z, Cheng A, Alzahrani S, Li B, Han Z, Ward BB. Elective neck dissection in T1N0M0 Oral squamous cell carcinoma: when is it necessary? J Oral Maxillofac Surg. 2020;78(12):2306–15. https://doi.org/10.1016/j.joms.2020.06.037. Epub 2020 Jul 4. PMID: 32730759.

Moe J, et al. Intraoperative depth of invasion is accurate in early-stage Oral cavity squamous cell carcinoma. J Oral Maxillofac Surg. 2019;77(8):1704–12.

Ebrahimi A, et al. Primary tumor staging for oral cancer and a proposed modification incorporating depth of invasion. JAMA Otolaryngol Head Neck Surgery. 2014;140(12):1138.

D'Cruz A, Dandekar M, Vaish R, Arya S, Pantvaidya G, Chaturvedi P, Chaukar D, Pai PS, Deshmukh A, Kane S, Nair D, Nair SV, Patil A, Hawaldar RW, Dhopeshwarkar M, Agarwal J. Elective versus therapeutic neck dissection in the clinically node negative early oral cancer: a randomised control trial (RCT). J Clin Oncol. 2015;33:1.

Hutchison IL, et al. Nationwide randomised trial evaluating elective neck dissection for early stage Oral cancer (Send study) with meta-analysis and concurrent real-world cohort. Br J Cancer. 2019;121(10):827–36.

Shah JP. Patterns of cervical lymph node metastasis from squamous carcinomas of the upper Aerodigestive tract. Am J Surg. 1990;160(4):405–9.

Brazilian Head and Neck Cancer Study Group. Results of a prospective trial on elective modified radical classical versus supraomohyoid neck dissection in the Management of Oral Squamous Carcinoma. Am J Surg. 1998;176(5):422–7.

Andersen PE, et al. The role of comprehensive neck dissection with preservation of the spinal accessory nerve in the clinically positive neck. Am J Surg. 1994;168(5):499–502.

Medina JE, Byers RM. Supraomohyoid neck dissection: rationale, indications, and surgical technique. Head Neck. 1989;11(2):111–22.

Brands MT, Brennan PA, Verbeek ALM, Merkx MAW, Geurts SME. Follow-up after curative treatment for oral squamous cell carcinoma. A critical appraisal of the guidelines and a review of the literature. Eur J Surg Oncol. 2018;44(5):559–65.

Gourin CG, Conger BT, Porubsky ES, Sheils WC, Bilodeau PA, Coleman TA. The effect of occult nodal metastases on survival and regional control in patients with head and neck squamous cell carcinoma. Laryngoscope. 2008;118(7):1191–4.

Rose BS, Jeong J-H, Nath SK, Lu SM, Mell LK. Population-based study of competing mortality in head and neck cancer. J Clin Oncol. 2011;29(26):3503–9.

Schneider U, Graß I, Laudien M, et al. Comparison of clinical examination and various imaging modalities in the diagnosis of head and neck cancer. Int Arch Otorhinolaryngol. 2020;25(02):e179.

Vaish R, Gupta S, D'Cruz AK. Elective versus therapeutic neck dissection in oral cancer. N Engl J Med. 2015;373(25):2475–7.

Chapter 24
Practical Tips in the Management of the N0 Neck: Sentinel Lymph Node Biopsy

Ashish Patel

Abstract The surgical management of the N0 neck in patients with oral squamous cell carcinoma (OSCC) has been long debated and evolved dramatically over the last century. Since the introduction of radical neck dissection by Dr. Crile in 1906, there has been a slow but steady trend to de-escalate surgical therapy to reduce morbidity without compromising oncologic safety. Cervical lymphadenectomy/elective neck dissection remains the gold standard in comprehensive pathologic interrogation and surgical staging of the regional lymph nodes in patients with oral cavity cancer. This, however, does come at a cost. Risks include injury to neurovascular structures, shoulder dysfunction, surgical scarring, and bleeding. In patients with early-stage, thin, oral cavity squamous cell carcinoma, elective neck dissection may be overtreatment in surgical staging and oncologic therapy. In this cohort of patients, sentinel lymph node biopsy (SLNB) may be an appropriate alternative to surgical staging.

Sentinel lymph node biopsy is a minimally invasive technique for staging OSCC and can potentially reduce the morbidity associated with selective neck dissection. The first published report of lymphatic mapping for cancer patients was completed by Seaman and Powers in 1955, in which they described the injection of breast tumors with radiolabeled colloidal gold and mapped the progression of the tracers through the regional lymphatics. Five years later, Gould et al. coined the term "sentinel node" when describing a level II cervical lymph node consistently identified during parotidectomy for malignant tumors – the status of which guided the operators to complete or forgo neck dissection.

The concepts of a "sentinel lymph node" and lymphatic mapping were first used to reliably and accurately predict regional cancer spread by Morton et al. in 1992. This

A. Patel (✉)
Head and Neck Surgical Oncology and Microvascular Surgery,
Providence Cancer Institute, Portland, OR, USA

Craniomaxillofacial and Neck Trauma, Legacy Emanuel Medical Center, Portland, OR, USA

Reconstructive Microsurgery, Head and Neck Surgical Associates, Portland, OR, USA
e-mail: patela@head-neck.com

D. Amin, H. Marwan (eds.), *Pearls and Pitfalls in Oral and Maxillofacial Surgery*, https://doi.org/10.1007/978-3-031-47307-4_24

group reported data from 223 patients with stage I cutaneous melanoma in which they performed a vital blue dye-directed sentinel node identification and regional lymphadenectomy. Since then, there have been many retrospective and prospective studies, and more recently, two randomized controlled clinical trials comparing SLNB to elective selective neck dissection in early-stage OSCC. In summary, the data suggest a negative predictive value of a negative sentinel node biopsy between 95 and 100%. Moreover, in a subset of early-stage oral cavity cancers, sentinel lymph node biopsy demonstrates oncologic equivalence at 2 and 5 years postoperatively compared to elective neck dissection with substantially reduced morbidity and hospital stay.

This chapter aims to discuss the practical pearls and pitfalls of sentinel lymph node biopsy for the N0 neck in managing squamous cell carcinoma.

Practical Tips

Preoperative Consideration

Patient Selection

- Patient selection for SLNB is critical. The primary site should be easily accessible for preoperative injection. Avoid oropharynx cancers, as the data is less clear on the role of SLNB for these.
- Patients with indurated tumors, evidence of high-risk features on biopsy, or T3/T4 tumors should not be considered for SLNB.
- Preoperative staging should include cross-sectional contrast-enhanced imaging of the neck. Computed tomography (CT) with contrast is our preference. Both the radiologist and surgeon should agree that the patient has a clinically N0 neck.
- Patients with previous radiotherapy or neck dissection may not be good candidates for SLNB as lymphatic drainage may be altered.
- Sentinel lymph node biopsy has a 96% negative predictive value and is a viable alternative to the observation of the cN0 neck in early stage oral cavity cancers. Two recent studies have demonstrated non-inferiority compared to elective selective neck dissection for early-stage oral cavity carcinoma.

Perioperative Technique

- For preoperative injection of a radiotracer, technetium Tc99m tilmanocept has replaced technetium Tc99m sulfur colloid at many US institutions. Both are acceptable radiotracers. A single dose should be divided into four equal aliquots drawn in tuberculin syringes (Fig. 24.1). Peritumoral injection in the submucosa at four quadrants around the tumor will allow accurate lymphatic drainage from the surgical site. Avoid "spillage" of the tracer into the oral cavity, as it can skew the lymphoscintigraphy.
- Some radiotracers, specifically Tc99m tilmanocept, have rapid transit time and can be detected in the sentinel node 12–21 h after injection. This affords a long

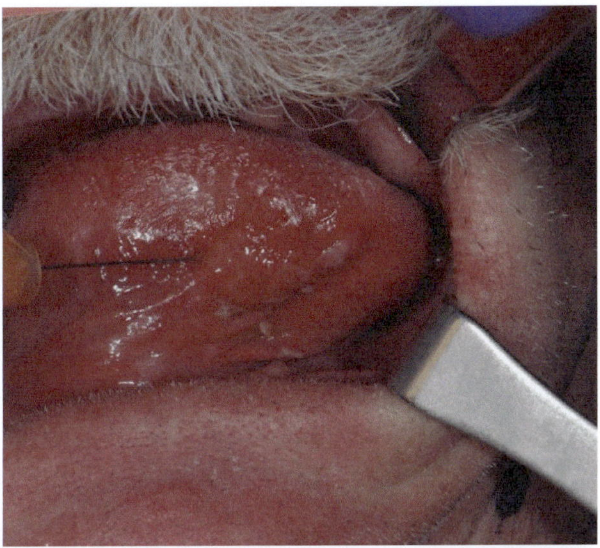

Fig. 24.1 mTc99 tilmanocept injection in the peritumoral submucosa. A total of four injections (0.25 mL each) were injected around the tumor

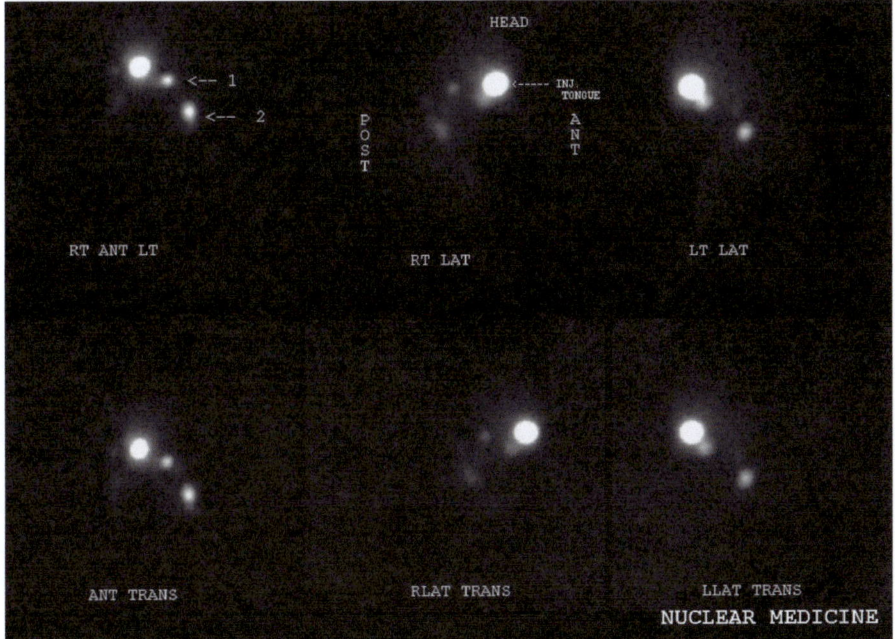

Fig. 24.2 Planar lymphoscintigram demonstrating the radiotracer at the tongue injection as well as two discrete sentinel lymph nodes

window for surgery. Depending on the Nuclear Medicine department, patients may undergo injection and lymphoscintigraphy the night before a morning surgery or 2–3 h before surgery on the same day (Fig. 24.2).

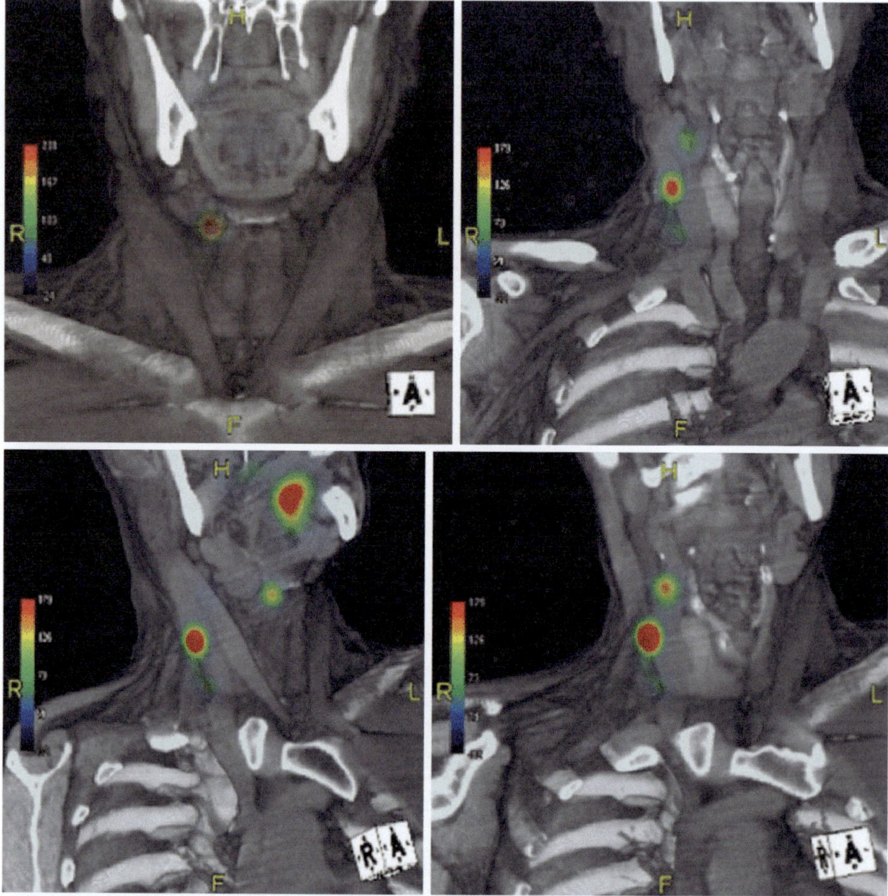

Fig. 24.3 SPECT scan localizing the sentinel nodes two both level 1 and level 2 of the ipsilateral neck

- It is preferable to order a single-photon emission computerized tomography (SPECT) scan for mapping; it is anatomically more accurate than planar lymphoscintigraphy. This allows for precise sentinel node localization with minimal access (Fig. 24.3).
- Some surgeons use blue dye (methylene blue, isosulfan blue) in addition to radiotracer injection to help localize the node, but this is optional and less accurate than radiotracer.

Intraoperative Consideration

- Using an intraoperative gamma probe is critical to accurate localization and identification of the sentinel node. Transcutaneous neck mapping with the gamma probe can help determine the skin incision.

- The primary tumor should be resected first as this can help reduce "shine-through" or excessive radiation noise from the primary site obscuring the radio-tracer in the neck.
- After studying the lymphoscintigraphy, SPECT scan, and gamma probe markings, a 2–3 cm skin incision should be made with short circumferential subplatysmal flaps. The gamma probe should be reintroduced into the wound to guide further dissection.
- A combination of blunt and sharp dissection directly to the most radioactive node can be accomplished quickly without the need for wide undermining or tissue disruption. Once the node is identified, care is taken to excise it in an extracapsular place. Some fascia can be left on the node as a "handle," as direct grasping of the node can crush and spill its contents (Fig. 24.4).
- Once removed, an ex vivo 10-s count of the node is accomplished with the gamma probe. It is best to rest the node directly on top of the gamma probe tip. This numerical value should be recorded. Another 10-s count of the wound is completed with the probe – this value should be 10% or less of the suspected sentinel node. If the wound bed count is greater than 10%, there may be more sentinel nodes to remove. This process is repeated until all the sentinel nodes are removed. In most cases, there is only one sentinel lymph node (Figs. 24.5 and 24.6).
- The sentinel lymph node should be labeled as such so the pathologist can examine it more closely than bisection. Often, sentinel nodes will be serially step-sectioned at 150-micron increments. Immunohistochemistry is also used to help detect micrometastatic deposits within a sentinel node. This is not routinely done in neck dissection specimens due to the massive burden of nodes but is standard practice for sentinel lymph node biopsy.
- After achieving hemostasis, the wound is closed in layers and generally does not require a drain. A sterile dressing is applied.
- If the final pathology demonstrates nodal metastasis, a completion modified radical neck dissection should be carried out.

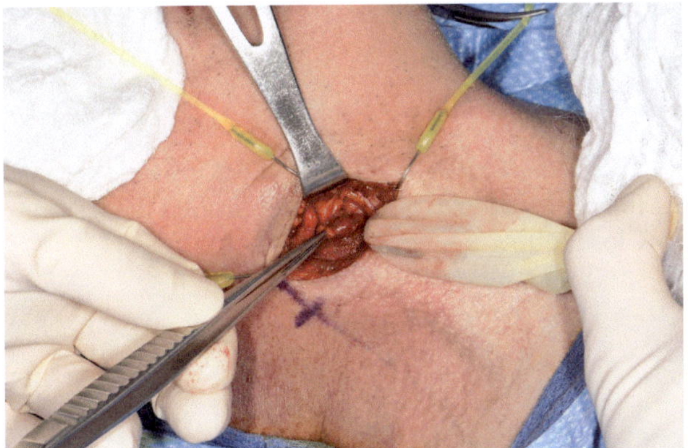

Fig. 24.4 Sentinel lymph node in level 2 identified and excised in an extracapsular fashion

Fig. 24.5 Ex vivo count of the sentinel nodes

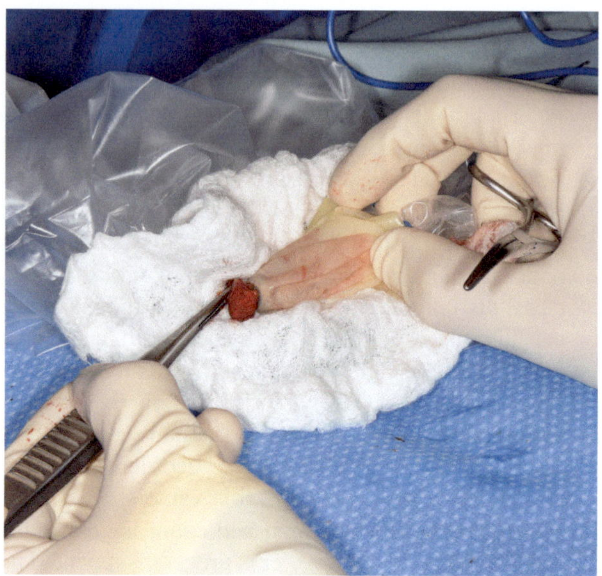

Fig. 24.6 A total of three sentinel lymph nodes were identified with gamma counts ranging in the 7000 s to 10,000 s. The final wound bed 10-s count was under 150

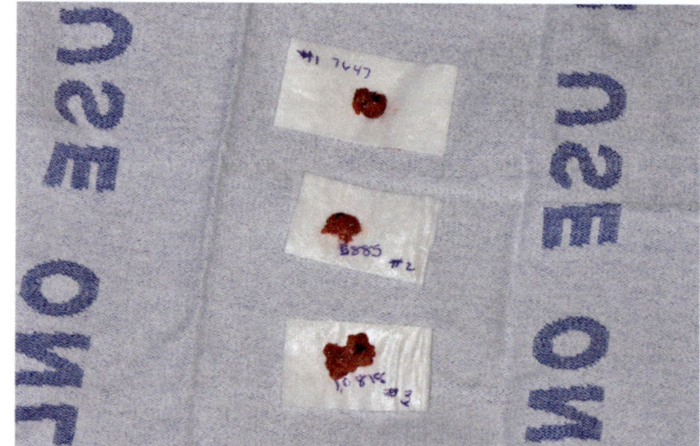

Pearls

- The primary site should be easily accessible for preoperative injection.
- Inject closely into normal tissue around the lesion.
- Close follow-up.

Pitfalls

- Avoid oropharynx cancers, as the data is less clear on the role of SLNB for these.
- Do not inject local anesthetics directly into the primary tumor.
- The sentinel lymph node should be labeled as such so the pathologist can examine it more closely than bisection.

Further Reading

Vaish R, Gupta S, D'Cruz AK. Elective versus therapeutic neck dissection in oral. Cancer. 2015;373:2477. https://doi.org/10.1056/NEJMc1511351.

Seaman WB, Powers WE. Studies on the distribution of radioactive colloidal gold in regional lymph nodes containing cancer. Cancer. 1955;8:1044–6. https://doi.org/10.1002/1097-014 2(1955)8:5<1044::aid-cncr2820080530>3.0.co;2-6.

Morton DL, Wen DR, Wong JH, Economou JS, Cagle LA, Storm FK, et al. Technical details of intraoperative lymphatic mapping for early stage melanoma. 1992;127:392–9. https://doi.org/10.1001/archsurg.1992.01420040034005.

Schilling C, Stoeckli SJ, Vigili MG, de Bree R, Lai SY, Alvarez J, et al. Surgical consensus guidelines on sentinel node biopsy (SNB) in patients with oral cancer. Head Neck. 2019;41:2655–64. https://doi.org/10.1002/hed.25739.

Hasegawa Y, Tsukahara K, Yoshimoto S, Miura K, Yokoyama J, Hirano S, et al. Neck dissections based on sentinel lymph node navigation versus elective neck dissections in early oral cancers: a randomized, multicenter, and noninferiority trial. J Clin Oncol. 2021;39:2025–36. https://doi.org/10.1200/JCO.20.03637.

Garrel R, Poissonnet G, Moya Plana A, Fakhry N, Dolivet G, Lallemant B, et al. Equivalence randomized trial to compare treatment on the basis of sentinel node biopsy versus neck node dissection in operable T1-T2N0 oral and oropharyngeal. Cancer. 2020;38:4010–8. https://doi.org/10.1200/JCO.20.01661.

Chapter 25
Practical Tips for Managing Cranial Nerves XI, XII, and Greater Auricular Nerve in Neck Dissection

Michael L. Winstead, Raymond P. Shupak, and Roderick Y. Kim

Abstract Preservation of neurovascular structures during cervical lymphadenectomy is critical to preserve future function. A mixture of both spinal and cranial nerves is routinely encountered during the procedure. The greater auricular nerve, which arises from the cervical plexus (C2, C3), provides sensory input to the skin over the parotid region, mastoid process, and portions of the ear, including the lobule. Cranial nerve XI, the spinal accessory nerve, supplies the motor innervation to the sternocleidomastoid (SCM) and trapezius muscles. Cranial nerve XII, the hypoglossal nerve, provides all the motor innervation to the intrinsic and extrinsic muscles of the tongue aside from the palatoglossus. Each of these nerves provides critical patient functions that require preservation if feasible from an oncologic standpoint. A careful understanding of the course and its relationship to other vital structures is imperative to recognizing and preserving these structures during dissection. The purpose of this chapter is to review pearls and pitfalls in managing cranial nerves XI, XII, and greater auricular nerve in neck dissection.

M. L. Winstead
Division of Maxillofacial Oncology and Reconstructive Surgery, Department of Oral and Maxillofacial Surgery, John Peter Smith Health Network, Fort Worth, TX, USA

R. P. Shupak
Department of Oral Medicine and Maxillofacial Surgery, Geisinger Commonwealth School of Medicine, Geisinger Medical Center, Danville, PA, USA

R. Y. Kim (✉)
Division of Maxillofacial Oncology and Reconstructive Surgery, Department of Oral and Maxillofacial Surgery, John Peter Smith Health Network, Texas Christian University Medical School, Fort Worth, TX, USA

D. Amin, H. Marwan (eds.), *Pearls and Pitfalls in Oral and Maxillofacial Surgery*, https://doi.org/10.1007/978-3-031-47307-4_25

Practical Tips

Greater Auricular Nerve

- The greater auricular nerve emerges from the posterior border of the SCM and travels superiorly toward the ear. As it travels superiorly, it is often found in close proximity to the external jugular vein (EJV). Identifying the EJV during dissection can help alert the surgeon to the location of the greater auricular nerve (Fig. 25.1).
- Care should be taken not to incise deeper than the superficial layer of the deep cervical fascia. Inadvertent injury or transection can occur if the incision is too deep over the SCM muscle.
- During the elevation of the subplatysmal flap, identification and protection of the external jugular vein often allows for easy identification of the greater auricular nerve as it is predictably located laterally and parallel to the path of the external jugular vein.
- Near the level of the auricle, the greater auricular nerve branches into an anterior and posterior branch.
- During ablative surgery, attempts should be made to spare the posterior branch as it can preserve sensation in the ear lobe.
- Luckily, most patients with damage or sacrifice of this nerve do not exhibit long-term interference with their daily quality of life. However, anesthesia of the lobule can be quite bothersome to those with ear piercings during attempted insertion of jewelry, and the risks should be discussed pre-operatively.

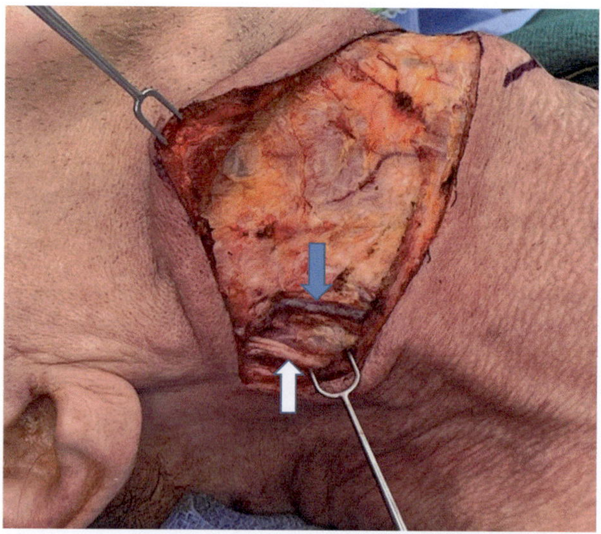

Fig. 25.1 Elevation of the subplatysmal flap in neck dissection. The blue arrow points to the external jugular vein, while the white arrow points to the greater auricular nerve

Cranial Nerve XI – The Spinal Accessory Nerve

- Locating and protecting the spinal accessory nerve is a critical step during a nerve-sparing neck dissection, as the sacrifice of the nerve can result in significant morbidity in the form of shoulder weakness, pain, and restricted range of motion (also referred to as "shoulder syndrome").
- Initial identification of the spinal accessory nerve often occurs superiorly as it crosses the internal jugular vein or laterally as it enters the SCM (Fig. 25.2).
- Superiorly, the nerve can be identified just anterior to the internal jugular vein (IJV), as it takes this route approximately 80% of the time. It will occasionally cross posterior to the IJV less than 20% of the time and rarely bifurcate around the IJV.
- The more predictable method of identifying the nerve is lateral. There are several maneuvers to identify the nerve in this location. One is blunt dissection with Metzenbaum scissors in a direction parallel to the path of the nerve, inferolaterally. This is done on the deep surface of the SCM while it is under lateral retraction, where the nerve enters the SCM near the junction of the superior and middle third of the muscle.
- An additional maneuver is to use a finger to palpate the fibrofatty tissue in this area with the SCM under lateral retraction. The spinal accessory nerve can be felt

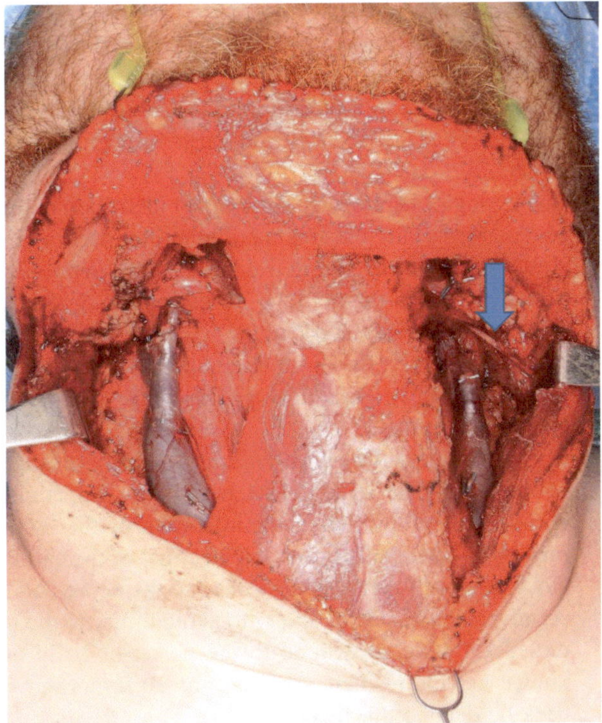

Fig. 25.2 Retraction of the subplatysmal flap and sternocleidomastoid muscles following bilateral selective neck dissections. The blue arrow points to the spinal accessory nerve coursing anterior to the internal jugular vein to enter the deep surface of the SCM

as taught structure running inferolaterally and is said to feel similar to a "guitar string."

- Yet another way of identifying the location of the nerve is at its entry into the deep surface of the SCM, which is approximately 1 cm superior to Erb's point. During a neck dissection, Erb's point can be identified by tracing the greater auricular nerve, which was identified earlier in the dissection, in a retrograde fashion to where it wraps around the SCM.
- Lateral retraction of the SCM should not be for prolonged periods during dissection, and care must be taken not to retract directly on the nerve as it enters the SCM, as an undue stretch or compression can result in neuropraxic injury or even avulsion.
- Should the spinal accessory nerve be injured or transected inadvertently during a nerve-sparing dissection, repair of the nerve with either an autogenous or allogeneic nerve is recommended. This is due to the inability to perform the primary repair by neurorrhaphy in a tension-free manner.
- Any known trauma to the nerve intraoperatively or signs of nerve injury postoperatively during cranial nerve exam should be followed by a prompt referral for physical therapy.

Cranial Nerve XII – The Hypoglossal Nerve

- The hypoglossal nerve must be identified during the dissection of the submandibular triangle and the removal of the submandibular gland to protect it from injury. While this nerve is relatively robust and can tolerate manipulation without injury, its dissection and retraction are rarely warranted during a neck dissection.
- The hypoglossal nerve is most easily identified in the floor of the submandibular fossa after freeing the submandibular gland from its fascia and retracting it inferiorly or posteriorly while retracting the lateral edge of the mylohyoid muscle anteriorly. Once this is done, three important structures are identified, running almost horizontally and parallel to one another. These structures are the lingual nerve superiorly, the submandibular duct in the middle, and the hypoglossal nerve inferiorly. Identifying the first two makes identifying the latter straightforward.
- The location of the nerve anteriorly can be easily identified by palpating the hyoid bone. The hypoglossal nerve lies immediately posterior to the greater cornu of the hyoid bone. Identification of the nerve in this area will not only prevent its iatrogenic injury but also that of the carotid system, which lies in very close proximity, immediately deep to the nerve and greater cornu of the hyoid.
- A universal measure of safety to avoid injury to the nerve is to maintain all tissue dissection at or superficial to the posterior belly of the digastric muscle (also known as "the resident's friend") as all important structures in this area of the neck lie deep to this muscle.

- Meticulous hemostasis during dissection of this area also helps ensure the safety of the nerve as attempted clamping, ligature, or cautery of the associated "Ranine vein" or veins, which often bleed if not carefully handled, can result in injury to the nerve.
- Careful dissection in this area must be performed in the irradiated neck, and those with a history of sialadenitis as fibrosis and scarring can result in the nerve becoming adherent to the duct or other structures in the submandibular fossa.
- Tongue deviation results from ipsilateral nerve injury. If noted by the clinician post-operatively, it should warrant exploration and attempted neurorrhaphy if indicated and/or referral for speech therapy as significant morbidity (i.e., dysarthria, dysphagia, obstructive sleep apnea) is associated with injury to this nerve.

Pearls

- Identifying the external jugular vein (EJV) can help locate the greater auricular nerve.
- Locating and protecting the spinal accessory nerve is critical during a nerve-sparing neck dissection.
- The hypoglossal nerve must be identified during the submandibular triangle's dissection and the submandibular gland's removal to protect it from injury.

Pitfalls

- Do not incise deeper than the superficial layer of the deep cervical fascia. Inadvertent injury to the greater auricular nerve can occur if the incision is carried too deep over the SCM muscle body.
- Erb's point can be used to locate the spinal accessory nerve.
- When the hypoglossal nerve injury is suspected, consider exploration and attempted neurorrhaphy if indicated and/or referral for speech therapy as significant morbidity.

Further Reading

George M, Karkos PD, Raghav CD, Leong SC, Kim D, Repanos C. Preservation of the greater auricular nerve during parotidectomy: sensation, quality of life, and morbidity issues. A systematic review. Head Neck. 2014;36:603–8.

Dziegielewski PT, McNeely ML, Ashworth N, O'Connell DA, Barber B, Courneya KS, Debenham BJ, Seikaly H. 2b or not 2b? Shoulder function after level 2b neck dissection: a double-blinded randomized controlled clinical trial. Cancer. 2020;126:1492–501.

Saman M, Etebari P, Pakdaman MN, Urken ML. Anatomic relationship between the spinal accessory nerve and jugular vein: a cadaveric study. Surg Radiol Anat. 2011;33:175–9.

Chapter 26
Practical Tips for the Management of the Advanced Head and Neck Infection

Stacey Nedrud and Laurent Ganry

Abstract

- Advanced head and neck infections can be fatal if not treated promptly and properly. This chapter will focus on the life-threatening head and neck infections that can be seen by the general oral and maxillofacial surgeon and otolaryngologist.
- Defining the anatomic subspaces is not the focus of this chapter, but the especially worrisome anatomic locations are highlighted. The deep space neck infections with fewer anatomical fascial barriers to spread are the most dangerous and can originate from odontogenic sources, the tonsils, the parotid, the middle ear, the sinuses, the cervical lymph nodes, and the skin.
- For advanced head and neck infections, prompt treatment with surgical intervention is often required.
- Discussions with the anesthesia team for the airway plan are paramount, and preparations are often made for difficult intubation and emergent awake tracheostomy/cricothyrotomy if needed.

Anatomy

- The anatomy of involved head and neck structures susceptible to infection can encompass the entire anatomy of the head and neck and thus will only be reviewed here.
- Anatomical spaces of the face.

S. Nedrud (✉)
Private Practice, Oral Maxillofacial Surgery, Jacksonville, FL, USA

L. Ganry
Head and Neck Surgery Department, Beth Israel Deaconess Medical Center, Harvard Medical School, Boston, MA, USA

D. Amin, H. Marwan (eds.), *Pearls and Pitfalls in Oral and Maxillofacial Surgery*, https://doi.org/10.1007/978-3-031-47307-4_26

- Buccal space.

  Anterior to the masticator space and lateral to the buccinator muscle.
  Composed of the buccal fat pad, Stenson's duct, the facial vasculature, lymphatics, minor salivary glands, and branches of the facial and glosso-pharyngeal nerve.
  From multiple sources, including maxillary and mandibular dentition, as there is poor fascial compartmentalization.

- Canine space.

  Between the levator anguli oris and the levator labii superioris muscles, spreading fast toward the orbito-palpebral region.
  Often from the root apices of the maxillary teeth.

- Masseteric space.

  Bordered by the fascia of the muscles of mastication: the masseter, temporalis, medial, and lateral pterygoid muscles.
  Contains the internal maxillary artery and inferior alveolar nerve.
  Typically of odontogenic origin (molars), with associated trismus.

- Pterygomandibular space.

  The space is bound by the mandible, medial pterygoid muscle, parotid gland, and the pterygomandibular raphe.
  Contains the inferior alveolar nerve, lingual nerve, and inferior alveolar vasculature.

- Parotid space.

  Encompassed by fascia of the investing layer of the deep cervical fascia.
  Composed of the parotid gland, lymph tissue, the branches of the facial nerve, branches of the external carotid arteries, and the retromandibular vein.
  Primary infection in this site is rare, typically from obstruction of the parotid duct.

- Temporal space.

  Includes the temporal fascia surrounding the temporalis muscle, splitting into deep and superficial layers.

• Anatomical spaces of the suprahyoid and infrahyoid levels of the neck.

- Sublingual space.

  Bordered by the mylohyoid and geniohyoid, and genioglossus muscles.
  Composed of the lingual artery, lingual, glossopharyngeal, and hypoglossal nerves, the sublingual gland, and Wharton's duct.
  From odontogenic sources perforating the mandible above the mylohyoid attachment.

- Submental space.

  Bound by the mandible, anterior bellies of the digastric muscles, and the mylohyoid muscle.
  Contains the submental arteries.
  The typical source is from the anterior mandibular dentition.

- Submandibular space.

  Bordered by the hyoid bone, the mandible, and the superficial layer of the deep cervical fascia.
  It is separated from the sublingual space by the mylohyoid but with free access between the spaces posteriorly. There is also potential to spread to the lateral pharyngeal spaces via the buccopharyngeal gap from the styloglossus muscle.
  Contains the submandibular gland, lingual and hypoglossal nerves, and facial vasculature.
  Often posterior dentition is the culprit, with periapical infections perforating the mandible.

- Lateral pharyngeal (or parapharyngeal) space.

  Bound by the base of the skull and hyoid bone, prevertebral fascia, the raphe of the buccinator and superior constrictor muscles, and the mandible and parotid fascia.
  Divided further into a prestyloid and retrostyloid compartment by the styloid process.

    Contains fat, lymph tissue, and muscle in the anterior (prestyloid) compartment.
    Contains the internal carotid artery, internal jugular vein, and the glossopharyngeal, vagus, spinal accessory, and hypoglossal nerves in the posterior (retrostyloid) compartment.

  Infection can spread from an odontogenic source, the tonsils, or other close proximity aforementioned fascial spaces.
  Lemierre syndrome involves bacterial spread to this space with internal jugular septic vein thrombosis, associated typically with right-side endocarditis and bilateral pulmonary septic emboli.
  The presentation of severe infections in this area can resemble Horner's syndrome.

- Peritonsillar space.

  Encompassed by the pharyngeal constrictors and includes the tonsils.
  The danger lies in the possibility of spreading to the lateral pharyngeal space.

• Anatomical spaces of the neck.

- Pretracheal space.

  Bound by the investing and visceral cervical fascia, the fascia to the thyroid cartilage and hyoid bone, and into the mediastinum to the sternum and the scalene fascia.
  The space contains the thyroid gland and infrahyoid muscles but can quickly communicate into the superior mediastinum.

- Retropharyngeal space.

  Bordered by the constrictor muscles and the alar fascia and connects posteriorly to the "Danger" space (see below).
  It can spread to the danger space and mediastinum down to the diaphragm and even more posteriorly to the prevertebral space.
  Involvement in this space can lead to mediastinitis, empyema, and pericardial effusions.

- "Danger" space

  Bound by the skull base, prevertebral fascia, and alar fascia, down to the diaphragm.
  It can pass from the neck to the mediastinum and pericardium, causing pericarditis.
  Figure 26.3 demonstrates an infection approaching the danger space.

- Prevertebral space.

  Bordered by the anterior cervical spine and the deep layer of the deep cervical fascia.
  Extends into the mediastinum and ends at the fourth thoracic vertebrae (T4).
  The space includes the prevertebral muscles, vertebral vessels, scalene muscles, phrenic nerve, and the brachial plexus.

- Carotid sheath space.

  Between the prevertebral fascia, pretracheal fascia, and the investing layer deep to the sternocleidomastoid muscle.
  It contains the common carotid artery, internal and external carotid arteries, internal jugular vein, vagus nerve, and sympathetic fibers.

- Emergent tracheostomy anatomical landmarks.

  - Palpate the laryngeal notch and the sternal notch, and feel the lateral borders of the trachea to palpate for any deviations of the trachea from the midline. This may not be possible in obese patients, irradiated patients, or edematous patients with diffuse multi-space infections.
  - The ideal incision is approximately two fingerbreadths above the sternal notch.
  - A vertical incision may be able to avoid the anterior jugular veins that can cross-communicate across the midline.

- In the emergent setting, a cricothyrotomy may be more expeditious and would require palpation of the cricoid, and the thyroid cartilage, to find the cricothyroid membrane between these two palpable structures.
- Equally satisfactory for the clinician that is comfortable in emergent and awake tracheostomies, an expeditious tracheostomy can be very rapid, utilizing bovie electrocautery and hemostats to dissect down to the trachea, and a blade and curved mayo scissors to access the trachea. Excellent retraction and assistance is paramount for the surgeon.

Preoperative Care

- As a general rule, smaller intraoral abscesses (such as mandibular or maxillary vestibular abscesses or peritonsillar abscess) can be drained bedside, but advanced multi-space head and neck infections or any transcutaneous approach is better served in the operating room in a controlled setting.
- It is paramount to understand the imaging and the anatomy prior to surgical intervention. The imaging will not only demonstrate which spaces are involved but also the proximity to important structures, such as the internal carotid artery that may pass just posterior to a peritonsillar abscess.
- For complex deep-space face and neck infections, a computed tomography (CT) image with intravenous (IV) iodine contrast is ideal. A magnetic resonance image (MRI) with gadolinium contrast can be an alternative in case of an allergy. A CT without contrast is the last option, which yields significantly less pertinent information.
- Complex deep posterior neck infections, especially if complicated with a severe sepsis presentation or compromised airway, should have a low threshold to benefit from a head and neck CT as well as a thoracic CT with IV iodine contrast to rule out an associated mediastinitis.
- Blood cultures and laboratory values for infectious markers, such as white blood cell count and CRP/ESR in severe scenarios, should be obtained prior to the start of empiric antibiotics.
- Empiric IV antibiotics should be started immediately, but should be de-escalated based on culture and sensitivities after a wound culture can be obtained, targeting both aerobic and anaerobic bacteria. The specifics of pharmacology and the ideal antibiotic regimen are outside of the scope of this chapter.
- It is important to recognize the dangers of the pharyngeal and deep spaces of the neck, as these spaces can have direct mediastinal communication.
- The treatment options for an advanced head and neck infection will depend on the spaces involved, size, patient presentation, and patient stability. A small, localized infection in a superficial space may be able to be treated with medical management only, but the majority of advanced head and neck infections are treated surgically. If there is the possibility of a malignancy with a superimposed infection as the cause, then an FNA or core biopsy would be preferred over surgical drainage, and/or an open node biopsy if necessary.

- The surgeon should always discuss the surgical plan with the anesthesiologist. In many cases, a surgical airway (tracheostomy) may be needed or prepared prior to anesthetizing the patient. Alternatively, the anesthesiologist may prefer awake intubation if there is a concern for obstruction and anticipated issues with ventilation. The anesthesia team and the operating room staff should all be apprised of the plan and ready for a speedy surgical airway should it be needed.
- If a surgical airway may be needed in an emergent fashion, prior to the patient being anesthetized, it is ideal to prepare the tracheostomy instruments, a wire-reinforced endotracheal tube, ready the suction, and sterilely prepare the neck. In such a scenario, the patient could be conscious but in severe respiratory distress and hypercapnic, not tolerating the supine position, and present with a higher risk of difficult conventional endotracheal intubation.

  - To avoid any form of sedation, start to ventilate the patient at 100% of FiO_2 in a sitting position with high-flow oxygen (>15 L of O_2) with or without the assistance of a bag-valve-mask ventilation. Anesthetize the anterior neck and transtracheal with Lidocaine with epinephrine, and start the tracheostomy procedure until the trachea is exposed and ready to be entered. At that time only, the patient can be placed in a supine position in cervical extension with a shoulder roll to allow an expeditious opening of the trachea and the placement of an endotracheal tube in the best respiratory conditions possible.

Incision and Drainage (I&D) Procedure

- Incision placement.
  - Incision placement should be ideal to access all involved spaces. More than one incision may be necessary.
  - Esthetics and local anatomy should be considered in incision placement, such as the marginal mandibular branch of the facial nerve for a submandibular or retromandibular approach.
  - The decision should be made on an intraoral versus transcutaneous approach to the infection. Often for advanced head and neck infection, a transcutaneous approach is necessary.

- Anatomical considerations.
  - As aforementioned, the local anatomy should be considered, including nerves and vasculature.

- Dissection.

  - For a deep neck infection, after transcutaneous incision through the skin and adipose tissue, as well as a transection of the platysma, the remainder of the access can be performed with a blunt tonsil or hemostat so as to decrease risk to neurovascular structures.
  - Once the space has been entered, a sterile culture swab should be taken of the purulent fluid.
  - Finger dissection is often adequate at this point to access all spaces involved. The CT scan will guide dissection to ensure adequate entrance to all loculations of the abscess. If all spaces are not properly drained, the patient's recovery may stagnate or worsen, necessitating another scan, and possibly another surgical drainage.
  - Irrigation may or may not be impregnated with an antibiotic. Irrigation should continue until flushing is clear, often over one liter.

- Drain placement.

  - Either Penrose drains or red rubber catheters can be placed in each involved space to ensure continued postoperative drainage, but also access to irrigation and flushing postoperatively.
  - Each drain should be secured with sutures.

- Odontogenic infections.

  - If the infection appears to be related to an odontogenic origin, then it may behoove the surgeon to remove the source of the infection (the tooth) at the time of the surgical drainage. This can also further decompress and drain purulent fluid.

Postoperative Care

- Postoperatively, pending the patient's stability and degree of airway compromise, typically, at least a progressive/intermediate-level unit will be required.
- The surgical team should continue to flush the surgical sites at least two to three times per day with normal saline to clear any continued purulence, as well as to be able to assess if the drainage is becoming clear or remains purulent.
- If the drains are both intraoral and extraoral, the intraoral drain should be removed first to allow the mucosa to heal prior to removing the extraoral drain.
- Postoperative antibiotics are integral, and empiric antibiotics should be de-escalated once culture and sensitivity results return.
- Discharge can be highly variable and depends on patient stability and improvement.

The Difficult Infection (Figs. 26.1, 26.2 and 26.3)

- The immunosuppressed patient under immunosuppression/immunomodulation therapy.

  - This situation can lead to severe infection with rapid head and neck diffusion without ever collecting into a drainable abscess due to the lack of immune response.

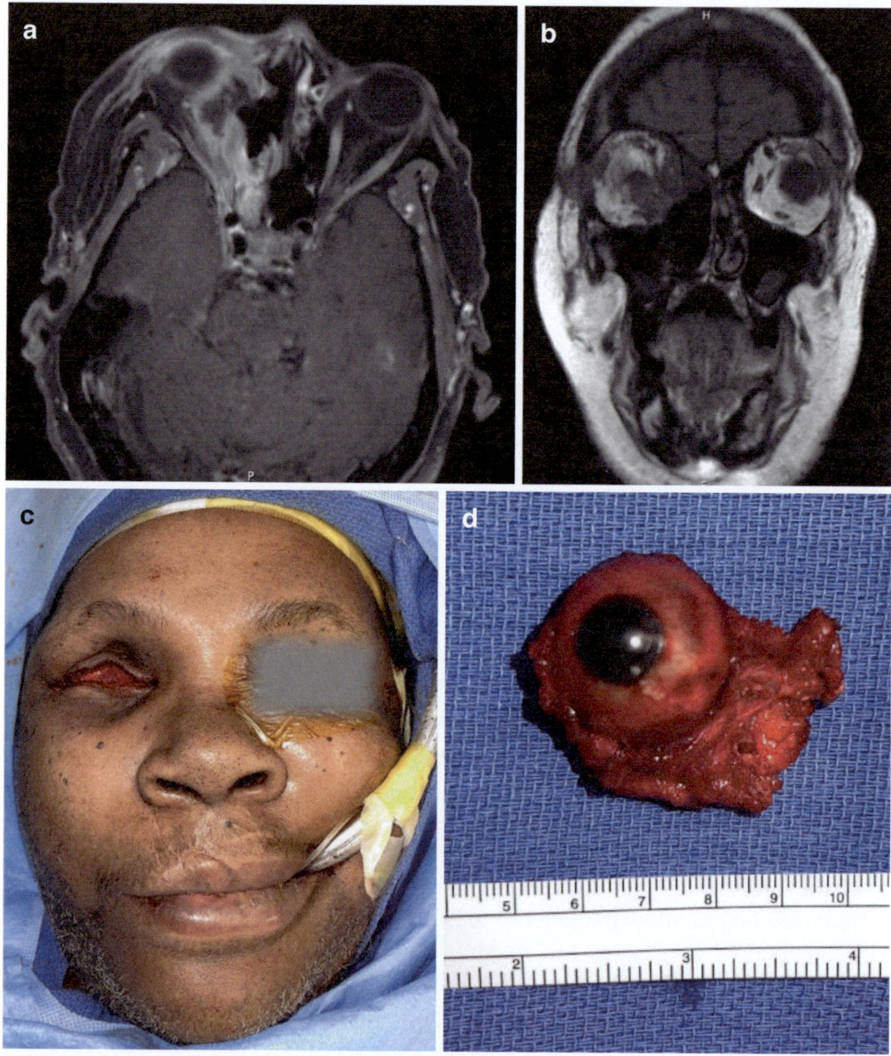

Fig. 26.1 An immunocompromised patient with rapidly progressing mucormycosis as seen in the MRI taken in the (**a**) axial plane (**b**) coronal plane. The patient underwent enucleation after the ophthalmology deemed the globe unable to be salvaged, as seen in (**c, d**)

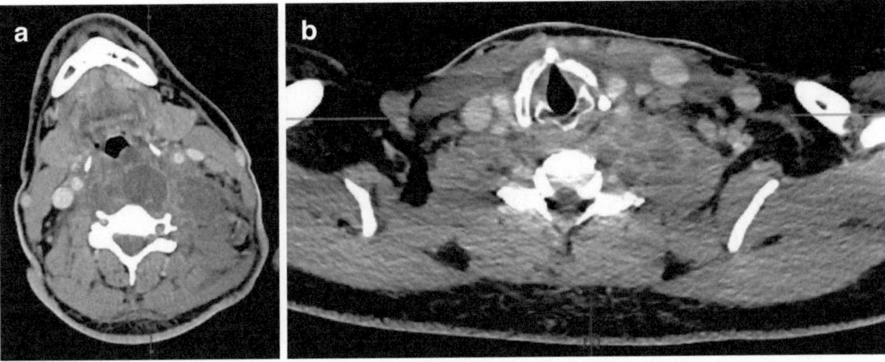

Fig. 26.2 This patient radiographically appeared to have an atypical infection versus a malignant process as seen in the CT scans (**a**, **b**), but clinically he did not present with an infectious picture, only airway compromise, thus, he was not surgically drained. Fine Needle Aspiration (FNA) and then subsequently an open node biopsy was performed. He was diagnosed with Castleman disease via biopsy and did well with treatment. Atypical infections and infections superimposed on malignancy can often be especially confounding, with tumor necrosis in the acute setting. The proper management can be very difficult

Fig. 26.3 This CT sagittal cut demonstrates a retropharyngeal abscess as it progresses toward the Danger space

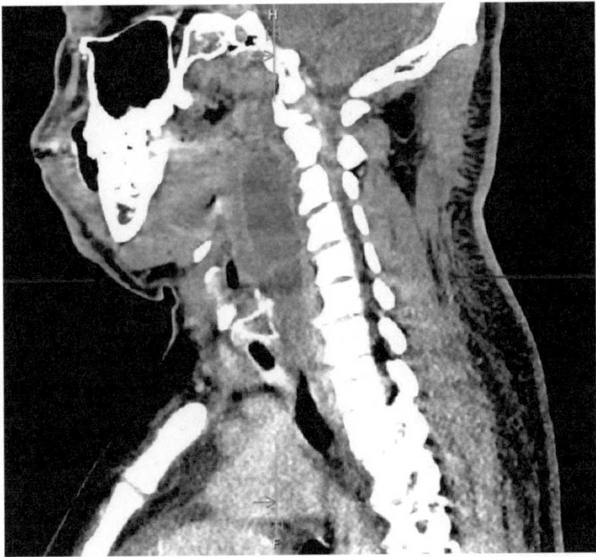

- This type of cellulitis can remain serious with underlying severe sepsis and edema.
- Care should be taken to select the right timing to perform surgical drainage: when a collection is starting to form under appropriate management (holding the causal treatment if possible and treating with broad-spectrum antibiotics) while protecting the upper airway.
- Repeat CT scans can be useful, as well as a serial clinical exam, to determine the right timing for the benefit of surgical intervention and to avoid performing

multiple incomplete procedures, which could lead to a higher rate of overall complications and longer stay in the intensive care unit.

- The persistent infection that requires multiple surgeries.

  - Case 1, Fig. 26.4: This was an 18-year-old patient referred by an outside private practitioner after routine third molar extractions. The patient was a poorly controlled diabetic with an Hba1c of >9%. The patient subsequently suffered from a postoperative infection, undergoing two separate surgical drainages via a transcutaneous approach by the outside provider, with failure to improve. The patient was then referred to our team, with the CT findings seen in Fig. 26.4a, b and the clinical presentation as seen in Fig. 26.4c, d, with the previous surgical debridement submandibular incision with purulence noted. The patient then underwent a third surgical debridement (the first with our team) via a transcutaneous submandibular approach, and she was on empiric antibiotics that were then de-escalated. She also was treated for her hyperglycemia. She was discharged by postoperative day three and did very well.

  - If a patient is not clinically improving after surgical debridement, then one must consider re-scanning the patient with a CT scan and possible re-

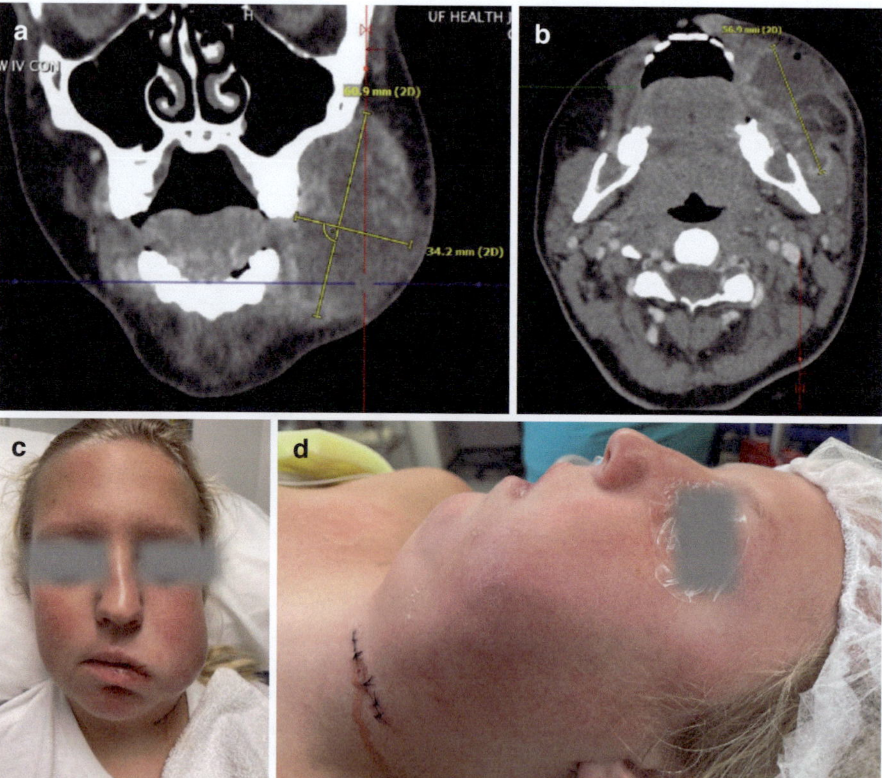

Fig. 26.4 This patient suffered a post-extraction infection refractory to antibiotics and initial surgical management. (**a, b**) Illustrate the persistent multi-space infection seen after two initial surgical debridements, with (**c, d**) illustrating the clinical presentation in this poorly controlled diabetic

operation. At the time of re-operation, ensure every possible space involved is entered and drained, obtain a new set of wound cultures, and adjust the antibiotic regimen as appropriate.

- The parotid abscess.

    - Case 2, Fig. 26.5: This severely immunocompromised patient had persistent parotitis with a parotid abscess seen on the CT scan, as seen in Fig. 26.5a, b. Initial medical management, with empiric antibiotics and local measures cannulating the parotid duct to extract a stone by another provider did not resolve the abscess. Repeat imaging showed a persistent infection, and thus the decision was made to take the patient to the operating room. A small incision was made in the preauricular area through the skin only, and then blunt dissection was taken to the involved space. Purulence was expressed, and cultures were taken. The facial nerve was intact thereafter. The patient improved clinically with a resolution of the abscess/parotitis.
    - The parotid abscess is inherently difficult to treat, as surgical intervention is not always straightforward, with a higher risk to the facial nerve. But if the infection does not respond to medical management, then one must surgically debride the area.

- The orbital infection.

    - Case 3, Fig. 26.1: During the COVID pandemic, possibly due to immunocompromise, this 82-year-old patient presented with altered mental status and an aggressive infection noted on CT/MRI, as seen in Figs. 26.1a, b. Initially, sinus surgery was performed to debride and obtain specimens, which returned as Mucormycosis. After serial debridements, the patient clinically improved, but her globe was not able to be preserved and was enucleated, as seen in Fig. 26.1c, d.
    - Orbital infections should be taken very seriously, as they can affect vision, and lead to cavernous sinus thrombosis. First, one must determine if the infec-

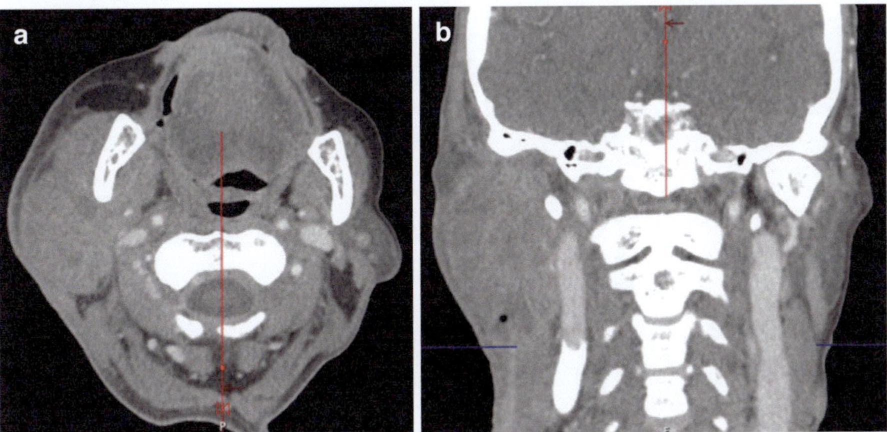

Fig. 26.5 This immunocompromised patient with a persistent parotid abscess with gas formation did not respond to medical management and required surgical debridement

tion is preseptal or postseptal. Postseptal infections can be especially devastating if they involve the optic nerve.

- The case seen in Fig. 26.6 is a patient with left preseptal orbitopalpebral cellulitis of lacrimal origin (dacryocystitis).
- The case presented in Fig. 26.7 is a left postseptal intraorbital subperiosteal abscess with left pansinusitis of odontogenic origin (teeth #12 and 14).

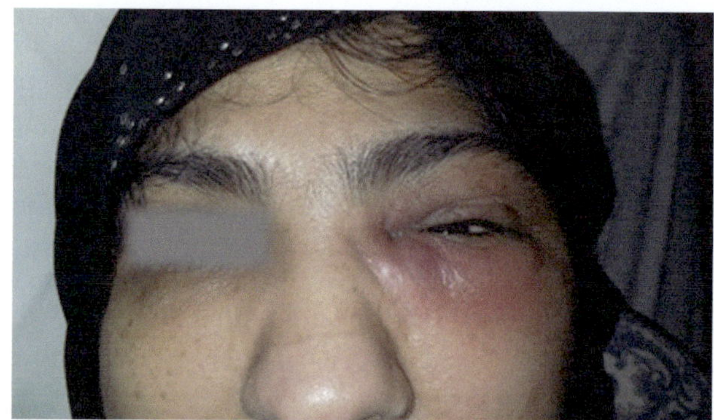

Fig. 26.6 Left preseptal orbitopalpebral cellulitis of lacrimal origin (dacryocystitis)

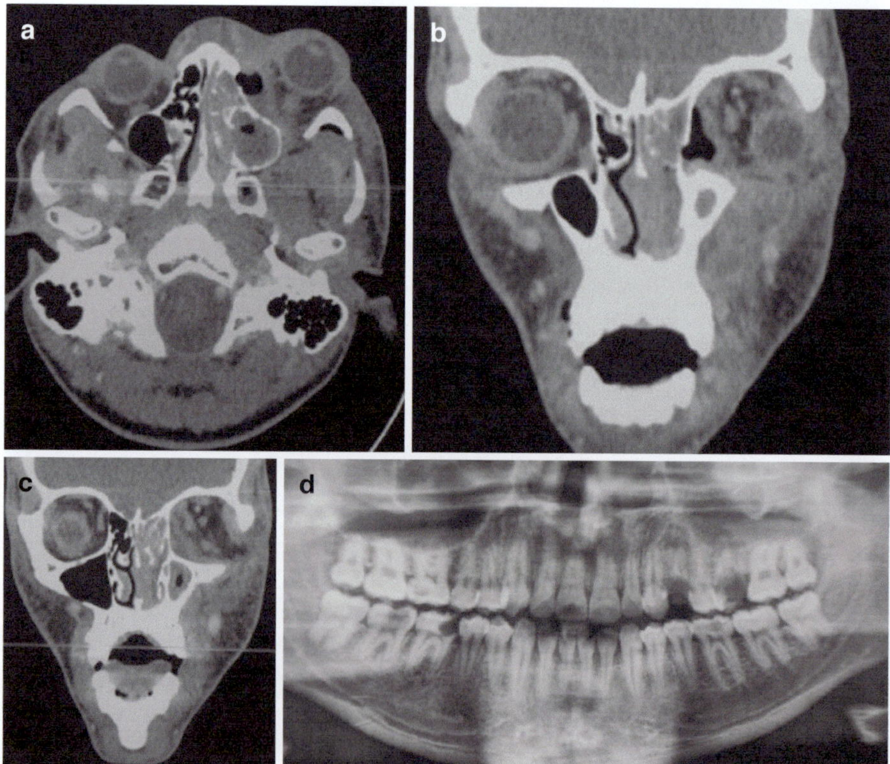

Fig. 26.7 (**a–c**) Show CT slices of a left postseptal intraorbital subperiosteal abscess with a left pansinusitis of odontogenic origin (teeth #12 and 14) seen in the panoramic radiograph in (**d**)

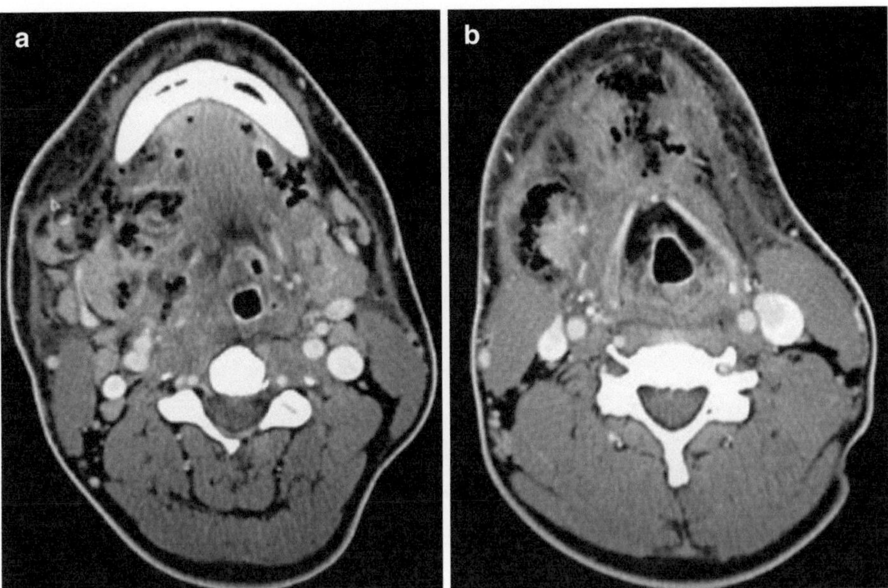

Fig. 26.8 (**a, b**) Illustrate CT axial slices of a neck necrotizing fasciitis with gas formation from an odontogenic origin (tooth #18)

- Neck necrotizing fasciitis:

  - Even if it is quite a rare clinical scenario, it should be managed like any other necrotizing fasciitis location in the human body: without any initial skin closure. It will allow the surgical team to perform serial aggressive surgical cleaning.
  - Typically, this aggressive process has odontogenic origins, and the patient presents with diffuse soft tissue gas, necrotic tissues, and brown fluid collections rather than frank purulence. Figure 26.8a, b demonstrates neck necrotizing fasciitis with gas formation from an odontogenic origin (tooth #18).
  - The treatment consists of opening all involved spaces, avoiding, if possible to open the lower aspect of the neck to prevent spreading the infection into the thorax.
  - The same indications for a tracheostomy remain. Tracheostomy ideally is avoided to preserve the pretracheal space.
  - A musculocutaneous cervical flap can be elevated and left open for further surgical cleaning (wash out six times per day). Figure 26.9 illustrates postoperative day one (A) and postoperative day seven (B), with the musculocutaneous cervical flap left open to allow further debridement if needed and sepsis control.
  - Once the necrotizing fasciitis disease process has been controlled, the patient may require locoregional rotational flaps or microvascular free flaps to reconstruct the defect.

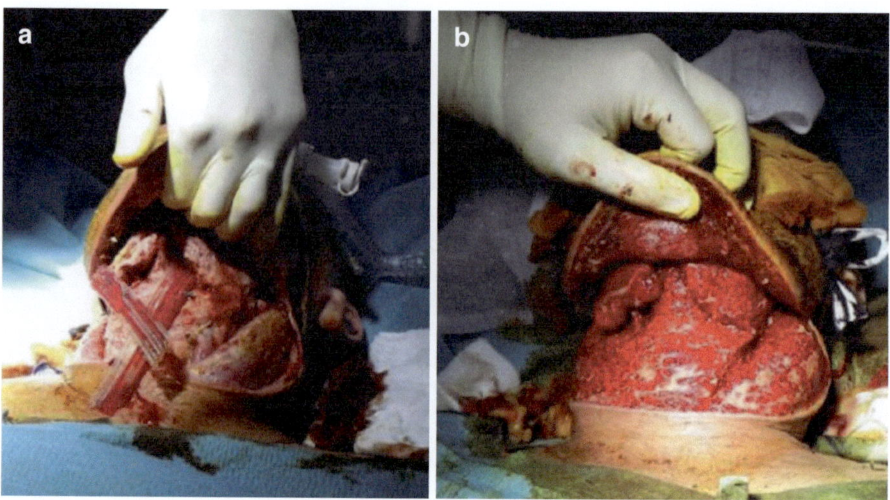

Fig. 26.9 Postoperative days 1 (**a**) and 7 (**b**) for treatment of neck necrotizing fasciitis, with the musculocutaneous cervical flap left open to allow healthy granulation and decrease necrosis. A washout was performed six times per day

Pearls and Pitfalls

- Infections can track to the mediastinum, causing empyema and pericardial effusions, or they can track posteriorly to the prevertebral space, causing spondylitis and epidural abscess with spinal cord compression.
- Infections in the anterior neck can make tracheostomy more difficult, blocking access to the trachea and ablating the surgical planes.
- Parapharyngeal infections can make intubation difficult or unachievable (the dreaded "cannot intubate, cannot ventilate" scenarios). The surgeon must anticipate and discuss this scenario with the anesthesia team prior to the situation and be prepared for an immediate surgical airway.
- The parapharyngeal and retropharyngeal spaces can quickly spread to the mediastinum.
- Signs and symptoms of a rapidly progressing airway are drooling, tripod posture, trismus, dyspnea, dysphonia or dysphagia, and using accessory respiratory muscles with increased work of breathing.
- Parotid abscesses can be difficult to treat surgically due to the risk to the facial nerve branches.
- Ludwig's angina involving the bilateral submandibular, sublingual, and submental spaces can quickly become an airway emergency.
- Necrotizing fasciitis is a surgical emergency and necessitates multiple surgical debridements and often results in large soft tissue defects if the patient survives.

- One must always consider oropharyngeal cancer in adult patients with recurrent peritonsillar abscesses and cancer risk factors.
- An immunocompromised patient with multiple medical comorbidities, such as uncontrolled diabetes, can have an atypically aggressive presentation and must be treated appropriately and promptly.

Further Reading

Flynn TR. Principles and surgical management of head and neck infections. In: Bagheri S, Bell R, Khan H, editors. Current therapy in oral and maxillofacial surgery. Amsterdam: Elsevier Saunders; 2012. p. 1080–91.

Cillo J. Fascial spaces of the head and neck. In: Kademani D, Tiwana P, editors. Atlas of oral and maxillofacial surgery. 1st ed. Amsterdam: Elsevier Saunders; 2016. p. 66–72.

Stein JM, Xian J. Imaging of head and neck infections. Neuroimaging Clin N Am. 2023;33(1):185–206. https://doi.org/10.1016/j.nic.2022.07.016.

Saibene AM, Allevi F, Ayad T, et al. Treatment for parotid abscess: a systematic review. Acta Otorhinolaryngol Ital. 2022;42(2):106–15. https://doi.org/10.14639/0392-100X-N1837.

Russell MD, Russell MS. Urgent infections of the head and neck. Med Clin N Am. 2018;102(6):1109–20. https://doi.org/10.1016/j.mcna.2018.06.015.

Rokkjaer MS, Klug TE. Tonsillar malignancy in adult patients with peritonsillar abscess: retrospective study of 275 patients and review of the literature. Eur Arch Otorhinolaryngol. 2015;272(9):2439–44. https://doi.org/10.1007/s00405-014-3186-0.

Chapter 27
Practical Tips for Performing Sialendoscopy

Hisham Marwan ⓘD

Abstract Sialendoscopy is a surgical technique that aims to assess and treat salivary ductal pathologies, including strictures and stones. Nahlieli et al. (Nahlieli and Baruchin, J Oral Maxillofac Surg 57:1394–401, 1999) were the first to describe the retrieval of salivary gland stones with a nasal endoscope. Subsequently, dedicated Sialendoscopy instruments were developed and applied to a larger scale.

Sialendoscopy can retrieve stones and treat strictures from recurrent sialadenitis or autoimmune diseases. In addition, Sialendoscopy dilation is particularly useful for treating radioiodine-induced sialadenitis. The purpose of this chapter is to explain the practical techniques in using sialoendoscopy.

Preoperative Assessment

- For suspected stones, a CT scan without contrast is the most sensitive imaging modality.
- Not all stones should be removed. Asymptomatic patient with a stone should be observed and followed up.
- In general, stones less than 6 mm in diameter can be successfully retrieved with Sialendoscopy (Fig. 27.1).

H. Marwan (✉)
Department of Surgery, The University of Texas Medical Branch, Galveston, TX, USA
e-mail: himarwan@utmb.edu

D. Amin, H. Marwan (eds.), *Pearls and Pitfalls in Oral and Maxillofacial Surgery*, https://doi.org/10.1007/978-3-031-47307-4_27

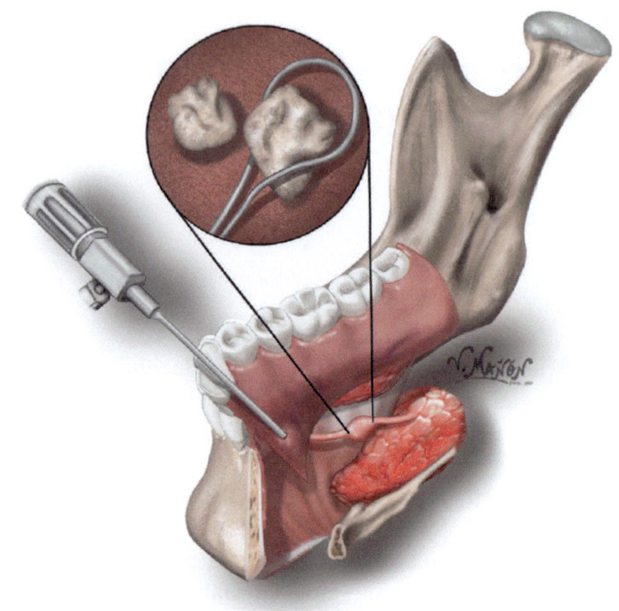

Fig. 27.1 The use of Sialoendoscopy for retrieval of submandibular gland stone

Intraoperative Pearls

- Magnification is beneficial in locating the papilla. Avoiding anti-sialagogue will help maintain the salivary flow and locate the papilla, particularly in Wharton's duct.
- Continuous irrigation is a key to successful dilation. However, avoid excessive irrigation due to the risk of swelling and airway compromise. Furthermore, avoid excessive pressure with irrigation to avoid inadvertent duct perforation.
- Start the dilation with the conical dilator to gently dilate the papilla without trauma.
- Dilate the duct with the salivary probes of increasing diameter. Avoid deep insertion into the duct to prevent false passage. There are 12 different sizes.
- If there are any problematic encounters with inserting the probe, go back to one or two smaller sizes and dilate more. Furthermore, straightening the duct (pullout) will help in inserting the probe.
- Sialoendoscopes: there are two types—multi-purpose and all-in-one. All the scopes are straight. They are susceptible to breakage if bent. The author recommends using a high-definition camera with those scopes.
- It is our preference to use the Storz-Marchal 1.3 mm Universal Sialoendoscope. This scope can be used for both diagnostic and intervention procedures. All the

intervention Sialoendoscopes have three ports with a working channel of 0.6 mm that allows the insertion of the basket or the forceps.

- Stone retrieval baskets are available in different sizes. You must pass the stone before opening the basket and pull the stone and basket outside the duct.
- The forceps are essential to break down the stone and directly grasp and retrieve small stones.
- If the stone is too large to be pulled out, a small papillotomy incision will help remove the stone.
- Holmium: YAG laser is used for large stones that cannot be crushed with forceps. Carefully aim at the center of the stone and avoid injuring the duct with the laser. The preferred setting for the lithotripsy is with a power of 2.5 W, a rate of 5 Hz/s, and an energy of 0.5 J.
- Approximately, 5% of patients will present with more than two stones. Examine the whole ductal system with the scope.

Postoperative Care

- Keep the stent in place for at least 4 weeks for submandibular glands and 8 weeks for the parotid to prevent stricture.
- The use of a specialized salivary stent is recommended. However, an angio catheter can be used if not available.
- Use a nonabsorbable suture to secure the stent in place.
- Assess the patient before extubation. Using excessive irrigation can result in elevating the floor of the mouth or swelling of the deep lobe of the parotid with resulting airway compromise.

Pearls

- Sialendoscopy can retrieve stones and treat strictures from recurrent sialadenitis or autoimmune diseases and is particularly useful for treating radioiodine-induced sialadenitis.
- Continuous irrigation is key to successful dilation.
- If the stone is too large to be pulled out, a small papillotomy incision will help remove the stone.
- Keep the stent in place for at least 4 weeks for submandibular glands and 8 weeks for the parotid to prevent stricture.

Pitfalls

- Avoid excessive irrigation due to the risk of swelling and airway compromise. Furthermore, avoid extreme pressure with irrigation to avoid inadvertent duct perforation.

Further Reading

Nahlieli O, Baruchi AM. Endoscopic technique for the diagnosis and treatment of obstructive salivary gland diseases. J Oral Maxillofac Surg. 1999;57:1394–401.

Part V
Head and Neck Reconstruction

Chapter 28
Practical Tips for Pectoralis Major Myocutaneous Flap

Cameron Lee, Eva Sidhu, Riya Gupta, Joshua Lubek, and Donita Dyalram

Abstract The pectoralis major myocutaneous flap was first described for head and neck reconstruction by Ariyan in 1979. Surgical innovations allowing for the harvest of composite tissue, including bone and multiple skin paddles, led to the widespread adoption of this flap in the late twentieth century. While free flaps have since supplanted regional flaps as the primary reconstructive option for head and neck defects, the pectoralis major flap is still a viable option as a salvage flap or as a primary reconstructive option for patients who are not candidates for free flaps. Benefits include excellent flap survival rates, ease of harvest, relatively short operative time, and abundant soft tissue allowing for various reconstructive options. The purpose of this chapter is to review pearls and pitfalls in harvesting pectoralis major myocutaneous flap.

C. Lee
University of Maryland Oral and Maxillofacial Surgery Fellowship Program, Baltimore, MD, USA

E. Sidhu · R. Gupta
University of Maryland Maxillofacial Surgery Residency Program, Baltimore, MD, USA

J. Lubek
Oral and Maxillofacial Surgery, University of Maryland Head and Neck Oncology/ Microvascular Reconstruction Fellowship, Baltimore, MD, USA

D. Dyalram (✉)
Oral and Maxillofacial Surgery, University of Maryland Maxillofacial Surgery Residency Program, Baltimore, MD, USA
e-mail: ddyalram@umaryland.edu

D. Amin, H. Marwan (eds.), *Pearls and Pitfalls in Oral and Maxillofacial Surgery*, https://doi.org/10.1007/978-3-031-47307-4_28

Practical Tips

Preoperative Consideration

- A thorough history and physical are imperative. This flap is contraindicated in patients with a history of trauma or surgery to the chest wall or those with congenital syndromes affecting the chest wall musculature.

Intraoperative Consideration

Flap Design

- The patient is positioned supine with the ipsilateral arm abducted to expose the anterior axillary fold. Surgical landmarks are marked, including the clavicle, sternum, xiphoid process, and humeral insertion of the pectoralis major.
- The patient is prepped and draped such that the clavicle, sternum, xiphoid process, axilla, and shoulder are accessible. This prep is included with the recipient site.
- The pectoralis major myocutaneous flap is an axial pattern flap based on the pectoral branch of the thoracoacromial artery. The pectoral branch is marked using either landmark-based techniques or a Doppler ultrasound.
- The origin of the pectoral branch is approximated by drawing a line from the acromion to the xiphoid process and transecting this line with one drawn perpendicular to the clavicle at the midclavicular line. The pedicle typically descends in the caudal-lateral direction within 1–2 cm of the perpendicular line.
- The skin paddle is drawn to approximate the size of the defect. The paddle is designed over the medial/inferior aspect of the pectoralis major adjacent to the sternal border (Fig. 28.1).
- Extending the skin paddle caudally past the sixth costal cartilage increases the risk of partial skin necrosis as the blood supply to the skin is random at this point.
- To ensure adequate pedicle length, the distance between the superior aspect of the skin paddle and the clavicle should be equivalent to the distance between the defect and the clavicle.
- A curvilinear incision is designed to start laterally at the anterior axillary line extending to the planned skin paddle. This part of the incision is usually superior to the nipple in males and within the inframammary fold in females.

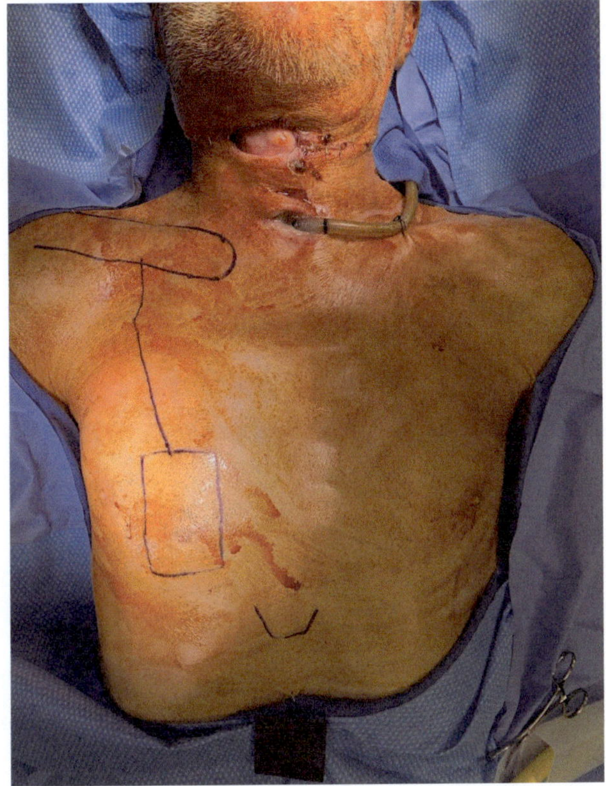

Fig. 28.1 Preoperative markings and flap design. Pectoralis major flap planned for a fistula closure in the right neck and skin defect. The clavicle, xiphoid process, skin paddle, and path of the pedicle are drawn. Note that the skin paddle remains superior to the level of the sixth costal cartilage, thus reducing the likelihood of partial necrosis

Flap Elevation

- The incision around the skin paddle should be beveled radially to leave a wide subdermal plexus and improve perfusion. Suturing the skin paddle to the muscle will help reduce the shearing of the blood supply (Fig. 28.2).
- Elevation of the pectoralis major begins inferolateral and proceeds toward the clavicle.
- Superolaterally, it is critical to clearly define the plane between the pectoralis minor and major muscles. This can often be accomplished with finger dissection.
- Medially, the pectoralis major must be freed from the sternum. Perforators from the internal thoracic artery are encountered here and should be clipped to prevent postoperative bleeding (Fig. 28.3).
- The vascular pedicle is identified on the deep surface of the pectoralis major once the flap is elevated and traced proximally (Fig. 28.4).

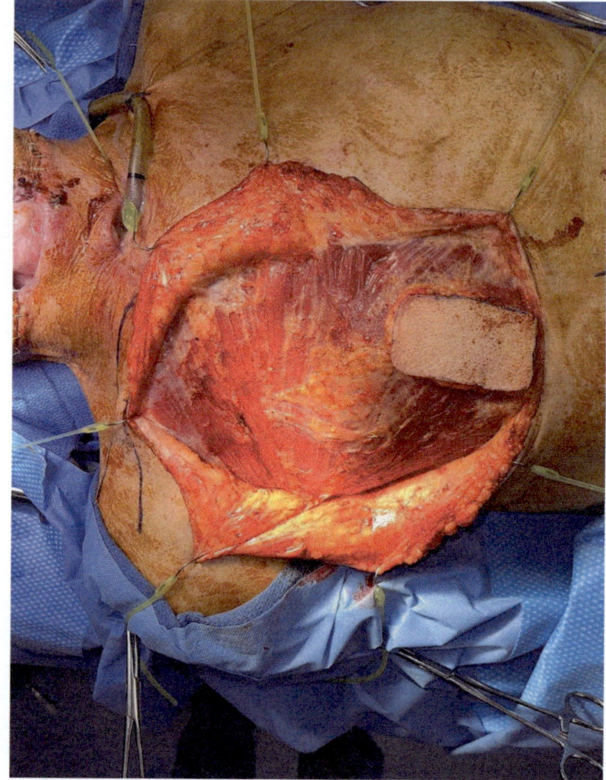

Fig. 28.2 Exposure of the pectoralis major. Skin flaps are raised to visualize the pectoralis major muscle. A cuff of subcutaneous tissue is maintained circumferentially around the skin paddle to maximize the quantity of perforators

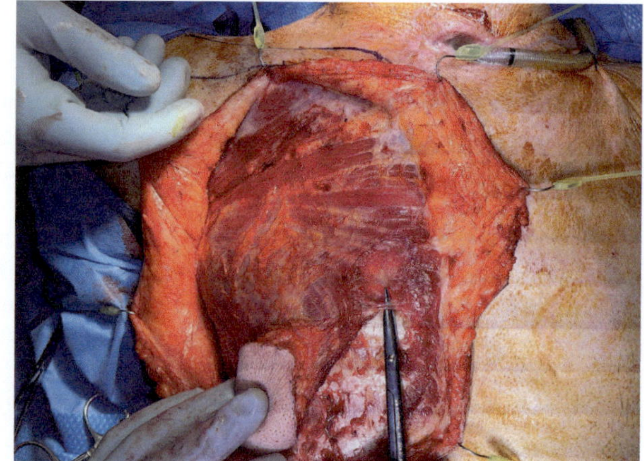

Fig. 28.3 Ligation of perforators from the internal thoracic artery. Perforators (isolated on the instrument) from the internal thoracic artery are encountered as the pectoralis major is dissected free from the chest wall and sternum

Fig. 28.4 Identification of the vascular pedicle. The pedicle can be seen running on the deep surface of the pectoralis major. Note the pectoralis minor muscle just deep into the pedicle

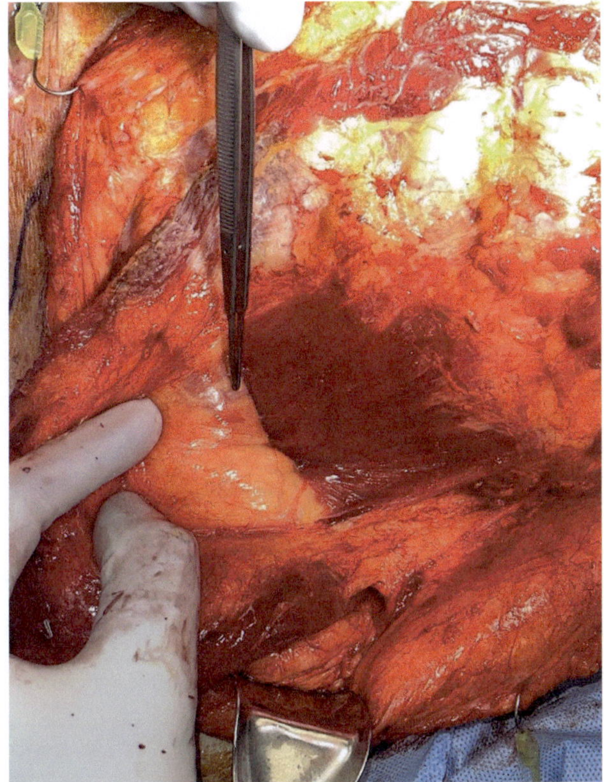

- The lateral thoracic artery descends laterally along the pectoralis minor and is traditionally sacrificed to improve pedicle length and arc of rotation. However, preservation of this artery may reduce the incidence of skin paddle necrosis.
- The lateral pectoral nerve and branches of the medial pectoral nerve are encountered entering the deep surface of the pectoralis major superolateral. These are also sacrificed.
- Finally, the pectoralis major insertion to the humerus is divided under direct visualization of the pedicle.

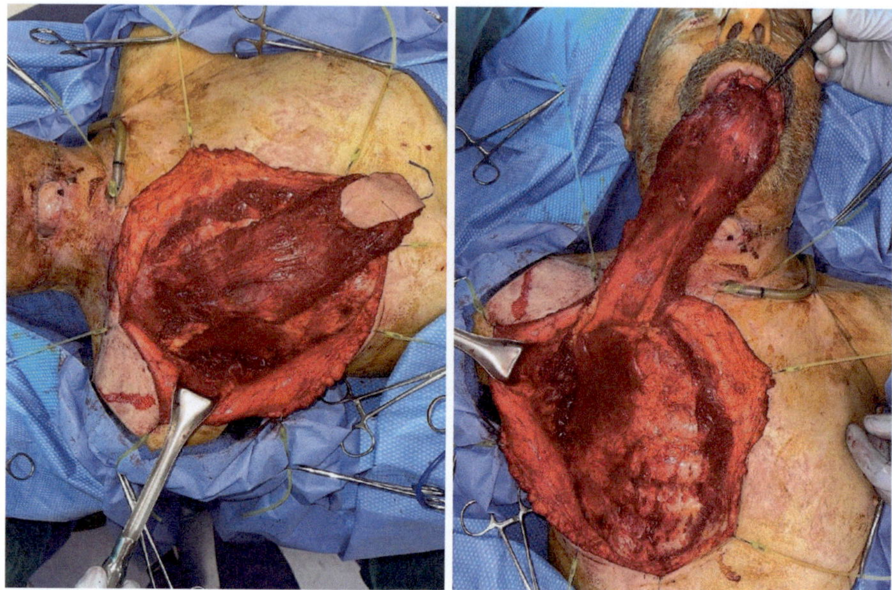

Fig. 28.5 Verification of flap length for reconstruction. Once fully mobilized, the flap is examined to determine the reach of the defect. Resection of muscle fibers at the insertion of the humeral head improves the reach superiorly. Both clockwise or counter-clockwise rotation of the flap is tolerated

Flap Inset

- The pedicled flap can be tunneled above or below the clavicle (Fig. 28.5). A wide subcutaneous tunnel is needed to prevent compression of the vascular pedicle regardless of the tunneling technique (Fig. 28.6).
- Depending on where the skin paddle is needed, the flap can be rotated 180 degrees or not (Fig. 28.7).

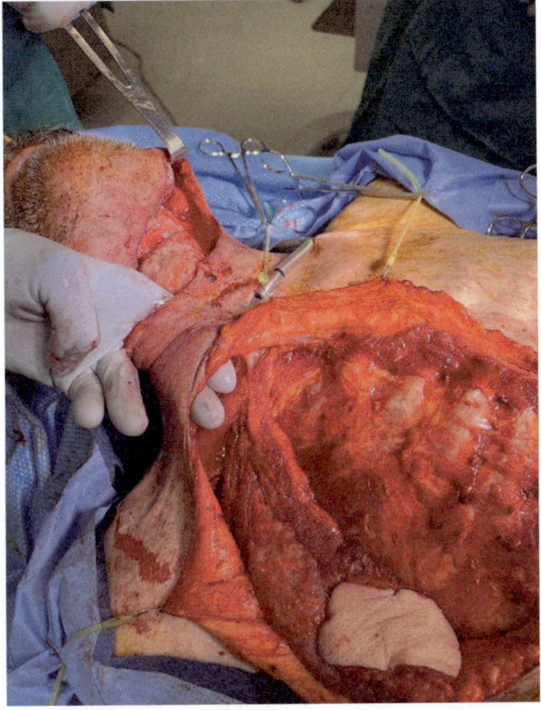

Fig. 28.6 Creation of subcutaneous tunnel. The tunnel should be wide enough to permit passage of the flap without compression of the pedicle. This tunnel is created above the clavicle

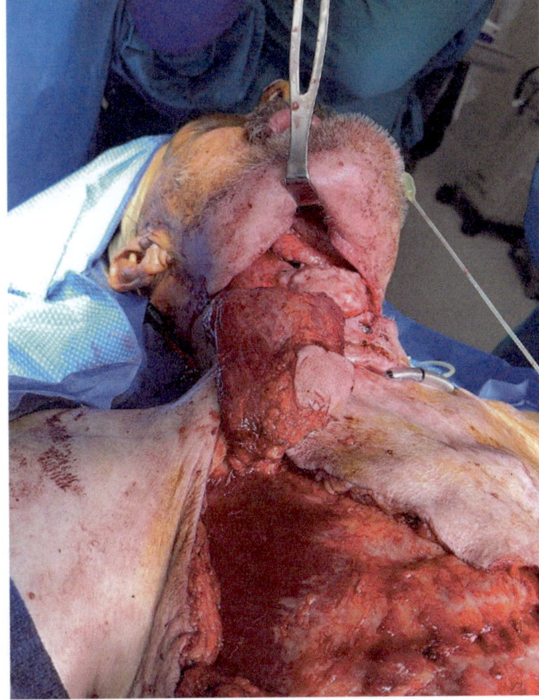

Fig. 28.7 Tunneling of the flap and inset. The flap is tunneled over the clavicle and below the subcutaneous tunnel into the defect. In this case, the flap was used to reconstruct a through-and-through defect of the anterior neck. Since the skin paddle needed to be placed intraorally, there was no need to rotate the flap

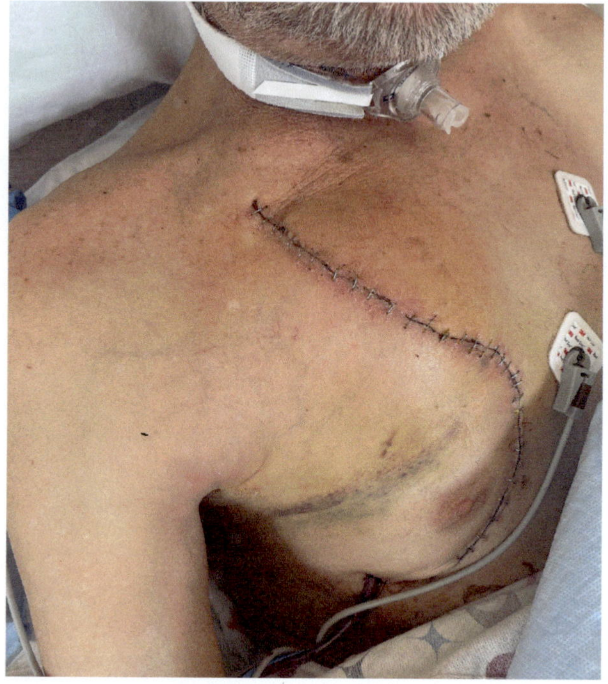

Fig. 28.8 Wound closure and cosmetic outcome. Primary closure is achieved with the placement of a single suction drain. Note the small supraclavicular bulge that is characteristic following pectoralis flap reconstruction

Closure

- A Valsalva maneuver can confirm the absence of any pleural tears.
- The chest is generally amenable to a primary layered closure. A large skin paddle may necessitate a split-thickness skin graft (Fig. 28.8).
- One or two suction drains are placed overlying the chest wall to help prevent hematoma formation.

Postoperative Consideration

- The flap can be monitored by checking viability with a scratch test, doppler, or clinical examination.
- The Doppler of the pedicle is more reliable if the flap is brought over the clavicle and rotated 180°.
- The most common complications are wound breakdown, orocutaneous fistula, and partial necrosis of the skin paddle. These are managed with local wound care measures. Skin grafting may be indicated in rare cases.
- The most common cosmetic issue is a supraclavicular bulge where the flap is rotated around the pedicle. This bulk can be reduced with muscle excision in this region once the flap is fully vascularized and integrated at the defect site.

Pearls

- Design the skin paddle over the medial/inferior aspect of the pectoralis major muscle and adjacent to the sternal border.
- Consider beveled incisions around the skin paddle to leave a wide subdermal plexus and improve perfusion.
- Suturing the skin paddle to the muscle will help reduce the shearing of the blood supply.

Pitfalls

- One or two suction drains are placed overlying the chest wall to help prevent hematoma formation.
- Consider Doppler of the pedicle when the flap is brought over the clavicle and rotated 180°.

Further Reading

Ariyan S. The pectoralis major myocutaneous flap. A versatile flap for reconstruction in the head and neck. Plast Reconstr Surg. 1979;63:73.
Cuono CB, Ariyan S. Immediate reconstruction of a composite mandibular defect with a regional osteomusculocutaneous flap. Plast Reconstr Surg. 1980;65:477.
Green MF, Gibson JR, Bryson JR, Thomson E. A one-stage correction of mandibular defects using a split sternum pectoralis major osteo-musculocutaneous transfer. Br J Plast Surg. 1981;34:11.
Milenovic A, Virag M, Uglesic V, Aljinovic-Ratkovic N. The pectoralis major flap in head and neck reconstruction: first 500 patients. J Craniomaxillofac Surg. 2006;34:340.

Chapter 29
Submental Artery Island Perforator Flap: Technique, Pearls, and Pitfalls

Lior Aljadeff and Anthony B. P. Morlandt

Abstract The submental artery island perforator flap (SIAPF) is a reliable and versatile axial pattern fasciocutaneous pedicled flap that can be used to reconstruct a variety of defects in the head and neck. Among several advantages are excellent skin color and texture match, rapidity and ease of harvest, and limited donor site morbidity. In our head and neck surgery practice, the SIAPF is used as a workhorse in treating elderly patients with multiple co-morbidities who may not be good candidates for free tissue transfer. Despite the advantages listed above, harvesting the submental artery flap requires a thorough understanding of the anatomy surrounding the submental artery and meticulous surgical technique. The purpose of this chapter is to review pearls and pitfalls for submental artery island perforator flaps.

Anatomy

The submental artery is the major cutaneous branch of the facial artery, consistently supplying the skin overlying the submandibular and submental triangles of the neck. It arises from the facial artery superficial to the submandibular gland or between the mandible's submandibular gland and inferior border over 95% of the time (69% superficial to the gland, 27% superior to the gland). In rare cases, the submental artery emerges from the facial artery from within the parenchyma of the

L. Aljadeff
Department of Oral and Maxillofacial Surgery, Head and Neck Surgery, University of Alabama at Birmingham, Birmingham, AL, USA

A. B. P. Morlandt (✉)
Department of Oral and Maxillofacial Surgery and Otolaryngology, University of Alabama at Birmingham, Birmingham, AL, USA
e-mail: morlandt@uab.edu

D. Amin, H. Marwan (eds.), *Pearls and Pitfalls in Oral and Maxillofacial Surgery*, https://doi.org/10.1007/978-3-031-47307-4_29

gland, which requires meticulous intraglandular dissection with attention to hemostasis. The origin of the submental artery is, on average, 23.8 mm (range 1.5–39 mm) anterior to the angle of the mandible and 5 mm (range 1.5–12 mm) below the inferior border of the mandible, with a mean diameter of 1.7 mm (range 1–2.3 mm) at its takeoff. After the submental artery branches off the facial artery, the facial artery crosses the inferior border of the mandible and takes a tortuous course superiorly over the face while the submental artery branches anteriorly along the medial aspect of the inferior border of the mandible, superficial to the mylohyoid muscle. After coursing over the mylohyoid muscle, the submental artery dives deep to the ipsilateral anterior digastric muscle 70–80% of the time (superficial 20–30%) and finally terminates deep to the mandibular symphysis, just ipsilateral to the midline. Along its course, the submental artery supplies one to four cutaneous perforators (diameter $\geq$ 0.5 mm) that pierce the overlying platysma to supply the subdermal plexus of the overlying skin. The largest perforator usually arises from the medial border of the ipsilateral anterior digastric muscle. The submental artery terminates by perfusing the mandibular periosteum, lower lip, and sublingual salivary gland. Its branches anastomose with the contralateral submental artery 92% of the time (Fig. 29.1).

The SIAPF is drained by the submental vein (mean diameter of 2.2 mm with a range of 1–2.9 mm), which runs superior to the submental artery and empties into the facial vein. The facial vein occasionally anastomoses with the external jugular vein, which can play an essential role in venous drainage of the flap. When harvesting a submental artery island flap, a critical consideration is the location of the marginal mandibular branch of the facial nerve. At the level of the submandibular gland, the marginal mandibular nerve is, on average, 12 mm superior to the submental artery (range 0–28 mm) within the superficial layer of deep cervical fascia that overlies the gland. However, the fact that the marginal mandibular nerve can be directly superficial to the submental artery should serve as a warning to surgeons and a rationale for identifying and protecting the nerve during harvest (Picture 29.1).

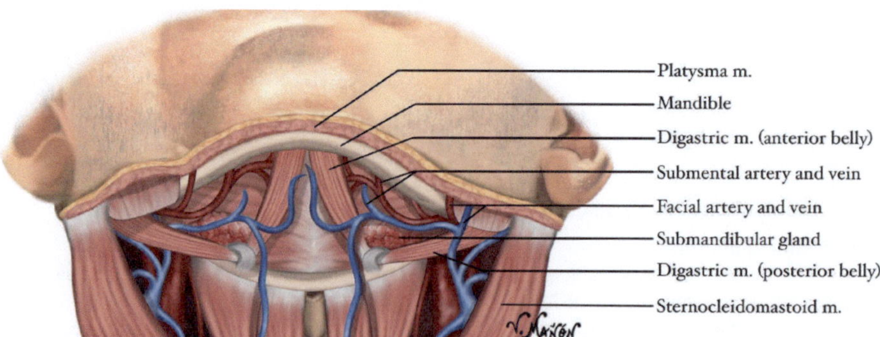

Fig. 29.1 Anatomical schematic from Magden et al. PRS, 2004

Practical Tips

Preoperative Consideration

- The cutaneous perforators of the submental artery supply the subdermal plexus of the submental and submandibular skin. This subdermal plexus has extensive anastomoses with the contralateral submental artery perforating branches and thus allows for the harvest of skin that extends mediolaterally as far as the contralateral angle based on only one submental artery.
- Practically speaking, the anteroposterior dimension of the skin flap that can be harvested is limited by the ability to achieve primary closure, which depends on the patient's skin laxity. Skin laxity can be estimated by marking out the desired anteroposterior dimension of the flap and attempting to passively pinch the marks together. A 6- to 8-cm anteroposterior defect in the submental region can usually be closed primarily with minimal tension. Primary repair of the donor site deformity takes the form of an inferiorly based platysmal myocutaneous advancement flap secured to the periosteum of the inferior border of the mandible to avoid dehiscence during neck extension.
- The anterior limit of the superior incision is the submental crease. This crease helps to hide the scar. Extending this incision superiorly beyond the submental crease onto the skin of the mentum can pull the chin down during repair of the donor site defect, potentially causing lip incompetence.
- Ideally, the posterior border of the skin paddle should connect to the neck dissection incision in a natural skin crease along a smooth and gentle curve. This allows the wound to be closed as a single smooth wound with minimal to no dog ear and avoids creating a "cobra neck" deformity (Picture 29.2).

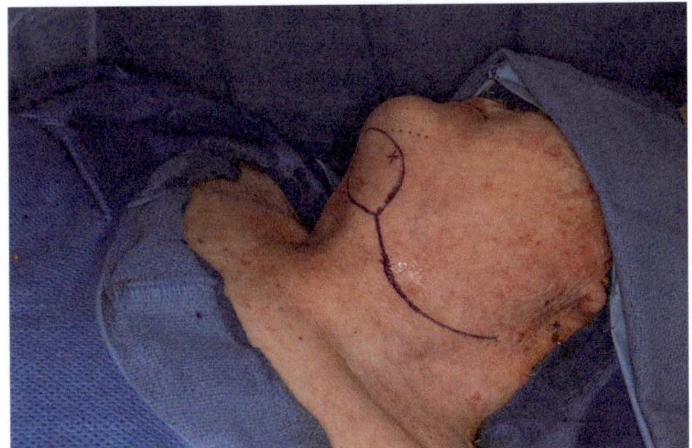

Picture 29.1 Notice how the posterior border of the skin paddle transitions smoothly into the neck dissection incision. Notes: notice how the posterior border of the skin paddle transitions smoothly into the neck dissection incision

Picture 29.2 Notice the marginal mandibular nerve identified and protected as it courses over the facial vein. Notes: Notice the marginal mandibular nerve identified and protected as it courses over the facial vein

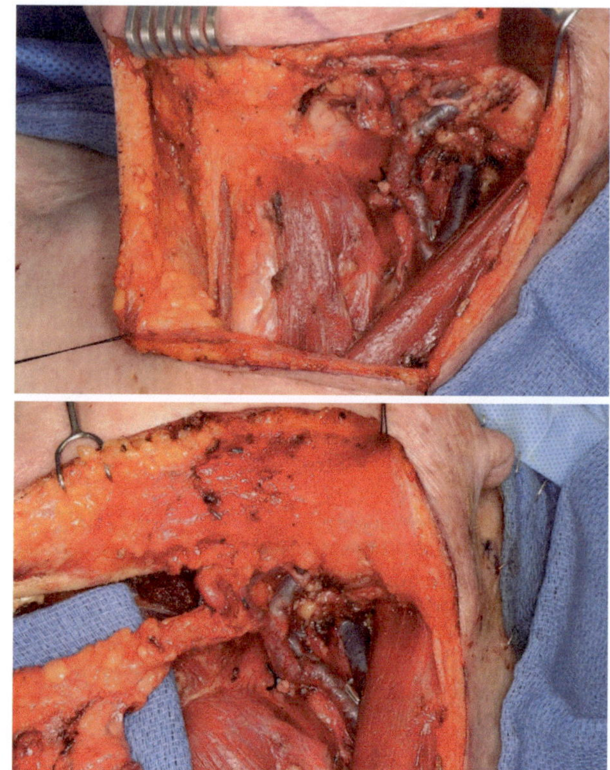

Intraoperative Consideration

- The marginal mandibular nerve is identified and protected.
- The needle-tip bipolar is helpful for safe, efficient, and clean dissection of the superficial layer of deep cervical fascia superiorly along the parenchyma of the gland and towards the inferior border of the mandible until the facial vessels are identified.
- The pedicle does not need to be cleaned entirely of surrounding fibrofatty tissue. Minimizing manipulation of the delicate vessels that supply and drain the submental flap reduces the risk of vasospasm and vessel injury. Clean and careful dissection of the pedicle may be necessary in the case of lengthening or when combined with a neck dissection that requires the removal of perifacial lymph nodes.
- When detaching the skin paddle from the anterior mandible, it is wise to leave a cuff of periosteum on the inferior border of the mandible to aid in the primary closure of the donor site.

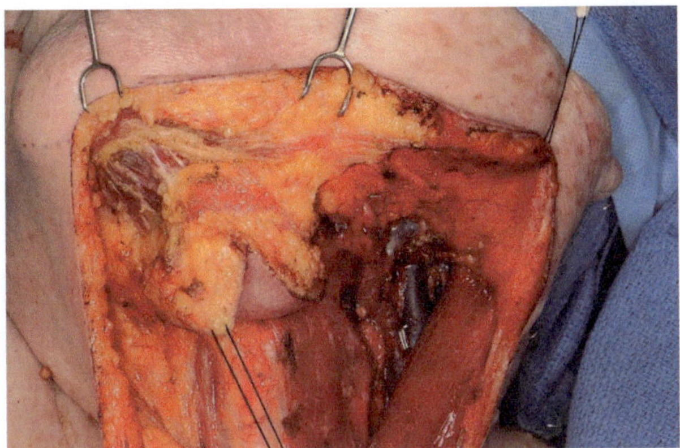

Picture 29.3 Notice the thin cuff of anterior digastric muscle and periosteum left on the inferior border of the mandible in the symphysis region to aid in the primary closure of the donor site defect. Notes: notice the thin cuff of anterior digastric muscle and periosteum left on the inferior border of the mandible in the symphysis region to aid in primary closure of the donor site defect

- The flap can be tunneled lateral or medial to the mandible for intraoral reconstruction, depending on the defect being reconstructed. If the defect is along the floor of the mouth, the flap should be tunneled medially, and a large cuff of mylohyoid muscle can be harvested with the flap to obturate the defect and minimize the risk of orocutaneous fistulae. However, for buccal mucosal or retromolar defects, tunneling lateral to the mandible in a subperiosteal plane is preferable as this minimizes the risk of leaking into the neck post-operatively. Tunneling under the periosteum, lateral to the mandible, may increase the risk of compressing the pedicle; thus, the tunnel must be large enough for a passive inset.
- The authors prefer to inset the flap before closing the neck, so there is adequate time to observe it for congestion in its final position while closing. Adjustments to the geometry of the skin paddle or pedicle geometry rarely need to be made after inset, but when they do, it's best to identify them in the operating room (Picture 29.3).

Postoperative Consideration

- The protocol at the authors' institution is to initiate a clear liquid diet on postoperative day 3, with some patients with small and more laterally oriented defects initiating a diet on postoperative day 1 (Picture 29.4).

Picture 29.4 The pedicle is dissected only as much as needed to achieve passive inset to the defect being reconstructed. Notes: the pedicle is dissected only as much as needed to achieve passive inset to the defect being reconstructed

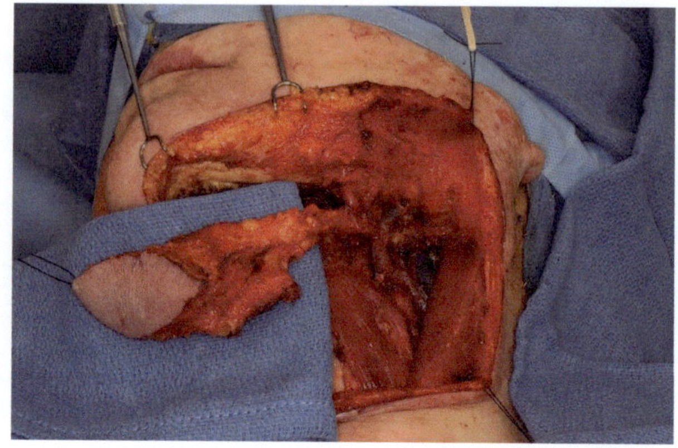

Pearls

- Consider submental artery island perforator flap (SIAPF) in treating elderly patients with multiple co-morbidities who may not be good candidates for free tissue transfer.
- A 6- to 8-cm anteroposterior defect can be closed primarily with minimal tension.
- During closure, consider developing an inferiorly based platysmal myocutaneous advancement flap secured to the periosteum of the inferior border of the mandible to avoid dehiscence during neck extension.

Pitfalls

- Consider leaving a cuff of periosteum on the inferior border of the mandible to aid in the primary closure of the donor site.
- Avoid extensive manipulation of the delicate vessels that supply and drain the submental flap.
- Consider flap inset before closing the neck; this will provide you with adequate time to monitor flap congestion in its final position while closing.
- There is no consensus on early oral intake following SIAPF for oromandibular reconstruction (Picture 29.5).

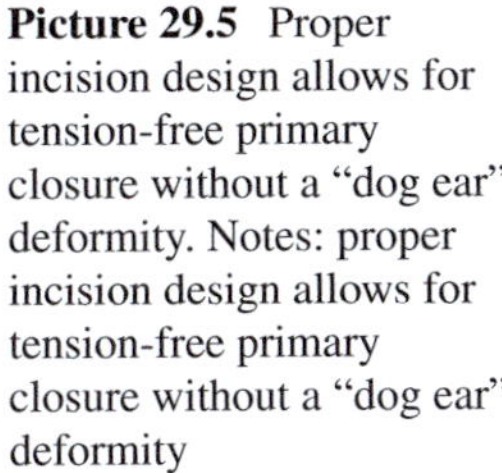

Picture 29.5 Proper incision design allows for tension-free primary closure without a "dog ear" deformity. Notes: proper incision design allows for tension-free primary closure without a "dog ear" deformity

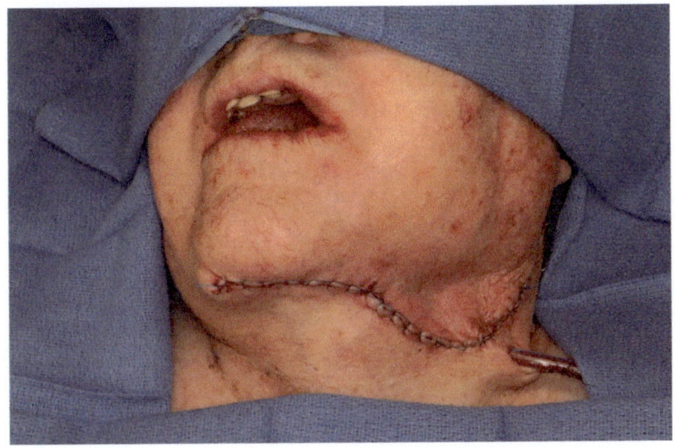

Further Reading

Cheng A, Bui T. Submental island flap. Oral and maxillofacial surgery clinics of North America. 2014;26(3):371–9.

Faltaous AA, Yetman RJ. The submental artery flap: an anatomic study. Plast Reconstr Surg. 1996;97:56–60.

Ishihara T, Igata T, Masuguchi S, Matsushita S, Sakai K, Ihn H. Submental perforator flap: location and number of submental perforating vessels. Scandinavian journal of plastic and reconstructive surgery and hand surgery. 2008;42(3):127–31.

Magden O, Edizer M, Tayfur V, et al. Anatomic study of the vasculature of the submental artery flap. Plast Reconstr Surg. 2004.

Patel UA, Bayles SW, Hayden RE. The submental flap: a modified technique for resident training. Laryngoscope. 2007;117:186–9.

Tang M, Ding M, Almutairi K, Morris SF. Three-dimensional angiography of the submental artery perforator flap. Journal of plastic, reconstructive & aesthetic surgery: JPRAS. 2011;64(5):608–13.

Chapter 30
Pearls and Pitfalls of Supraclavicular Flap

Srinivasa Rama Chandra

Abstract Supraclavicular flap or supraclavicular island flap is based on the skin and fascia of the supraclavicular area, which is of an axial pattern recently popularized for head and neck reconstruction and server comment scar contractures.

The supraclavicular flap is a fascio-cutaneous locoregional flap on the supraclavicular artery. The flap may be rotated around the base of its pedicle to reconstruct a diverse range of mucosal and cutaneous defects of the deep neck spaces, larynx, trachea, mid and lateral face, oral cavity, and oropharynx. The purpose of this chapter is to review the anatomy of the flap and explain the pearls and pitfalls while harvesting the supraclavicular flap for head and neck reconstruction.

Anatomical Landmarks

The supraclavicular artery is found in the triangle formed by the posterior border of the sternomastoid muscle of the ipsilateral side, the inferior border is formed by the clavicle, and the External jugular vein is the lateral border. The trapezius muscle forms the posterior border of the triangle (Fig. 30.1).

S. R. Chandra (✉)
Oregon Health and Science University, Portland, OR, USA
e-mail: chandrsr@ohsu.edu

D. Amin, H. Marwan (eds.), *Pearls and Pitfalls in Oral and Maxillofacial Surgery*, https://doi.org/10.1007/978-3-031-47307-4_30

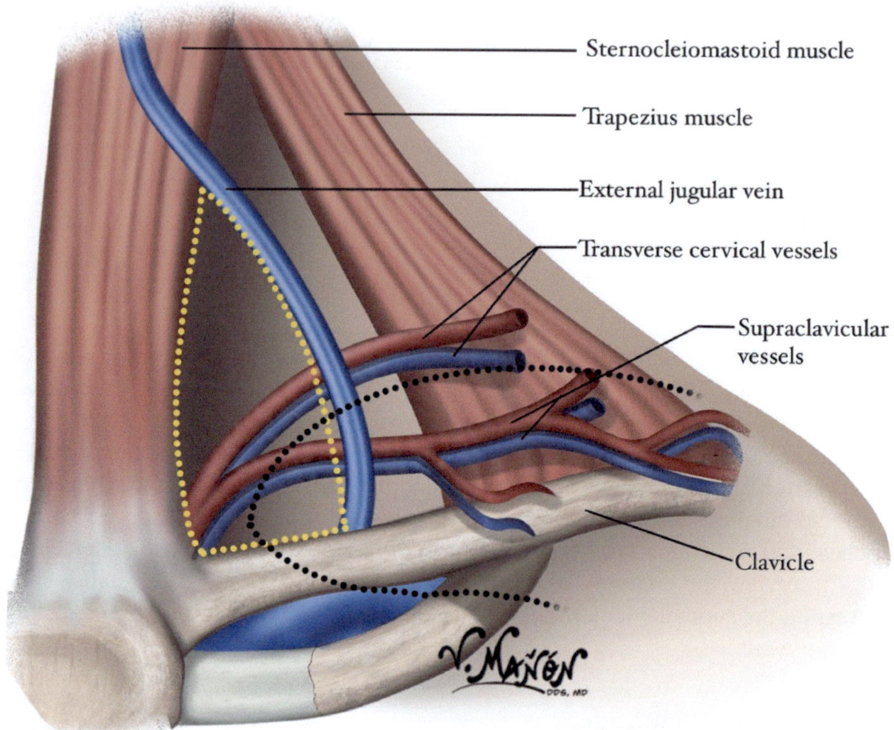

Fig. 30.1 Vascular anatomy, innervation, and the localization of the pedicle for the Supraclavicular flap

Localization of Pedicle

The common location of the supraclavicular artery is approximately 8 cm lateral to the sternoclavicular joint, 2 cm posterior to the edge of the sternomastoid muscle, and 3 cm superior to the upper border of the clavicle.

The dominant pedicle is the supraclavicular artery, and venous drainage is a paired venae comitantes that joins the cervical vein or the external jugular vein. The vein diameter is at least 2.5 mm. Supraclavicular nerves C3 and C4 supply the sensory area on the supraclavicular fossa in the middle and the sternoclavicular joint area medially and the acro-clavicular area laterally.

In most cases, the supraclavicular artery is a distinct branch of the transverse cervical artery and occasionally a branch of the suprascapular artery in the neck.

Technique of Harvesting

Elliptical to a rectangular design flap after isolation of the pedicle in the triangle using a pencil Doppler is ideal. The harvest begins distal 2 medium with a super muscular and subfascial dissection using monopolar electrocautery or knife. Anteroposterior or base of the neck identification of the pedicle is not necessary. Transillumination can be done by elevating the flap to the mid-dimension or Doppler confirmation about 2 cm above the clavicle superior border and 8 cm lateral to the sternoclavicular joint intraoperatively. The pedicle is thin, small, and tortuous. The C4 and C5 infraclavicular nerves are usually encountered, which can be divided with no significant concern. Defatting can be carefully completed if the donor site is significantly thick with much fibrofatty tissue. Based on the defect, the skin island can be tailored by trimming the distal edge of the flap to bleeding healthy tissue. Intraoperative microscopy-based indocyanine green angiography can be utilized.

Tunneling of the flap should be performed after the full harvest to the base of the neck and the 180-degree arc of rotation is confirmed. Damage to the accessory nerve or the subclavian system is a potential pitfall.

No drain is needed, and the most optimal flap dimensions can be closed primarily (Fig. 30.2).

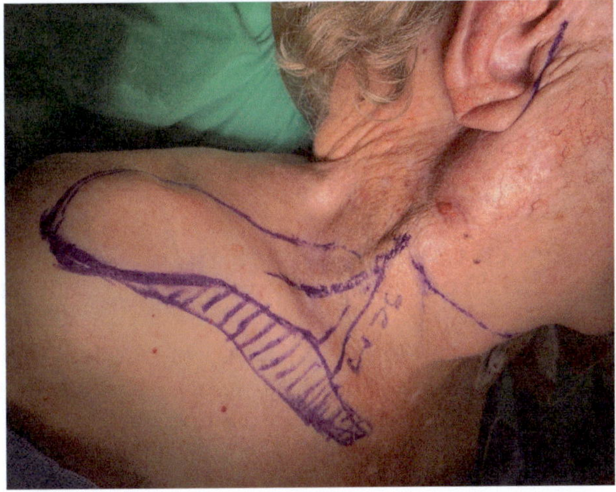

Fig. 30.2 Patient marking, including the clavicle and the location of the thyrocervical trunk

Clinical Applications

The lower third of the face, neck, chest, and lower oral and pharyngeal defects, including the base of the tongue and lateral skull base, are potential reconstructive options for the supraclavicular-based flap.

This elliptical flap with an arc of rotation situated in the ipsilateral base of the neck can reach the surface head and neck defects up to the zygomatic arch on the external surface of the face.

Intraoral mucosal defects- lower aspects like the posterior tongue, the floor of the mouth, and lateral buccal mucosa. Lower pharyngeal and laryngeal defects. Anterior and posterior chest, and lateral skull base, including mastoid, occiput, laryngeal, and tracheal fistula defects, can be reconstructed with a supraclavicular flap. Tissue expansion and dual flap approach can increase reconstructive options. Skin grafting of the donor site with a large flap harvest can be considered if the angiosome perfusion is confirmed.

Practical Tips

1. Rectangular-shaped flap from the base of the ipsilateral neck to the deltoid prominence of the upper arm and shoulder area.
2. The flap can be raised as a fascial or fasciocutaneous flap with de-epithelialization of portions of the flap skin[9,14].
3. The maximum width is approximately 6–7 cm anterior posteriorly and about 25–30 cm from the fulcrum point at the base of the neck.
4. Patient position in the supine placement with a shoulder bump or support for the base of the neck access with the entire neck and arm prepped for access his ideal.
5. Dissection is initiated after a pencil Doppler identification of the pedicle in the triangular fossa location described above in the anatomical landmarks section.
6. Dissection begins distal to proximal, just about the deltoid muscle and a subfascial region off the flap.
7. Doppler, angiogram, interoperative transillumination, and indocyanine green angiography intraoperatively are all easy modalities to confirm pedicle presence based on the complexity of the individual case.

Pearls

1. Perform a 'pinch test' on the supraclavicular area to assess for the width, which is never more than 7–8 cm.
2. Identify the supraclavicular artery with the Doppler probe or occasionally with transillumination (after the elevation of the distal half of the subfascial dissection).

3. Resist the efforts to skeletonize the vascular pedicle. If left around the pedicle, fibrofatty tissue helps prevent kinks in rotation and tunneling.
4. Never tunnel under a band of radiation, burn-induced scar tissue, or skin bridge.
5. Use bipolar cautery while dissecting the acromion and clavicle, preserving the periosteum of the bones to avoid delay and dehiscence of the harvest wound.
6. Monopolar cautery or scalpel is used to harvest the distal edge of the subfascial plane elevation from the underlying deltoid muscle. Perforators from the posterior circumflex humeral artery, when found, are cauterized.
7. Indocyanine green angiography intraoperative can be a good tool in determining the flap viability at its borders prior to inset; this technique reduces flap edge necrosis and reconstruction failures.
8. There are options for other free tissue transfers with better success than supraclavicular free flaps, so they should not be considered for such reconstruction.

Pitfalls

1. Previous modified or any type of radical neck dissection or level 5 neck dissection, where the thyrocervical trunk has been sacrificed or accessed.
2. Prior history of neck radiation, including the base, increases the complexity of flap harvest.
3. Previous history of clavicle and shoulder injuries associated
4. Flap harvest of wider dimension- dorsal to ventral, may lead to difficulty in primary closure. Approximately 6–7 cm or less.
5. Even with undermining and primary closure, the bony prominences of the shoulder may get exposed. See illustration number ##.
6. Harvest past the deltoid muscle (or even mid-deltoid) insertion into the arm compromises flap viability at the distal margin.
7. Donor site closure should be done after adequate undermining to prevent tension and would not break down, especially over the bony prominences. Multi-layered closure is important. Skin grafting in these areas results in a painful experience for most patients.
8. High rate of fistula (20–30%) formation inferential reconstruction in salvage situations with multiple previous failures after radiation, chemotherapy, previous tracheostomies, tumor, infection, and prior flap failures.
9. Tank top and tight shoulder strap dressing is avoided in the initial phase of the healing.
10. Excessive proximal defatting and de-epithelization with dermal plexus damage will compromise the distal skin paddle dermal plexus perfusion (Table 30.1).

Table 30.1 Fine points in supraclavicular flap harvest

Longer than wider flap design
Mucosal and cutaneous defects in the lower oropharyngeal and face-neck-chest
No difference in stay; complications between the free flap and SAI for pharyngeal fistula reconstruction
Review previous levels of neck dissection and radiation
Doppler, ICG angiogram, and intraoperative transillumination
Tension-free closure, in layers
24 × 8 cm maximum dimension for optimal results

Further Reading

Pallua N, Machens HG, Rennekampff O, Becker M, Berger A. The fasciocutaneous supraclavicular artery island flap for releasing postburn mentosternal contractures. Plast Reconstr Surg. 1997;99(7):1878–84; discussion 1885-6. https://doi.org/10.1097/00006534-199706000-00011.

Mutter TD. Cases of deformity from burns, relieved by operation. Am J Med Sci. 1842;4(7):66.

Granzow JW, Suliman A, Roostaeian J, Perry A, Boyd JB. The supraclavicular artery island flap (SCAIF) for head and neck reconstruction: surgical technique and refinements. Otolaryngol Head Neck Surg. 2013;148(6):933–40.

Tayfur V, Magden O, Edizer M, Menderes A. J Craniofac Surg. 2010;21(6):1938–40.

Su T, Pirgousis P, Fernandes R. Versatility of supraclavicular artery island flap in head and neck reconstruction of vessel-depleted and difficult necks. J Oral Maxillofac Surg. 2013;71(3):622–7.

Chapter 31
Principles of Microvascular Surgery

Victoria A. Mañón, Hisham Marwan, and Dina Amin

Abstract During the last three decades, the development of microvascular surgical techniques has been considered the most significant contribution to reconstructive surgery. The success of microvascular surgery depends on many factors, such as careful selection and preparation of the recipient and donor's vessels, avoiding pedicle tension and kinking, and preventing hematoma around the vascular anastomosis. The purpose of this chapter is to review the essential principles of microvascular surgery.

Practical Tips

Preoperative Consideration

- Avoid designing bulky flaps when reconstructing the anterior oral cavity.

Intraoperative Consideration

- Avoid using monopolar/bipolar coagulation in areas near to the flap vascular pedicle because coagulation causes thermal injury of the vascular pedicle. Instead, use micro-clips with magnification to control the bleeding.

V. A. Mañón
Department of Oral and Maxillofacial Surgery, University of Texas Health at Houston, Houston, TX, USA

H. Marwan
Department of Surgery, The University of Texas Medical Branch, Galveston, TX, USA

D. Amin (✉)
Department of Oral and Maxillofacial Surgery, University of Rochester, Rochester, NY, USA

D. Amin, H. Marwan (eds.), *Pearls and Pitfalls in Oral and Maxillofacial Surgery*, https://doi.org/10.1007/978-3-031-47307-4_31

- Consider harvesting a long vascular pedicle. Ideally, the vascular pedicle should reach the (1) mid-internal jugular vein, (2) superior thyroid artery, (3) facial artery, and/or (4) transverse cervical artery.
- Consider placing the arterial and venous anastomoses at some distance from each other.
- When selecting a donor artery, consider the following: (1) proximity of the donor artery to the defect, (2) adequate access to perform the anastomosis, (3) diameters of the flap and neck arteries, (4) the length of the flap vascular pedicle, and/or (5) presence of atherosclerosis, scarring from previous surgery, and/or irradiation.
- Once the artery is selected, assess the flow by releasing the clamp and using heparinized saline. The most important factor for choosing the recipient's vessel is the amount and the strength of blood flow through the vessel.
- Dividing the posterior belly of the digastric and the stylohyoid muscle may improve access to the stump of the facial artery.
- Do not traumatize the endothelium when dilating the artery.
- Additional trimming is indicated when the endothelium is separated from the mesothelium.
- To decrease ischemia time, divide and ligate the vascular pedicle of the flap after the recipient's vessels in the neck have been prepared.
- Partially secure bone flaps to mandible/maxilla and/or suture skin flaps to mucosa or skin before anastomosis to avoid unintentional traction to the microvascular anastomoses. However, do not entirely suture a skin flap before the flap revascularization to have access to bleeding control once the flap is revascularized.
- Avoid kinking, twisting, or rotating the vascular pedicle. Marking the anterior edge of the pedicle with blue ink or suture will help to avoid twisting the pedicle when it is transferred.
- Be aware that the pedicle elongates after it has been revascularized due to the vessels distending with blood.
- It is easier to suture toward yourself. During microvascular suturing, consider the following:

  - Avoid constricting the lumen or catching the back walls of the vessels with the sutures.
  - Include the endothelial layer with the suture, especially if separated from the mesothelium.
  - Space the sutures to compensate for vessel discrepancy.

- To relieve arterial spasms, apply a Raytec gauze soaked in 10% lidocaine or papaverine for a few minutes.
- Minor bleeding at the anastomosis will settle within a few minutes.
- Significant bleeding should be sutured with a single 8/0 or 9/0 nylon suture at the bleeding point and ligate to seal the bleeding area.

- Always check the following after the anastomosis:
  - Ensure an adequate blood pressure.
  - Observe and feel the pulsation of the arterial anastomosis. Vertical pulsation of the artery indicates good anastomosis.
  - Check for spontaneous bleeding from the flap edges.
  - Prick the skin flap with a needle:

    No bleeding suggests arterial inflow obstruction.
    Dark blood suggests venous outflow obstruction.

  - Intra- and postoperative Doppler of the vascular pedicle.

Postoperative Consideration

- Flap monitoring is critical during the first 48–72 h. Careful examination of the flap skin turgor, color, and Doppler is essential to detect any early changes to the flap.
- Don't delay any exploration, particularly with a congested flap. The best chance to save the flap is to take it back immediately.
- The use of postoperative anticoagulation is controversial. However, most studies have shown that it will increase the risk of postoperative hematoma.

Pearls

- Avoid significant size discrepancies between the donor's and the recipient's veins.
- Avoid tension at the anastomosed pedicle.
- Consider vein graft if severe size discrepancies or tension is anticipated at the anastomosis.
- Meticulous hemostasis of the flap and at the surgical bed (around the anastomosis) is key to avoiding hematoma and subsequent postoperative congestion of the flap.

Pitfalls

- Short pedicle length is anticipated in the following scenarios: (1) contralateral neck is used for the vascular anastomoses, (2) with revision flaps following previous neck dissection and/or irradiation, and/or (3) midface or maxilla reconstruction.

- Atherosclerotic arteries are rigid and cannot be curved toward the donor artery. Consider preparing a longer donor artery to reach across to the flap artery.
- Additional trimming to the artery is indicated when the endothelium is separated from the mesothelium. Alternatively, care to include the endothelial layer during suturing of the artery. So it prevents dissection of the endothelial layer, formation of an endothelial flap, and thrombosis.
- Trim loose adventitial strands around the tip of the vessel to prevent adventitial prolapse into the arterial lumen and thrombosis.
- To mitigate flap failure, consider monitoring and/or correcting the following: (1) reduced cardiac output, (2) hypotension, (3) hypovolemia, (4) hypercoagulability, (5) hypothermia, (6) anemia or polycythemia, (7) external compression on the neck, (8) hematoma, (9) neck position, which may kink the pedicle, and/or (10) wound infection or salivary leak.

Further Reading

Pannucci CJ, Kovach SJ, Cuker A. Microsurgery and the hypercoagulable state: a hematologist's perspective. Plast Reconstr Surg. 2015;136(4):545e.

Spiegel JH, Polat JK. Microvascular flap reconstruction by otolaryngologists: prevalence, postoperative care, and monitoring techniques. Laryngoscope. 2007;117(3):485–90.

Blackwell KE. Unsurpassed reliability of free flaps for head and neck reconstruction. Arch Otolaryngol Head Neck Surg. 1999;125(3):295–9.

Free tissue transfer flaps in head and neck reconstruction. https://vula.uct.ac.za/access/content/group/ba5fb1bd-be95-48e5-81be-586fbaeba29d/Principles%20and%20technique%20of%20microvascular%20anastomosis%20for%20free%20tissue%20transfer%20flaps%20in%20head%20and%20neck%20reconstructive%20surgery.pdf. Accessed 27 Jan 2023.

Reddy TJ, Sham E, Ganesh MS, Menon PS, Gowda KV, Malick R. Feasibility and reliability of microvascular reconstruction in the vessel-depleted previously operated neck. Ann Maxillofac Surg. 2020;10(1):96–101.

Chapter 32
Practical Tips for Harvesting Radial Forearm Free Flap

James C. Melville, Salah Al Din Al Azri, Brian D. Rethman, Jonathan Shum, and Simon Young

Abstract The radial forearm free flap (RFFF) has been used to reconstruct head and neck defects since it was first described by Yang et al. over 30 years ago. Although it is commonly used as a fasciocutaneous flap, it has also been described as an adipofascial and/or osteocutaneous flap by harvesting a portion of the radius. Due to its predictable anatomy, the RFFF is considered a relatively easy flap to harvest, and the location on the extremity allows for the feasibility of a two-team approach. Various surgical sequences have been described; however, the main principles remain the same. The purpose of this chapter is to review pearls and pitfalls for harvesting radial forearm free flap.

J. C. Melville (✉)
Department of Oral and Maxillofacial Surgery, Oral, Head and Neck Oncology and Microvascular Reconstructive Surgery, University of Texas Health Science Center at Houston, Houston, TX, USA

UTHealth|The University of Texas Health Science Center at Houston Houston's Health University, Houston, TX, USA
e-mail: james.c.melville@uth.tmc.edu

S. A. D. Al Azri
Katz Department of Oral and Maxillofacial Surgery, School of Dentistry, The University of Texas Health Science Center at Houston, Houston, TX, USA

B. D. Rethman
Katz Department of Oral and Maxillofacial Surgery, The University of Texas Health Science Center at Houston Houston's Health University, Houston, TX, USA

Oral and Maxillofacial Surgery, Bayne-Jones Army Community Hospital, Fort Johnson South, LA, USA

J. Shum · S. Young
UTHealth|The University of Texas Health Science Center at Houston Houston's Health University, Houston, TX, USA

Department of Oral and Maxillofacial Surgery, The University of Texas Health Science Center at Houston, Houston, TX, USA

D. Amin, H. Marwan (eds.), *Pearls and Pitfalls in Oral and Maxillofacial Surgery*, https://doi.org/10.1007/978-3-031-47307-4_32

223

Practical Tips

Preoperative Consideration

- A thorough history and physical examination are essential. Significant concerns would include any previous history of trauma or surgery to the donor extremity under consideration for harvest. A previous history of deep venous thromboembolism or any obvious deformities should also be noted.
- The use of the dominant versus nondominant hand should be kept in mind when selecting the side to be harvested.
- A modified Allen's test (MAT) can be used to determine the adequacy of collateral circulation. The use of pulse oximetry to complement MAT has also been described.
- No specific imaging is routinely required preoperatively.

Intraoperative Consideration

- Positioning of the donor's arm on an operating arm board abducting the shoulder at 45–90° to the patient.
- Identification of important landmarks, including the distal radial artery and its proximal course, scaphoid tubercle, and the center of the antecubital fossa. The line drawn from the center of the antecubital fossa to the scaphoid tubercle corresponds to the surface anatomy of the radial artery and the anterolateral intermuscular septum.
- The size and shape of the skin harvest are marked. The flap design is centered on the radial artery unless the cephalic vein is to be used for venous drainage, in which case the flap is centered on both the radial artery and cephalic vein.
- The use of a tourniquet is operator dependent.
- Collateral circulation can be confirmed intraoperatively prior to ligating the radial artery and flap harvest by clamping the radial artery and releasing the tourniquet. This is especially useful in cases when the MAT is equivocal.
- The use of the superficial venous system with or without the deep venous system for venous drainage has been controversial. However, it is recommended to harvest the cephalic vein whenever possible.
- The RFFF can be safely harvested using either suprafacial or subfascial dissection, with the former leaving more tissue on top of tendons with less associated postoperative tendon exposure.
- The palmaris longus is included in the flap if a tendon graft is needed.
- If the bone is needed, a portion of the distal radius can be harvested. However, there is a risk of bone fracture, and one should consider immobilization postoperatively with or without prophylactic plating.

Postoperative Consideration

- Closure techniques contribute to both functional and aesthetic outcomes of the donor site. Different donor site defect coverage techniques have been described, including split or full-thickness skin grafting, local flaps, tissue expanders, and dermal substitutes.
- Postoperative immobilization is crucial for the success of the skin graft. That is usually achieved using either a prefabricated volar splint or a custom-made ortho-glass splint.
- Using a static pressure wound dressing (SPD) and negative pressure wound dressing (NPD) over the skin graft is controversial; however, the use of NPD has been found to improve hand and wrist function in the immediate postoperative period.
- Continuous physical therapy is an important part of postoperative care to maintain strength and wrist range of motion.

Pearls

- Consider harvesting the flap from the nondominant hand.
- Modified Allen's test can be used to determine the adequacy of collateral circulation.
- Can be harvested with extended subcutaneous tissue for bulk and/or with 7–9 cm of the radius bone.

Pitfalls

- Donor site complications include skin graft loss (partial or complete) with or without tendon exposure, poor appearance, neurosensory alterations, and reduced grip strength. Recipient site complications include flap loss (partial or complete), fistula formation, wound dehiscence, or hematoma.
- Neurosensory complications include persistent hypoesthesia, hyperesthesia, allodynia, and neuroma formation. Nerves at higher risk of injury include the lateral antebrachial cutaneous nerve, the radial sensory nerve, the medial antebrachial cutaneous nerve, and the palmar cutaneous branch of the median nerve. Transected sensory nerves should be ligated and/or implanted in adjacent muscles to prevent neuroma formation. If a neuroma is formed postoperatively, surgical excision is required, especially if symptomatic.
- Postoperative tendon exposure can be minimized with suprafascial dissection, appropriate defect grafting, and wound care.
- Evaluation of collateral circulation preoperatively is essential to avoid permanent vascular compromise.

Further Reading

Yang GF, Chen PJ, Gao YZ, Liu XY, Li J, Jiang SX, He SP. Forearm free skin flap transplantation: a report of 56 cases. Br J Plast Surg. 1997;50(3):162–5. https://doi.org/10.1016/s0007-1226(97)91363-1. PMID: 9176001.

Jeremić JV, Nikolić ŽS. Versatility of radial forearm free flap for intraoral reconstruction. Srp Arh Celok Lek. 2015;143(5-6):256–60. https://doi.org/10.2298/sarh1506256j. PMID: 26259395.

Urken ML, Cheney ML, Blackwell KE, Harris JR, Hadlock TA, Futran N. Atlas of regional and free flaps for head and neck reconstruction: flap harvest and insetting. Philadelphia: Lippincott Williams & Wilkins; 2012.

Strauch B, Yu HL. Atlas of microvascular surgery: anatomy and operative techniques. New York: Georg Thieme Verlag; 2006.

Al-Azri SA, Galbraith BS, Melville JC. The use of pulse oximetry in conjunction with the modified Allen's test prior to the radial forearm free flap. Adv Oral Maxillofac Surg. 2021;2:100077.

Patel R. Reducing morbidity in radial forearm free flap donor site: a review of closure techniques. Curr Opin Otolaryngol Head Neck Surg. 2022;30(5):363–7. https://doi.org/10.1097/MOO.0000000000000834.

Melville JC, Bennetts NA, Tijerina L, Shum JW. The use of acellular urinary bladder matrix as coverage for fasciocutaneous free flap donor sites: an alternative to traditional grafting procedures. J Oral Maxillofac Surg. 2017;75(10):2254–60. https://doi.org/10.1016/j.joms.2017.03.011. Epub 2017 Mar 18. PMID: 28399392.

Clark JM, Rychlik S, Harris J, Seikaly H, Biron VL, O'Connell DA. Donor site morbidity following radial forearm free flap reconstruction with split-thickness skin grafts using negative pressure wound therapy. J Otolaryngol Head Neck Surg. 2019;48(1):21. https://doi.org/10.1186/s40463-019-0344-9. PMID: 31113481; PMCID: PMC6528371.

Chen CM, Lin GT, Fu YC, Shieh TY, Huang IY, Shen YS, Chen CH. Complications of free radial forearm flap transfers for head and neck reconstruction. Oral Surg Oral Med Oral Pathol Oral Radiol Endod. 2005;99(6):671–6. https://doi.org/10.1016/j.tripleo.2004.10.010. PMID: 15897852.

Chapter 33
Practical Tips for Harvesting Microvascular Fibula Flap

Brent B. Ward and Paul L. Shivers

Abstract First described by Hidalgo in 1989 for use in the head and neck, the fibula osteomyocutaneous free flap hsa become a workhorse reconstructive option for composite maxillofacial defects. Following improvements in the understanding of pertinent surgical anatomy, surgeons can expect predictable outcomes with multiple bony segments and the use of a corresponding skin paddle. The distant nature of the fibula facilitates a two-team approach, which yields a shorter operating time for both the patient and surgical team. Donor site morbidity is generally mild and does not preclude patients from resuming an active lifestyle following recovery. Recent advances in computer-assisted surgical planning have paved the way for guided "jaw-in-a-day" modalities, which provide the most complete immediate restoration of function. The purpose of this chapter is to review pearls and pitfalls for harvesting microvascular fibula flap.

Practical Tips

Preoperative Consideration

- Preoperative planning generally involves the acquisition of a computed tomography angiogram (CTA) of the aorta with a three-vessel runoff to assess for vascular abnormalities (such as peronea magna, stenoses, or atherosclerosis) and

B. B. Ward (✉)
Chalmers J. Lyons Professor of Oral and Maxillofacial Surgery, University of Michigan, Ann Arbor, MI, USA
e-mail: bward@med.umich.edu

P. L. Shivers
Oral and Maxillofacial Surgery/Hospital Dentistry, University of Michigan, Ann Arbor, MI, USA

D. Amin, H. Marwan (eds.), *Pearls and Pitfalls in Oral and Maxillofacial Surgery*, https://doi.org/10.1007/978-3-031-47307-4_33

prevent ischemic damage to the foot following harvest. Advances in perforator identification allow skin paddle positioning integration into computer-assisted surgical planning. Perforators can also be detected with Doppler ultrasound. Patients should be questioned regarding a history of trauma, surgery, and clotting disorders such as deep venous thrombosis (DVT) in the lower extremities.

- Fibula osteomyocutaneous flaps offer 22–26 cm of bone, an up to 25 × 14 cm skin paddle, and varying degrees of muscle bulk. The flap can typically accommodate all mandibular bone defects and moderate through-and-through soft tissue defects. Additionally, a partial thickness segment of the peroneus longus tendon can be harvested for lip suspension.
- The flap vasculature is based on the peroneal artery (2–3 mm) and venae comitantes (2–4 mm), often an excellent match for recipient vessels in the neck. The minimum pedicle length is 5–6 cm, which can be extended if a distal bone segment is selected for harvest.
- Positioning is accomplished by placing an ipsilateral hip roll, knee in a flexed position, and heel on a bump. Utilization of a Zimmer "WalterLorenz" arm can facilitate retraction for one to two operators.
- Anastomosis geometry generally favors a posterior pedicle course into the neck for easy access to the facial vessels. For oral cavity defects, the contralateral leg will most easily place the skin paddle intraorally with a posteriorly positioned pedicle. Ipsilateral leg use will accommodate extraoral defects or allow for an anterior course of the pedicle for oral defects. There is typically sufficient flexibility of the skin paddle septum to accommodate situations where the ideal leg is not an option. Optimally, the pedicle will course anteriorly for condylar reconstruction as a hairpin turn at this level can result in the vessels' kink. Alternatively, a devascularized fibula segment is expected, which in some cases may be acceptable. All else being equal, the authors favor using the left leg by convention to limit restrictions in motor vehicle operation postoperatively.

Intraoperative Consideration

- A tourniquet can be set to 325 mg Hg with an Esmarch wrap to exsanguinate the leg. Tourniquet times are controversial, but the authors are typically limited to 70 min or less for harvest. Surgeons should allow time off the tourniquet before ligating the pedicle for transfer to the head and neck. Fifteen minutes is generally adequate.
- Incision design is made by drawing a line from the fibular head to the lateral malleolus. To avoid damage to skin perforators, care must be taken to stay anterior to the posterior intermuscular septum. Of proximal and distal fibula, 6–8 cm should be preserved for knee and ankle joint stability. Preservation of additional length is unnecessary as this is not a load-bearing bone. Skin incisions can extend slightly more proximal and distal for access, but extending too far proximally can compromise the common or deep peroneal nerves.

- Most oral cavity defects require a skin paddle width of 5 cm or less. If a larger paddle is anticipated, the initial incision may be designed anteriorly to prevent challenges in harvesting a skin paddle from the posterior leg.
- Initial dissection is carried sharply into the lateral compartment to expose the peroneus longus muscle. First, identifying this muscle superiorly can limit the risk to perforators in the distal aspect of the leg, which tends to provide the most predictable perforator options.
- At this time, the posterior intermuscular septum can be exposed bluntly, and perforators are selected. Choosing a perforator that will allow for appropriate skin paddle positioning, particularly for hemi-mandibular reconstructions with large ramus segments, is critical. Septocutaneous and septomuscular perforators are typically available in the distal aspect of the leg, while musculocutaneous perforators are more frequently encountered proximally. Additionally, there are instances of skin perforators branching from the posterior tibial vasculature. Utilizing a distal septocutaneous or septomuscular perforator is favored for increased pedicle length and greater reliability of the skin paddle.
- Once the perforator(s) are identified, electrocautery is used to elevate the lateral compartment muscles from the fibula while maintaining a 3 mm cuff of attached muscle to protect the underlying periosteal vasculature. Excessive muscle thickness can complicate surgical guide fit if one is used for contouring.
- The superficial peroneal nerve is often exposed during this portion of the procedure and should be retracted superomedially to avoid injury. The nerve and its distal branches have a variable course that can traverse either or both of the anterior and lateral compartments and can closely approximate the fibula near the distal osteotomy site.
- Dissection of the lateral compartment musculature continues until the anterior septum is reached. It is helpful to isolate this septum for the entire harvest length before sharply incising into the anterior compartment to avoid inadvertent injury to the anterior tibial pedicle and deep peroneal nerve.
- The extensor muscles can then be swept medially with a broad periosteal elevator, exposing the interosseous septum. A full-guard retractor or other broad retractors are used to protect the pedicle medially during osteotomies. Creating space medially with the retractors is necessary to accommodate a reciprocating saw for the cut.
- With proximal and distal osteotomies complete, Dingman clamps apply lateral pressure to the fibula, and an incision is made through the interosseous septum with #15 blade. Once the interosseous septum is completely released, an additional 2–3 cm exposure will be appreciated.
- The peroneal vascular pedicle is now identified in the distal aspect of the dissection. The distal pedicle is clamped and ligated with 2-0 silk sutures. Additional application of surgical clips on the distal stump may avoid recalcitrant bleeding from the pedicle, particularly if it retracts medially to the distal fibular stump.
- Incision through the posterior tibialis muscle then ensues. This muscle has a varying thickness, and finger dissection can be used to appreciate the plane between the posterior tibialis and underlying fascia to accelerate this portion of

the operation. At the superior aspect of this step, a large branch can often be found coursing laterally from the main pedicle. Clear identification of the main trunk of the peroneal vessels before ligating this branch can avoid inadvertent transection of the pedicle.

- The fascia underlying the posterior tibialis can be disrupted bluntly and then sharply incised with scissors to limit risk to the pedicle. Before completing the medial aspect of the dissection, the surgeon should be able to identify the posterior tibial nerve medially and the takeoff of peroneal vessels from the tibioperoneal trunk.
- Attention is then turned to the lateral aspect of the dissection, where the posterior septum and soleus muscle are sharply released from the superior aspect of the fibula. It is critical to release this muscle without dissecting medially into the soleus muscle, which can lead to catastrophic injury of the vascular pedicle on the medial aspect of the fibula. The soleus attachment varies, but the release should continue inferiorly until the flexor hallucis longus muscle can be identified. At this time, blunt dissection with a finger can be used to create a plane between the two muscles in preparation for the elevation of the skin paddle.
- Following the release of the posterior septum to the level of planned skin paddle harvest, an incision is made through the septum extending superficially toward the skin. The A-P limbs of the skin paddle are generally made first, which confirms the capture of the septum and perforators in the skin paddle. The skin incisions are completed, and sharp dissection is carried to the underlying soleus muscle. The shape of the skin paddle is designed according to the defect to be closed. Care should be taken to avoid injury to the sural nerve and saphenous vein in the posterior compartment.
- When released appropriately from the underlying fascia, the surgeon should be able to flip the skin paddle anteriorly to view the posterior aspect of the septum and the soleus muscle unless a musculocutaneous perforator is required. With a finger placed deep in the plane between the soleus and flexor hallucis longus, a 0.5–1 cm cuff of the soleus muscle is maintained during the release of the septum to avoid perforator injury.
- The flap is now attached strictly to the flexor hallucis longus muscle and vascular pedicle. To further release the fibula, the fascia overlying the posterior aspect of the flexor hallucis longus (FHL) is incised. With a finger beneath the posterior aspect of the fibula to protect the course of skin perforators, the FHL is transected medially. At least 0.5–1 cm of muscle cuff should be preserved.
- Contouring of the fibula begins with either careful dissection of the vascular pedicle from the proximal aspect of the fibula graft extending to the level of planned osteotomy or subperiosteal dissection of all soft tissue from the proximal fibula. Dissection of the pedicle requires additional time but does limit soft tissue bulk surrounding the vasculature during inset and anastomosis. Once the most proximal osteotomy is made, excess bone can be preserved if bone particulate is needed for gaps between fibular segments.
- A surgical guide can be applied for complex reconstructions, and all additional contouring can be completed in the leg before ischemia if desired. Estimating the

defect with transfer and revision at the recipient site is an alternative, especially for single-piece reconstructions. The pedicle and perforators should be carefully protected prior to contouring osteotomies, either with a malleable retractor or the #9 periosteal elevator. Individual segment length is generally no less than 2 cm to limit the risk of devascularization. Smaller segments can be viable, though, as free grafts.

- If dental implants are to be placed during the flap harvest, computer-assisted planning and guides may help identify a meaningful position for final prosthodontic restoration. Care should be taken to avoid both pedicles and perforators during planning. The drilling sequence often requires a dense bone protocol to accommodate the fibular cortices. Implants are slightly countersunk, and healing abutments instead of cover screws are used to ease future exposure. Bone stock is more predictably sufficient for implants in the distal third of the fibula and male patients, with evidence that a 1 cm minimum thickness optimizes implant success.

- Gentle separation of the peroneal artery and venae comitantes at the release level can be done in the leg to facilitate microsurgical dissection in the neck. 2-0 silk ties and surgical clips control the peroneal pedicle stump following transfer to the head and neck.

- In the leg, the FHL is suspended to the residual interosseous membrane with care to avoid excess tension. The great toe should be positioned passively. A10 flat Jackson-Pratt suction drain or equivalent is placed in the wound bed, and closure is accomplished with 3-0 deep resorbable and 4-0 skin sutures. A split-thickness skin graft is necessary for coverage except in narrow skin paddles for which tension-free closure can be achieved. A compression dressing or a wound vac may be applied for the first 5 days following surgery before switching to daily Xeroform dressing changes. A novel technique to circumvent grafting involves the elevation of a propeller flap from a proximal musculocutaneous perforator to achieve primary closure for distal wounds.

- Reconstruction plates with two mono-cortical screws per fibular segment are used for mandibular reconstruction. Mini-plates or thinner patient-specific reconstruction plates are typically sufficient to suspend the fibula for maxillary reconstruction. An alternative technique utilizes a single long screw through the pterygoid plate as a dowel rod to position the graft for posterior maxillary alveolar reconstruction.

- If immediate prosthodontic reconstruction is planned, the inset should allow for abutment emergence along a suture line between the skin paddle and native mucosa. Designing the skin paddle position buccally can also create a neo-vestibule.

Postoperative Consideration

- Careful monitoring of distal pulses and signs of compartment syndrome is critical in the immediate postoperative period, particularly for patients with primary wound closure.
- The authors favor early ambulation with an Aircast boot as early as postoperative day 1. Patients may continue boot use for comfort following discharge, though this seldom exceeds 1 month after surgery.
- Common complications include partial or total skin graft loss, neurosensory deficits, claw toe or limited dorsiflexion of the great toe, and gait abnormality/ankle instability.

Pearls

- Two-team approach can be utilized.
- Fibula osteomyocutaneous flaps offer 22–26 cm of bone, an up to 25 × 14 cm skin paddle, and varying degrees of muscle bulk.
- During dissection, flex the leg to relax the muscles of the posterior compartment of the leg.
- A partial thickness segment of the peroneus longus tendon can be harvested for lip suspension.

Pitfalls

- Ipsilateral leg use will accommodate extraoral defects or allow for an anterior course of the pedicle for oral defects.
- Avoid extensive periosteal dissection when multiple osteotomies are necessary.
- Surgeons should allow time off the tourniquet before ligating the pedicle for transfer to the head and neck. Fifteen minutes is generally adequate.

Further Reading

Hidalgo DA. Fibula free flap: a new method of mandible reconstruction. Plast Reconstr Surg. 1989;84(1):71–9.

Kim DUCKSOO, Orron DE, Skillman JJ. Surgical significance of popliteal arterial variants. A unified angiographic classification. Ann Surg. 1989;210(6):776.

Ettinger KS, et al. Accuracy and precision of the computed tomographic angiography perforator localization technique for virtual surgical planning of composite osteocutaneous fibula free flaps in head and neck reconstruction. J Oral Maxillofac Surg. 2022;80(8):1434–44.

Wei F-C, et al. Fibula osteoseptocutaneous flap for reconstruction of composite mandibular defects. Plast Reconstr Surg. 1994;93(2):294–304.

Wheeless CR. Wheeless textbook of orthopedics. Extremity tourniquets. http://www.wheelesson-line.com/ortho/extremity_tourniquets.

Jones NF, Monstrey S, Gambier BA. Reliability of the fibular osteocutaneous flap for mandibular reconstruction: anatomical and surgical confirmation. Plast Reconstr Surg. 1996;97(4):707–16.

Wei F-C, et al. Fibular osteoseptocutaneous flap: anatomic study and clinical application. Plast Reconstr Surg. 1986;78(2):191–200.

Schusterman MA, et al. The osteocutaneous free fibula flap: is the skin paddle reliable? Plast Reconstr Surg. 1992;90(5):787–93.

Urken ML, et al. Oromandibular reconstruction using microvascular composite flaps: report of 210 cases. Arch Otolaryngol Head Neck Surg. 1998;124(1):46–55.

Barrett SL, et al. Superficial peroneal nerve (superficial fibular nerve): the clinical implications of anatomic variability. J Foot Ankle Surg. 2006;45(3):174–6.

Fry AM, Laugharne D, Jones K. Osteotomized the fibular free flap: an anatomical perspective. Br J Oral Maxillofac Surg. 2016;54(6):692–3.

Williams FC, et al. Immediate teeth in fibulas: expanded clinical applications and surgical technique. J Oral Maxillofac Surg. 2021;79(9):1944–53.

Moscoso JF, et al. Vascularized bone flaps in oromandibular reconstruction: a comparative anatomic study of bone stock from various donor sites to assess suitability for endosseous dental implants. Arch Otolaryngol Head Neck Surg. 1994;120(1):36–43.

Shpitzer T, et al. Leg morbidity and function following fibular free flap harvest. Ann Plast Surg. 1997;38(5):460–4.

Kaleem A, et al. Use of soleus musculocutaneous perforator-based propeller flap for lower extremity wound coverage after osteocutaneous fibula free flap harvest. Microsurgery. 2021;41(3):233–9.

Fodor L, et al. Severe compartment syndrome following fibula harvesting for mandible reconstruction. Int J Oral Maxillofac Surg. 2011;40(4):443–5.

Ling XF, Peng X. What is the price to pay for a free fibula flap? A systematic review of donor-site morbidity following free fibula flap surgery. Plast Reconstr Surg. 2012;129(3):657–74.

Momoh AO, et al. A prospective cohort study of fibula free flap donor-site morbidity in 157 consecutive patients. Plast Reconstr Surg. 2011;128(3):714–20.

Shindo M, et al. The fibula osteocutaneous flap in head and neck reconstruction: a critical evaluation of donor site morbidity. Arch Otolaryngol Head Neck Surg. 2000;126(12):1467–72.

Chapter 34
Pearls and Pitfalls in Anterolateral Free Flap Harvest

Neel Patel, Hisham Hatoum, Arshad Kaleem, and Ramzey Tursun

Abstract The anterolateral thigh (ALT) flap is a robust soft tissue flap first described in 1984 by Song and colleagues. The ALT flap has expanded use and has become one of the most used flaps in reconstructive surgery. This chapter aims to discuss the pearls and pitfalls of harvesting ALT flaps for head and neck reconstruction.

Pearls in Flap Harvesting

Optimize the position of the leg. This is especially important in patients with loose skin in order not to alter the orientation and direction of the perforators and the location of the intermuscular septum in relation to the skin perforators. Avoid internal or external rotation and keep the leg neutral before marking.

Skin dimensions depend on skin tone, quality, and patient body habitus. Flap length ranges from 4 cm to 35 cm and width from 4 cm to 25 cm. The ALT flap is based on the descending branch of the lateral circumflex femoral artery (LCFA) and venae comitantes.

N. Patel
HCA Florida Head and Neck Oncology and Reconstructive Surgery, Nova Southeastern University College of Medicine, Miami, FL, USA

H. Hatoum
Oral and Maxillofacial Surgery, Head and Neck Oncology and Microvascular Reconstructive Surgery, School of Dentistry, Louisiana State University, New Orleans, LA, USA

A. Kaleem
High Desert Oral and Facial Surgery, El Paso, TX, USA

R. Tursun (✉)
Security Forces Hospital, Riyad, Saudi Arabia

Due to variable anatomy, take note that 43% of the time, the dominant perforator comes from the descending branch of the lateral circumflex femoral artery. However, it can also come off the ascending, transverse, or oblique branches of the lateral circumflex femoral artery or rarely directly off the main trunk of the lateral circumflex femoral artery or from the profunda femoris itself.

We start with flap marking. A line is marked connecting the ASIS to the lateral patella (Fig. 34.1). We mark the midpoint of this line. A circle is drawn with a radius of 3 cm around the midpoint. This delineates the predominant location of the skin perforators. A Doppler probe is used to mark the skin perforators within the circle and can be done or verified with ultrasound or CTA alternatively.

Palpate the intermuscular septum between the rectus femoris and vastus lateralis muscles with your fingertips in a mediolateral direction. A more precise way to locate the perforators is by lifting the leg straight up (Fig. 34.2). Additional perforators can be found with the Doppler probe over or slightly posterior to this septum. Mark these skin perforators as well. Once this is done, confirm that the leg is still positioned in a neutral position.

Flap dimensions are marked based on the recipient defect. Initially, including more than one perforator in the flap design is important. However, as we proceed with the surgery, we can choose to keep one or more perforators based on the design and size of the recipient soft tissue defect or the need for separate skin paddles, such as in chimeric flaps. Also, the surgeon can include the TFL perforator and muscle with the design of the flap (Fig. 34.3).

On the other hand, the surgeon may choose the largest perforator with the shortest intramuscular path requiring less dissection or may choose to include a cuff of the vastus lateralis muscle, especially if we need more bulk at the recipient side. We design the flap longitudinally to allow for primary closure of the donor site. A pinch test is done before the flap to help estimate how much skin can be taken to allow primary closure at the end. Remember, flap design may change intraoperatively based on the location of the skin perforators.

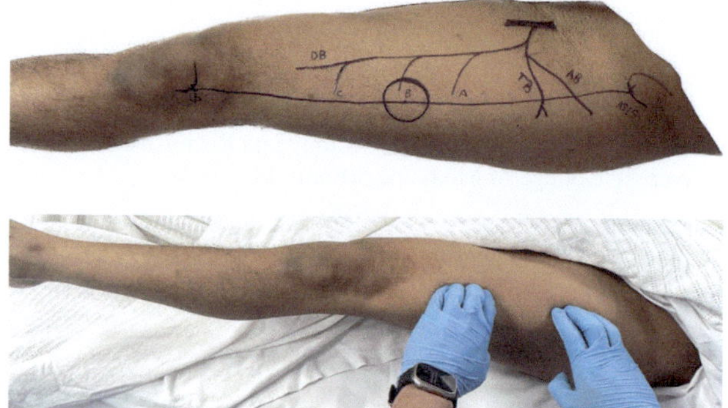

Fig. 34.1 Anatomical landmarks for ALT flap

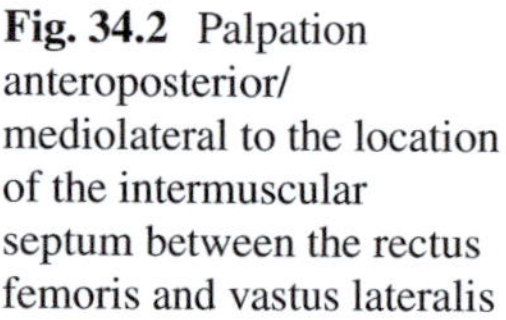

Fig. 34.2 Palpation anteroposterior/mediolateral to the location of the intermuscular septum between the rectus femoris and vastus lateralis

Fig. 34.3 DB to ALT and TFL perforators were dissected to supercharge the perfusion of a large flap

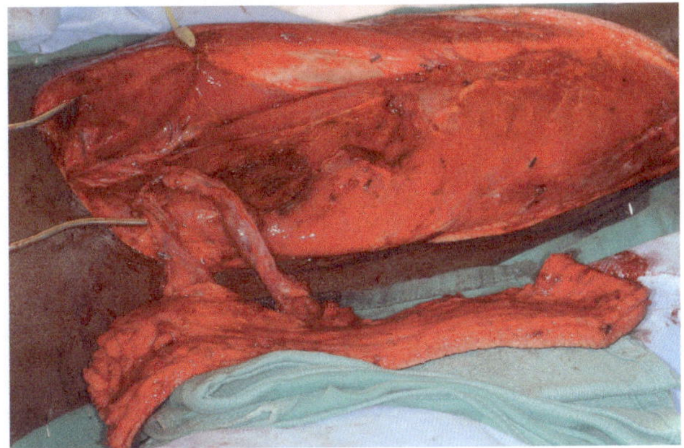

Fig. 34.4 Medial incision and sub-facial dissection to identify the rectus femoris and the intermuscular septum

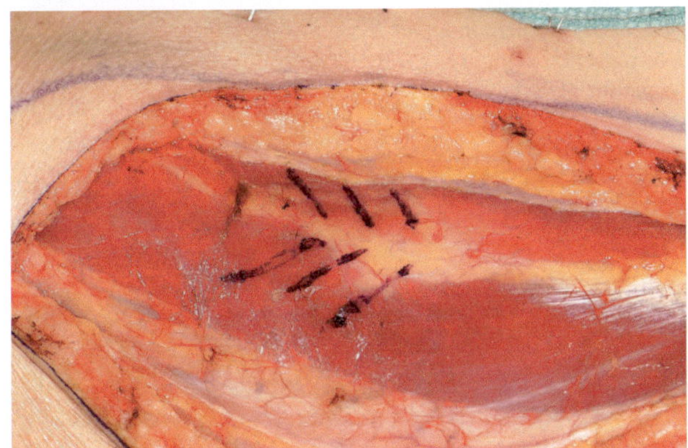

Anterior Incision

Bovie electrocautery or sharp scalpels can be used to incise through the skin and subcutaneous tissue of the medial skin marking. The author's preference is to start with the distal one-half of the medial skin incision to identify the septum first and to confirm that the septum is medial to the skin perforators. If we note that the incision is too lateral, we can adjust it at this time. Extend the medial skin cut a few centimeters proximally to have better exposure of the pedicle in cases where a small skin paddle is needed. Continue incising down to the Scarpa's fascia in the middle by pushing with two fingers, one lateral and one medial to the cut. Dissect through the subcutaneous tissue, Scarpa's fascia, and the muscular fascia along the whole length of the incision. This will expose the septum between the rectus femoris and VL muscle (Fig. 34.4).

Continue with lateral subfascial dissection to expose laterally until we visualize the perforators (Fig. 34.5). At this time, if the size of the skin paddle of the recipient site is confirmed and the chance of modifying it after the ablative part is low, then the posterior or lateral incision is carried out, and a subfascial dissection toward the

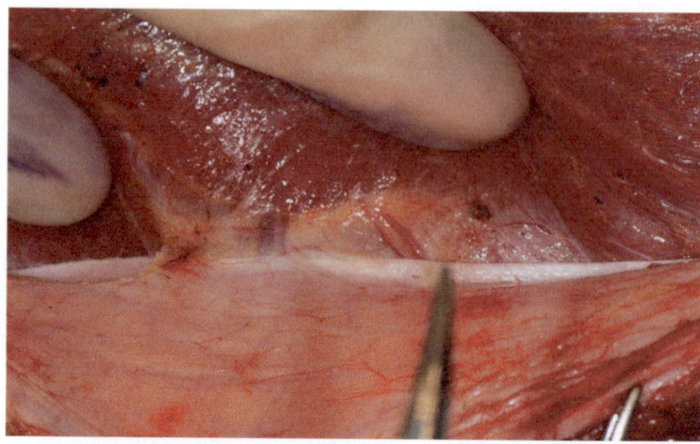

Fig. 34.5 Identification of the skin perforators

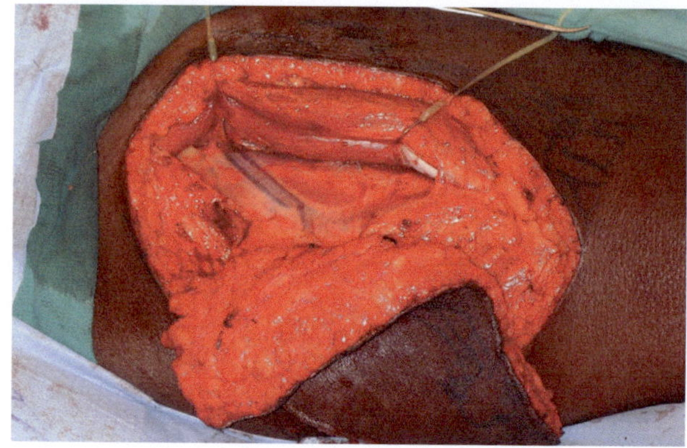

Fig. 34.6 Proximal dissections through the intermuscular septum to locate the pedicle

perforators is performed; otherwise, the posterior incision can be made at a later stage to allow for modification of the skin paddle.

If more bulk is needed, the fascia is kept attached to the muscle, and there will be no need to identify the perforators subfascially. On the contrary, if immediate debulking is desired, extreme care must be taken to (a) protect the entry point of the perforator(s) and (b) ensure the integrity of the subdermal plexus. Alternatively, the flap can be elevated supra-fascially to decrease bulk substantially but should only be done after significant experience with this flap. The intermuscular septum separating the vastus lateralis and rectus femoris muscles is dissected by retracting the rectus femoris medially and clipping all small muscular branches; dissecting proximally through the septum, we can locate the pedicle and its junction with the profunda (Fig. 34.6).

Branches of the descending branch of the LCFA are observed either within the septum to reach the skin perforators (septal cutaneous) or penetrating through the vastus lateralis muscle (muscular cutaneous branch) (Figs. 34.7 and 34.8).

For septocutaneous perforators, the dissection is performed in a retrograde fashion. Open the fascia medial and lateral to the pedicle and ligate all the muscular branches of the descending branch of the LCFA. Dissect the nerve to the vastus

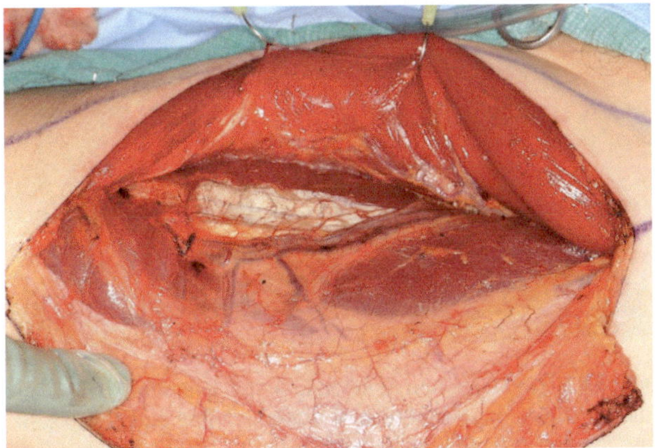

Fig. 34.7 Septocutaneous perforators

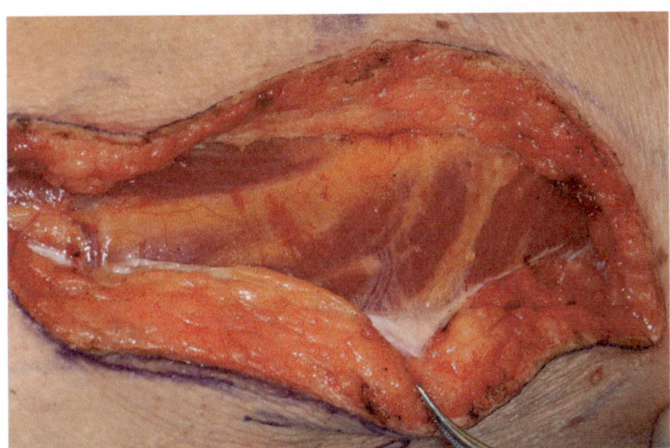

Fig. 34.8 Musculocutaneous perforators

lateralis away from the pedicle unless the vastus lateralis muscle is utilized as a functional muscle (Fig. 34.9a).

If the skin perforator is musculocutaneous, then intramuscular dissection is performed first, from the skin paddle to the pedicle. Unroof the perforator by lifting the muscle overlying the perforator up with tooth forceps. Tenotomy scissors are used next to spread the muscle fibers gently, which is then cut by a bipolar cautery (Fig. 34.9b).

All blood vessels branching laterally and deep from the pedicle are ligated with micro-clip. Dissect from a distal to a proximal fashion until all the muscular fibers attaching to the pedicle are cleared. Perforator dissection proceeds proximally until its takeoff from the descending branch of the LCFA; generally, a single perforator is enough to perfuse the flap. However, some surgeons prefer to dissect multiple perforators as a backup in case one of the perforators gets injured during dissection or when the design of the flap requires more than one perforator, or if a chimeric flap is needed (Fig. 13).

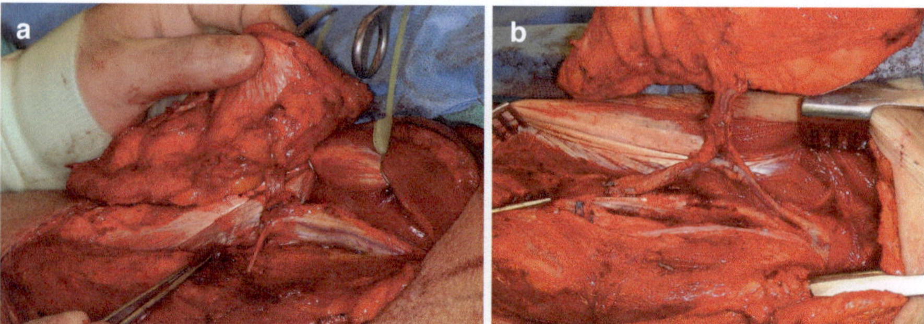

Fig. 34.9 (**a**) Dissection of nerve to vastus lateralis. (**b**) The nerve to vastus lateralis is freed from the pedicle, and the distal end of the descending branch is ligated, in this case with some length to use the flap as a flow-through flap

Fig. 34.10 Unroofing the perforator and clipping lateral muscular branches

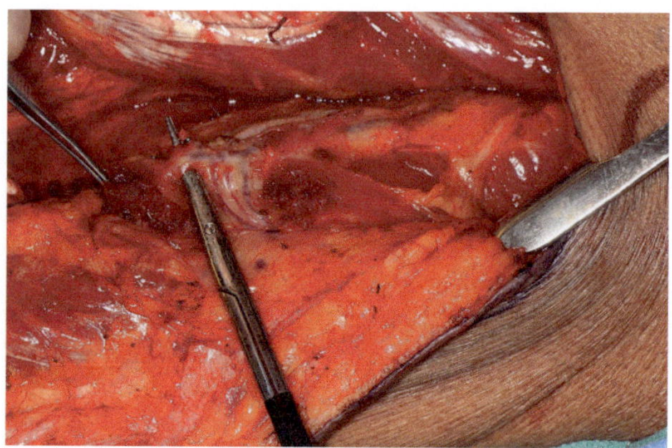

Sometimes ligation of the distal part of the descending branch can aid in pumping more blood to the perforators, which makes the dissection much easier. Finally, proximal dissection of the pedicle is performed. If more length of the pedicle is needed, one of the branches to the rectus femoris can be ligated after confirming the presence of a more proximal branch to the rectus femoris muscle in order to prevent muscle necrosis (Figs. 34.10 and 34.11); in rare occasions, when more length is needed, both branches can be clamped. The muscle is evaluated for perfusion; if the perfusion is good, both large branches can be ligated (Fig. 34.10). The pedicle is then ligated for the flap inset, or the flap is secured to the skin edges of the thigh until the ablative team is ready for the inset. Only divide the pedicle once ablation is completed; you might need more length to the pedicle or want a better size match of the vessels. Mark the superior surface of the pedicle with a marking pen to prevent the pedicle from kinking or twisting during the inset.

In some cases, the perforator to ALT may not be ideal, such as (A) there is only a small perforator, (B) the perforator got damaged during dissection, or (C) the medial incision was lateral to the septum, especially in cases with excess loose thigh

Fig. 34.11 Clamping the distal branch to the rectus femoris to add more length to the pedicle prior to ligating the branches

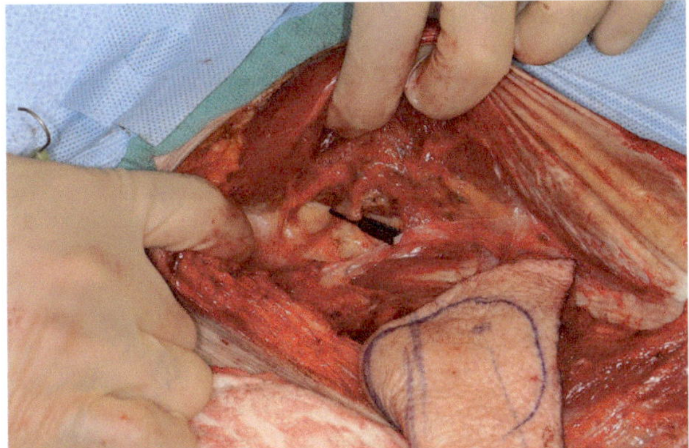

Fig. 34.12 (**a**) Ascending and transverse branches supplying the TFL flap. (**b**) An AMT flap was harvested following injury to the ALT perforators

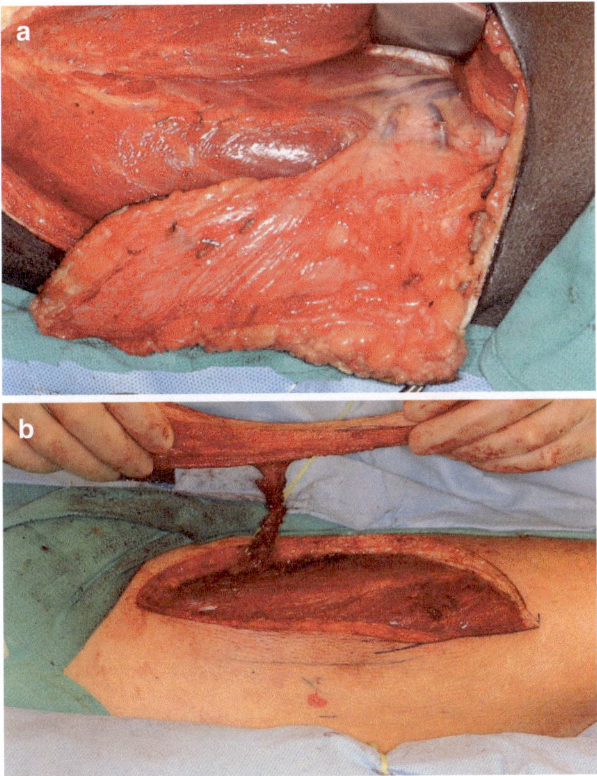

skin, switching to an AMT or TFL flaps utilizing the same incision without added morbidity or Pifferent surgical site can be used to salvage the flap (Fig. 34.12a, b).

ALT flap can be dissected as a chimeric flap with separate skin paddles and muscle components (vastus lateralis, vastus intermedius, TFL, rectus femoris). The nerve to vastus lateralis and lateral femoral cutaneous nerves can be used as vascularized nerve grafts.

Further Reading

Tursun R, et al. Combined anterolateral thigh and tensor fascia latae flaps: an option for reconstruction of large head and neck defects. J Oral Maxillofac Surg. 2017;75:1743–51.

Wong C-H, Ong Y, Wei F-C. Revisiting vascular supply of the rectus femoris and its relevance in the harvest of the anterolateral thigh flap. Ann Plast Surg. 2013;71(5):586–90.

Chapter 35
Practical Tips for Deep Circumflex Iliac Artery Free Flap

Ashleigh Weyh, Marina Morante, Sat Parmar, and Rui Fernandes

Abstract Taylor and Sanders described the first bone containing free flap in the literature in the late 1970s. Deep circumflex iliac artery (DCIA) free flap is a well-accepted reconstruction option for composite bone and soft tissue defects of the mandible and maxilla. No other flap can provide the same large quantity of cancellous bone, with regard to both the width and height, for dental rehabilitation with endosseous dental implants. Harvesting composite flaps with a skin paddle, muscle (internal oblique), and bone is possible if a chimeric design or extra bulk is desired. Vessels are usually unaffected by atherosclerosis and are consistently of sufficient caliber for successful microvascular anastomosis. The donor site can generally be closed primarily, and the incision can be well hidden with proper placement. The purpose of this chapter is to review pearls and pitfalls for deep circumflex iliac artery free flap.

Practical Tips

Anatomy

- Surface landmarks (Fig. 35.1):

  - Anterior superior iliac spine and the iliac crest.

A. Weyh · M. Morante · R. Fernandes (✉)
University of Florida Jacksonville, Jacksonville, FL, USA
e-mail: rui.fernandes@jax.ufl.edu

S. Parmar
University Hospital Birmingham, Birmingham, UK

D. Amin, H. Marwan (eds.), *Pearls and Pitfalls in Oral and Maxillofacial Surgery*, https://doi.org/10.1007/978-3-031-47307-4_35

Fig. 35.1 Surface anatomy
for the DCIA free flap

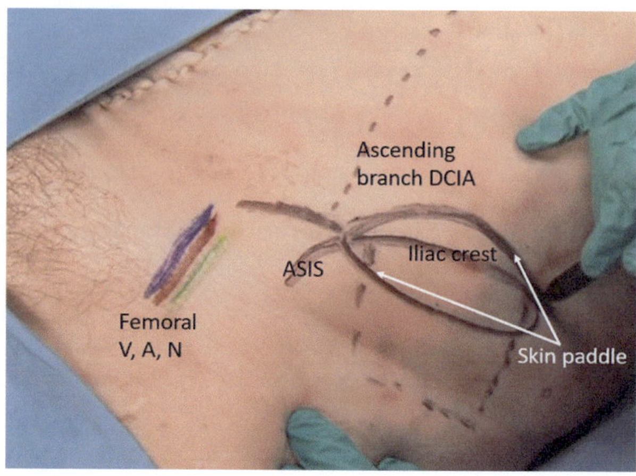

- Palpate the femoral pulse, and the incision will begin just laterally to these vessels.

  Note: the femoral nerve lies lateral to the artery and vein.

- The bone and skin paddle are based on the DCIA, usually with two comitant veins, but there may just be one vein, all originating from the external iliac vessels.
- The vascular supply to the internal oblique muscle is via the ascending branch of the deep circumflex iliac vessels:

  - Can be found running along the inner surface of the muscle, 2 cm medial to the anterior superior iliac spine (ASIS)
  - In most cases, a 2 cm muscle cuff for perforators to the skin paddle of transversus, internal, and external oblique. However, a perforator paddle would require no muscle cuff.
  - The blood supply for the bone of the iliac crest is the transversus branch which is a continuation of the DCIA after the ascending branch is given off.

- The skin paddle is obliquely oriented and centered over the iliac crest:

  - The greatest concentration of musculocutaneous perforators is 6–8 cm behind the anterior superior iliac spine.
  - The most common anatomical variations of the DCIA are as follows:

    Duplication of the DICA and/or ascending branches
    Ascending branch arising from the main trunk of the external iliac artery
    Multiple small ascending branches instead of a single dominant artery
    A dominant ascending branch supplying the iliac crest bone with a non-dominant DCIA

- Sensory innervation to the skin over the iliac crest mostly from T12, as the ilio-inguinal nerve (L1), which gives sensation to the groin.

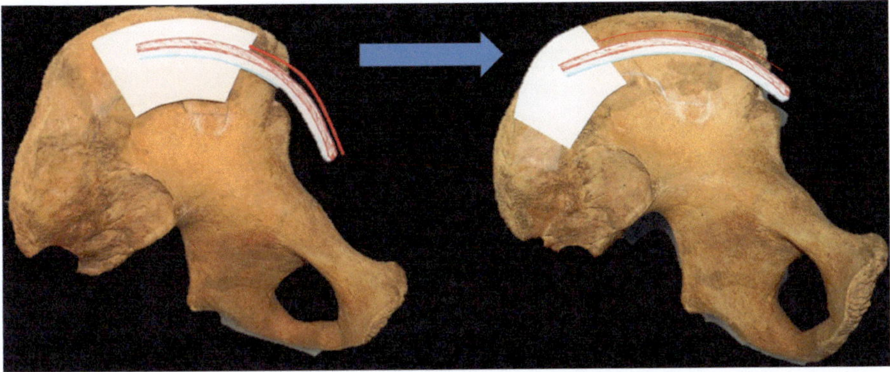

Fig. 35.2 Demonstration of how to lengthen the pedicle for DCIA free flap by positioning the osteotomies further posterior on the crest

- It is possible to create a sensate flap based on the lateral femoral cutaneous nerve; the DCIA will cross over this nerve near the ASIS.
- No uniformity in the description of the perforators and high variability in location and size.
- Relatively short pedicle length (5–7 cm), but one can lengthen the pedicle by not including the anterior superior iliac spine and making the anterior cut more posterior/lateral to the ASIS (Fig. 35.2). However, going too far posterior results in poorer bone quality, makes dissection more complex, and risk of harvesting non-vascularized bone.

Preoperative Consideration

- Preoperative virtual surgical planning can be performed to reduce operative time and increase accuracy through the fabrication of stereolithic models, cutting guides for the ilium, and patient-specific implants (Fig. 35.3).
- Using computed tomography angiography (CTA) may help in the safe design of the skin paddle.
- A two-team approach is possible and will reduce total operating and anesthetic time.

Intraoperative Consideration

- The best position for harvest is supine with a small hip bump.

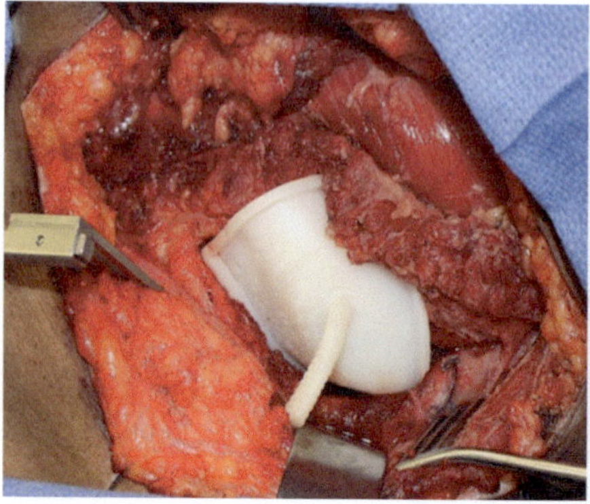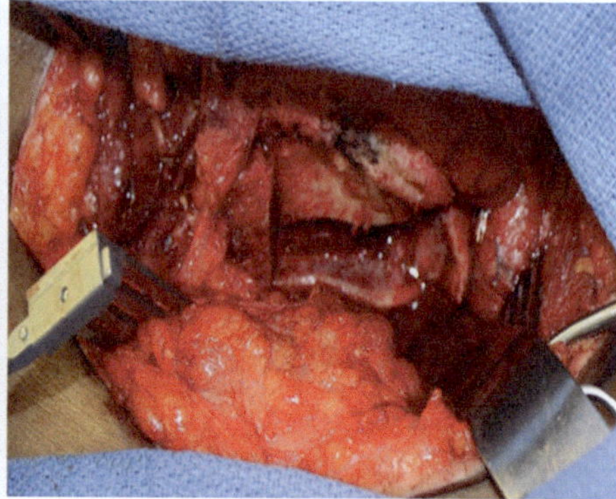

Fig. 35.3 Custom cutting guides for the DICA osteotomies

Fig. 35.4 View of external oblique muscle; note the direction of muscle fibers traveling medial and inferior

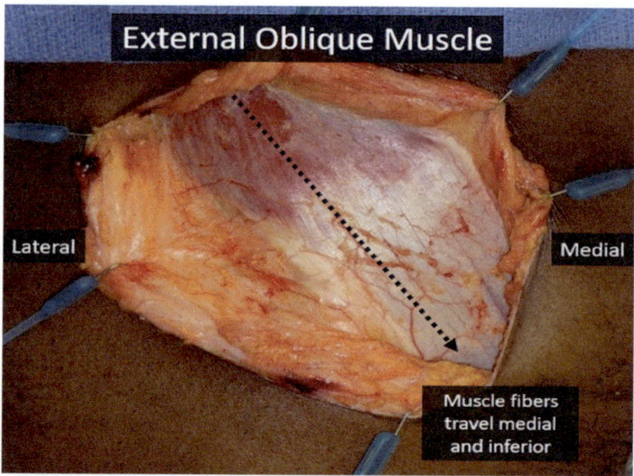

- In general, the side of the reconstruction will be determined by the preference side of the pedicle, the flap is usually raised with bone and muscle, and the pedicle comes out posteriorly, and the curvature of the bone, in general:

  - If reconstructing the mandible is bone only, or if the skin paddle will be extraoral and muscle intraoral, then use the ipsilateral hip. If reconstructing intraoral with the skin paddle, select the contralateral hip.

- Identification and dissection of the pedicle:

  - If including a skin paddle, begin the incision on the superior aspect.
  - The incisions of the skin and subcutaneous tissues are performed just lateral to the femoral pulse and taken deep to expose the external oblique muscle and its aponeurosis (Fig. 35.4).

    Note the direction of muscle fibers running medial and inferior from the origin on the lateral abdominal wall.

Fig. 35.5 View of internal oblique muscle; note the direction of muscle fibers perpendicular to the external oblique muscle

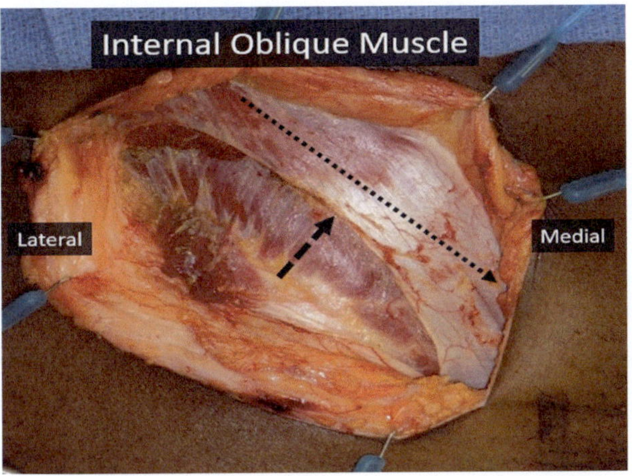

- Here, between the external oblique and subcutaneous tissues, it is possible to identify dominant musculocutaneous perforators.
- Next, an incision is made through the full thickness of the external oblique muscle to expose the entire internal oblique muscle (Fig. 35.5). Elevate the external oblique muscle off the internal oblique, dissecting up to the palpable costal margin where the 12th rib becomes palpable.

   Note again the change in the direction of muscle fibers in this region being opposite the external oblique.

- Once the internal oblique muscle is exposed, it should be separated from the transversus abdominis muscle (Fig. 35.6).

   The coastal margin is an excellent place to start this plane of dissection. Again, looking for a change in the direction of muscle fibers, transversus abdominis muscle fibers run horizontally to delineate the layers.

- Completely elevate the internal oblique muscle from cephalad to caudal, with care to preserve the ascending branch of the DCIA.
- The DCIA and veins can be located by following the ascending branch found in the internal oblique muscle inferior and medial, as the ascending branch will join the DCIA in the region medial to the ASIS (Fig. 35.7).

Flap Harvest

- Once the pedicle is identified, the remaining skin paddle incisions can be performed, cutting down onto bone at the external surface of the ilium.

   - If we preserve the ASIS, we can raise the flap posteriorly to the tensor fascia lata; if not, we will need to cut through both tensor fascia lata and gluteus medius muscle (unless you leave ASIS intact and raise posterior).

Fig. 35.6 View of transversus abdominis muscle

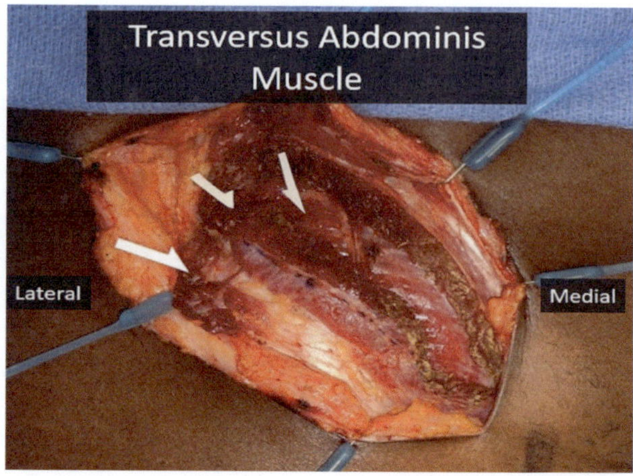

Fig. 35.7 View of DICA and ascending branch

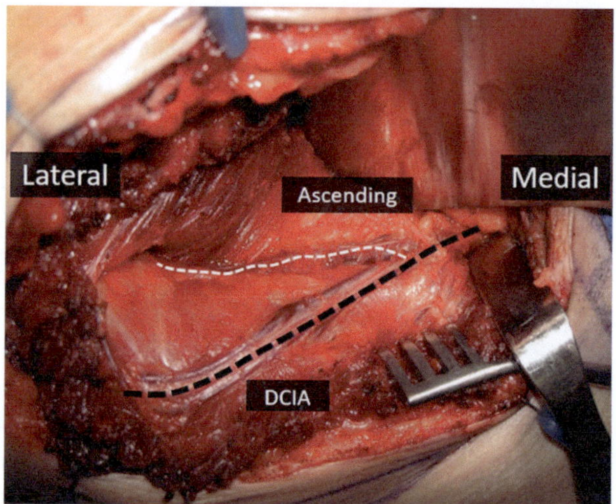

- Medial to the crest, preserve a 2 cm cuff of internal oblique muscle; oblique abdominal muscles are transected from caudal to cranial, taking care to preserve the DCIA, which will be 1–3 cm inferior to the inner rim of the ilium.
- Once DCIA is identified, the iliacus muscle can be transected 1–2 cm below the artery down to the periosteum.
- Sartorius muscle is detached at the ASIS (again, unless one chooses to leave the ASIS intact).
- We can then dissect the pedicle at this time toward takeoff from external iliac vessels before the osteotomies.
- Osteotomies with an oscillating saw should be done on the lateral surface to protect the pedicle medially, starting distally. The distal vascular pedicle can be ligated after this distal osteotomy (Fig. 35.8).

Fig. 35.8 The iliac crest was dissected and visualized before osteotomy

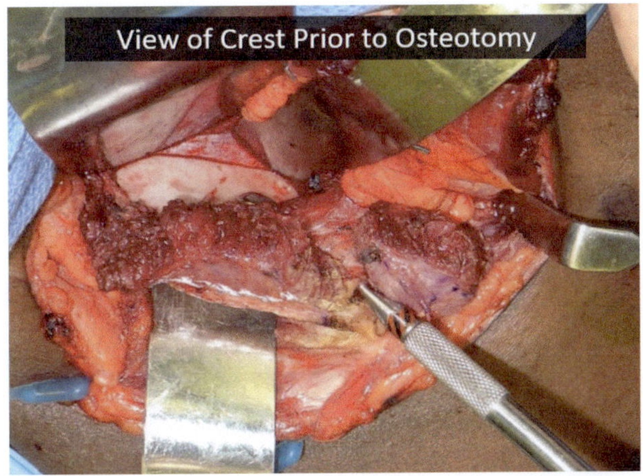

Fig. 35.9 Final dissection of DICA free flap

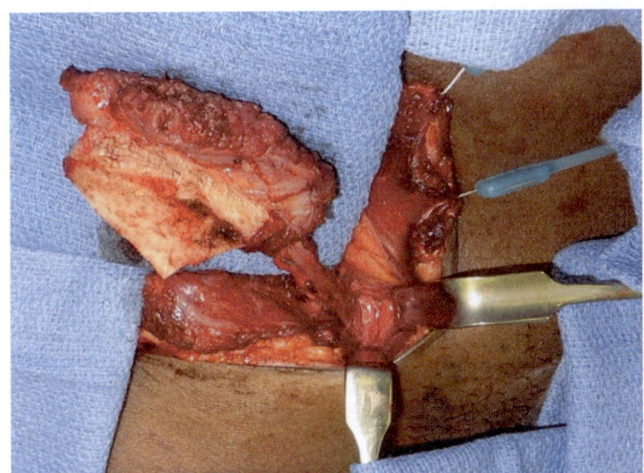

- The cuts should be made to facilitate the in-fracture of the bone flap. If angled, so the outer table is larger than the inner table, in-fracture will not be possible.
- The osteotomy is continued anteriorly, and once complete remaining muscle fibers can be detached from the osteotomized bone.
- The flap can then be harvested when the recipient's vessels are ready for anastomosis. It can be preferred to do all dissection of the pedicle prior to the osteotomies, as the surgical field will be much less hemostatic after bone cuts (Fig. 35.9).
- Patient-specific titanium implants to reconstruct the donor site at the iliac crest can prevent aesthetic deformities, and the risk of hernia decreased.
- Proper closure is critical to avoid complications like hernia, and the use of mesh is recommended to minimize this risk.
- Before closure, meticulous hemostasis must be achieved; it may help to use bone wax on the iliac crest donor site, as well as two drains, one on each side of the iliac crest.

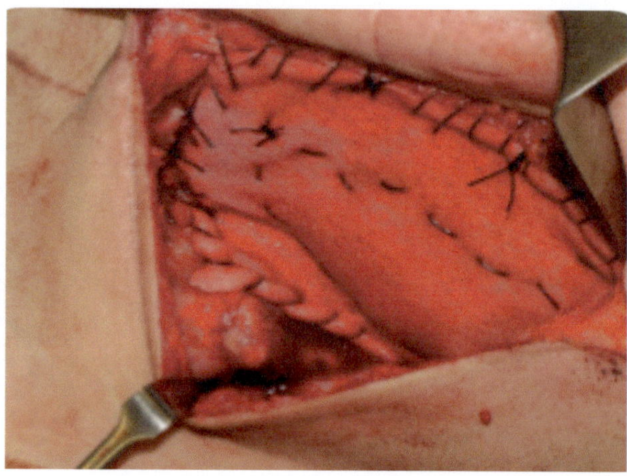

Fig. 35.10 Layered closure of DICA donor site, using a mesh to prevent hernia

- Multilayered closure with large sutures placed to obtain a tight seal as follows:

  - Remnants of the transversus abdominis muscle and fascia are closed to the cut ends of the iliacus muscle:

      Closure can be strengthened by passing suture through drilled holes along the cut edge of the iliac bone.

      For internal oblique muscle closure, one may need to bolster muscle layer closure with an abdominal surgical mesh cut to fit the defect. By widely exposing the internal oblique muscle and portions of the more solid aponeurosis anterior, the closure with mesh becomes much easier (Fig. 35.10).

  - Internal and external oblique muscles are re-approximated with the tensor fascia lata and gluteal muscles.
  - The final muscle layer should be the closure of the external oblique muscle edges onto itself.
  - Recommend the use of a local anesthetic catheter.
  - Closure of the subcutaneous and skin layers.

Variations of Iliac Flap

- *Unicortical bone flap*: The surgeon may choose to harvest the inner table only if less bone is needed. The plane between the inner iliac cortical bone and the outer table is created with curved osteotomes. However, only one cortex of bone may not be as beneficial for supporting dental implants.
- *Split lateral iliac crest chimeric flap*: Will give more freedom of movement among the different components of the flap as it provides longer pedicles, also provides for easier closure, and does not result in iliac crest deformity (Fig. 35.11).

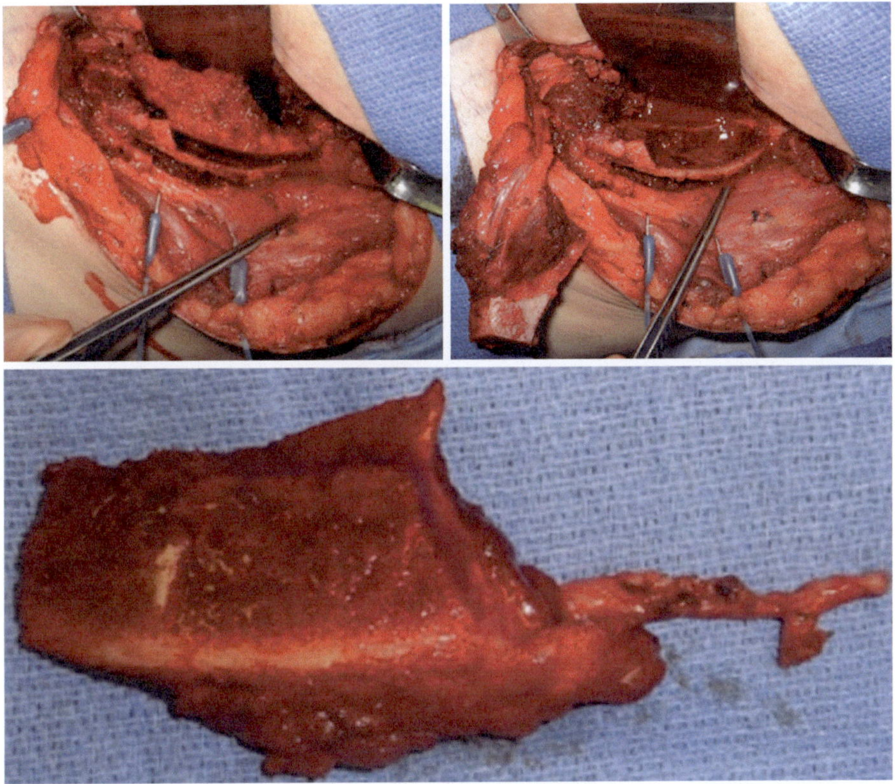

Fig. 35.11 Split lateral iliac crest chimeric flap, preserving the outer cortex of the iliac crest

- *Skin paddle via a groin flap*: The skin paddle for DCIA is often quite bulky, so the skin paddle can be harvested as a groin flap within the same surgical field, which is thinner and easier to inset. Unfortunately, frequently, this groin flap may have a separate origin from DCIA, requiring two separate anastomoses.

Postoperative Consideration

- Routine flap monitoring, if the bone-only buried flap can utilize a Doppler ultrasound probe (Cook-Swartz probe).
- Three to five days of bed rest with the thigh slightly flexed, and then ambulation with assistance from the physical therapy team as well as respiratory physiotherapy.
- Use of an indwelling analgesia catheter that slowly releases bupivacaine, or equivalent, for the first 3 days can reduce donor site pain and help with earlier ambulation and opioid reduction.

- Maintain suction drain until acceptably low output and after ambulation, which can temporarily increase output.
- Abdominal binders can improve patient comfort and prevent dehiscence/hernia.
- Donor site morbidity includes chronic hip pain, ventral hernias, persistent lateral femoral paresthesia, and sexual impotence.
- Patients should be monitored for gastrointestinal ileus; starting a diet with liquids slowly can help.

Case Presentation

An 18-year-old female presented with biopsy-proven osteosarcoma of the right mandible. The preoperative CT scan of her head, neck, and face showed an extensive lesion with mixed osteolytic lesions around the mandibular anterior incisors and apical region with cortical expansion (Fig. 35.12). She was planned for resection and reconstruction with an osseous flap from the iliac crest. The patient underwent surgery with hemimandibulectomy and a DCIA free flap from the left hip (Fig. 35.13). The iliac crest free flap was osteotomized and fixated with the reconstruction bar to create the new mandible. The patient did well in the postoperative period and was followed up with a surveillance CT (Fig. 35.14). The patient was

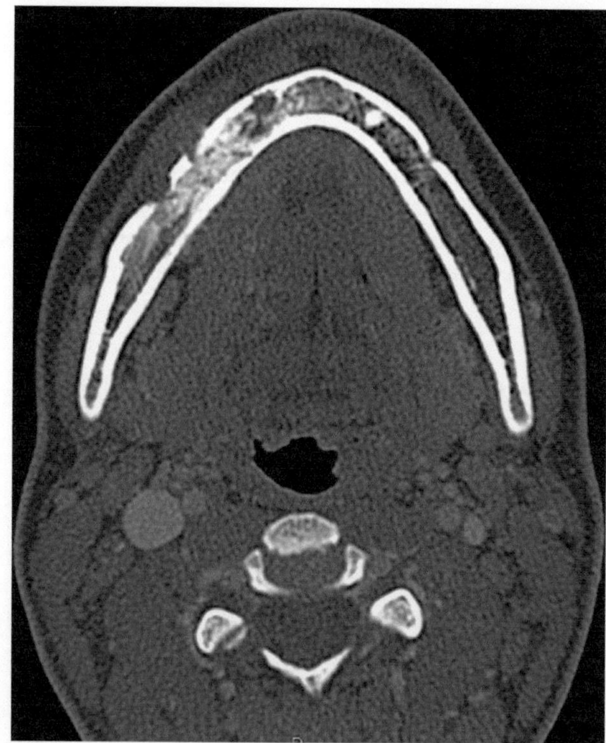

Fig. 35.12 Preoperative CT showing osteosarcoma of the right mandible

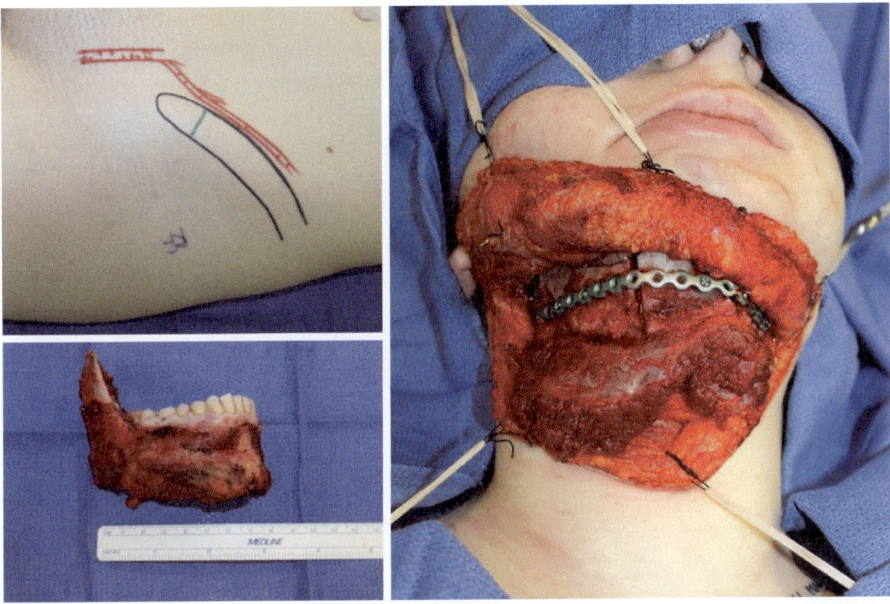

Fig. 35.13 Intraoperative photos. (Top left) Surface marking showing the relationship of DCIA and the iliac artery, (bottom left) resection specimen, and (right) final inset and plating of the DCIA flap

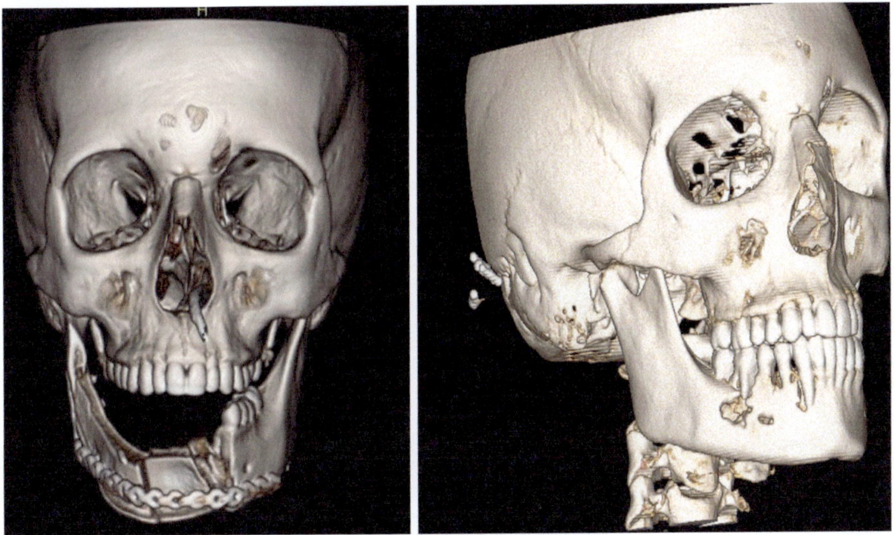

Fig. 35.14 Immediate postoperative CT 3D reconstruction

followed up for 5 years, achieving disease-free state and good mandibular contour and function, including full dental rehabilitation with implants (Figs. 35.15, 35.16, and 35.17).

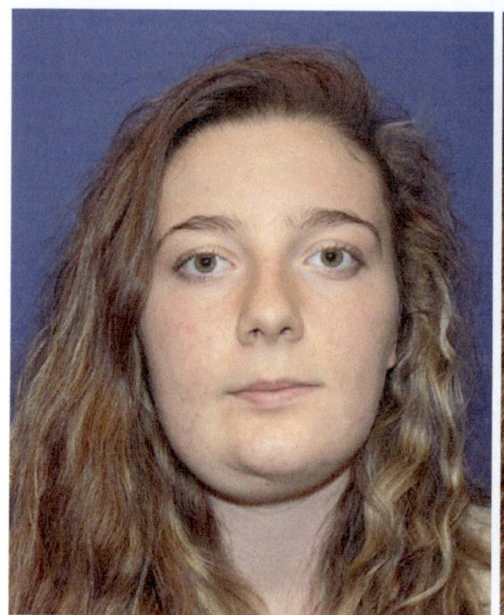
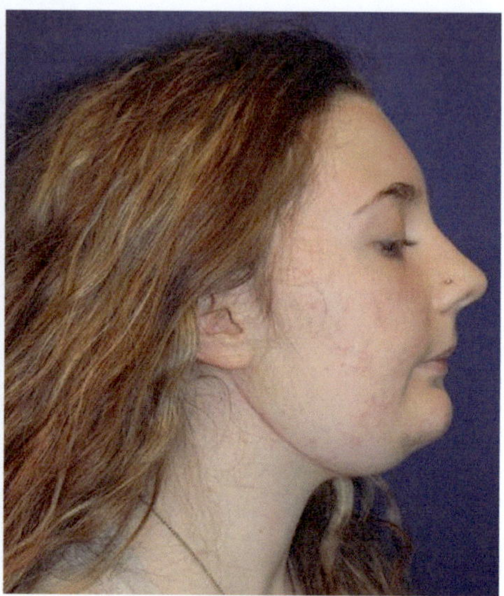

Fig. 35.15 Face photo of postoperative healing

Fig. 35.16 1-year postoperative CT showing good bony fusion and position of neomandible

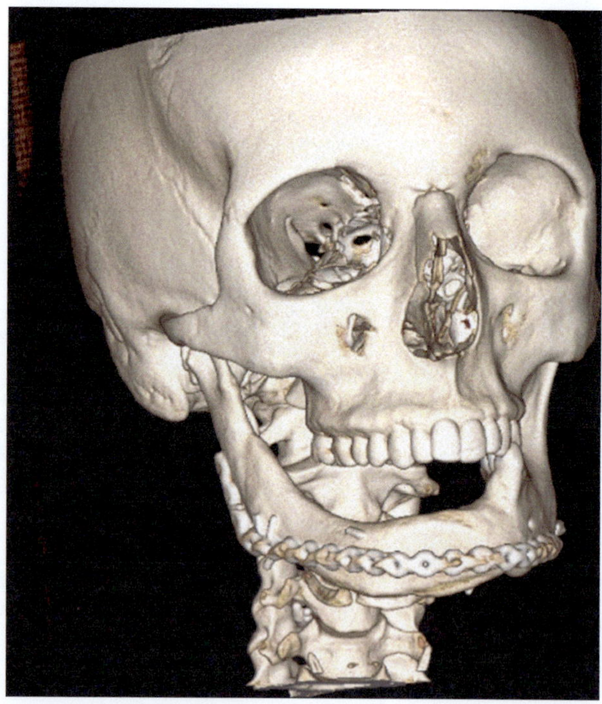

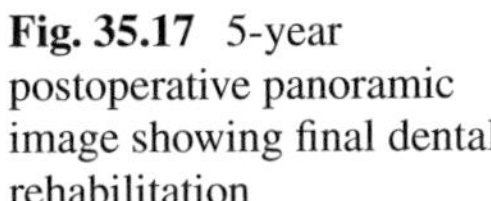

Fig. 35.17 5-year postoperative panoramic image showing final dental rehabilitation

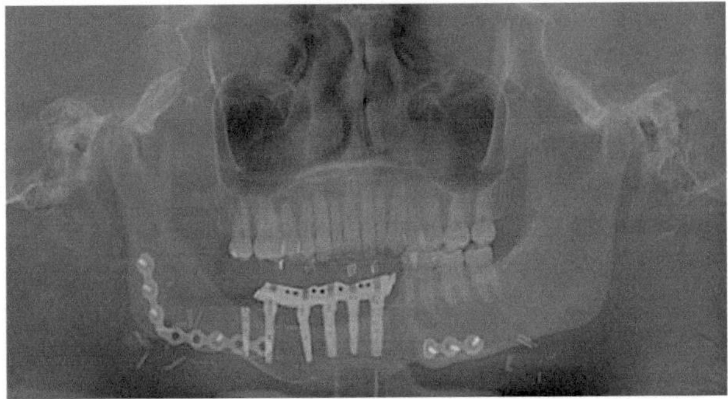

Pearls

- Deep circumflex iliac artery (DCIA) can increase harvest time, especially for obese patients.
- DCIA is often quoted as a much less favorable donor site to the fibula or scapula; however, newer studies show this was likely an exaggeration, and morbidity is acceptable.
- Flap has a shorter vascular pedicle and bone length when compared to other osteocutaneous free flaps.
- There is a risk of a postoperative hernia. To minimize this complication, using appropriate layered closure and the use of mesh is recommended.

Pitfalls

- No uniformity in the description of the perforators and high variability in location and size.
- Pedicle length (5–7 cm) can be lengthened by not including the anterior superior iliac spine and making the anterior cut more posterior/lateral to the anterior superior iliac spine (ASIS).
- It is essential when harvesting this flap to maintain the ascending branch to the internal oblique to ensure blood supply to the bone through this muscle.
- One should not rely solely on using the ascending branch to find the DCIA, as in a small percentage of patients, DCIA and the ascending branch will have two separate origins, or even there may be no ascending branch.
- Avoid this flap in women of childbearing age, as this flap harvest can weaken the abdominal wall and cause problems during delivery.

- Try to avoid in patients with previous abdominal surgeries due to increased risk for hernia or compromised vascularity:

  - The history of abdominal surgeries, such as appendectomy, can compromise the ascending branch of the DCIA. This will compromise the blood supply to the internal oblique muscle—only the left DCIA should be used in this situation.
  - Past surgeries can also lead to abdominal wall weakness, predisposing patients to developing a hernia. A synthetic mesh may need to be used during the closure if the internal oblique muscle is harvested.
  - Bowel perforation.

- The skin paddle often has little mobility due to short perforators unless a perforator paddle is used.

Further Reading

Taylor GI, Watson N. One-stage repair of compound leg defects with free, revascularized flaps of groin skin and iliac bone. Plast Reconstr Surg. 1978;61(4):494–506.

Sanders R, Mayou BJ. A new vascularized bone graft transferred by microvascular anastomosis as a free flap. Br J Surg. 1979;66(11):787–8.

Barbera G, Della Monaca M, Manganiello L, Battisti A, Priore P, Cassoni A, Terenzi V, Valentini V. Reconstruction of the mandibular symphysis: pilot study compares three different flaps. Minerva Dent Oral Sci. 2022;71(3):139–48. https://doi.org/10.23736/S2724-6329.21.04597-6. Epub 2021 Dec 1.

Ling XF, Peng X, Samman N. Donor-site morbidity of free fibula and DCIA flaps. J Oral Maxillofac Surg. 2013;71(9):1604–12. https://doi.org/10.1016/j.joms.2013.03.006. Epub 2013 Jun 27.

Wei F, Mardini S. Flaps and reconstructive surgery. 2nd ed. Amsterdam: Elsevier; 2016.

Wolff K, Holzle F. Raising of microvascular flaps: a systematic approach. 3rd ed. Cham: Springer; 2018.

Dorafshar AH, Seitz IA, DeWolfe M, Agarwal JP, Gottlieb LJ. Split lateral iliac crest chimera flap: utility of the ascending branch of the lateral femoral circumflex vessels. Plast Reconstr Surg. 2010;125(2):574–81. https://doi.org/10.1097/PRS.0b013e3181c83013.

Chapter 36
Practical Tips for Harvesting Scapula Osteocutaneous Flap

Camila Franco-Mesa, Victoria A. Mañón, and Hisham Marwan

Abstract Scapular flaps have a versatile nature that allows numerous combinations of skin, muscle, and bone. Additionally, atherosclerosis rarely affects the pedicle, which offers further advantages in patients with peripheral artery disease. Given the anatomical location, scapular flaps favor early patient ambulation and are not associated with long-term movement limitations in the lower extremity. Both scapular and parascapular osteocutaneous flaps are associated with acceptable postoperative morbidities, allowing for primary closure without skin graft and a well-hidden scar. Nonetheless, several key points or pitfalls must be carefully addressed to avoid surgical complications and undesired outcomes. One of the main limitations of harvesting the scapula flap is positioning. A two-team approach is usually difficult, and additional time is required for patient positioning. The purpose of this chapter is to review pearls and pitfalls for harvesting scapula osteocutaneous flap.

Practical Tips

Preoperative Consideration

- A thorough physical exam to assess baseline upper extremity musculoskeletal function, including the range of motion and strength.

C. Franco-Mesa
University of Texas Medical Branch at Galveston, Galveston, TX, USA

V. A. Mañón
McGovern Medical School, UTHSC School of Dentistry at Houston, Houston, TX, USA

H. Marwan (✉)
Department of Surgery, The University of Texas Medical Branch, Galveston, TX, USA
e-mail: himarwan@utmb.edu

- Patients with previous neck dissection are at greater risk of postoperative shoulder dysfunction after harvesting the scapula.
- Patients with axillary lymph node dissection are at increased risk of vascular compromise. CTA shoulder should be considered to evaluate the blood vessels before surgery.
- Overlooking flap considerations regarding tissue composition, quantity, pedicle length, and vessel anastomosis before proceeding to surgery. Every flap should be tailored to the patient's specific needs.

Intraoperative Consideration

- Inadequate patient positioning limits exposure during the dissection of vascular structures in the axillary fossa. Positioning of the patient in lateral decubitus with chest and pelvis at a vertical position and arms properly abducted. Avoid hyper-abduction and over-rotation of the arm to prevent injury to the brachial plexus.
- To ease the transition from ablation to reconstruction, the patient should be prepped with a beanbag at a slightly lateral decubitus position. The patient should be securely strapped. The table can be rotated to help position the ablation part of the surgery.
- Identifying the triangular fossa is the key to identifying the circumflex scapular vessels. The fossa is bounded superiorly by the teres minor, inferiorly by the teres major, and laterally by the long head of the triceps muscle (Fig. 36.1).
- Once the triangular fossa is identified and confirmed with Doppler, the flap design must incorporate the triangular fossa. The skin flap design can be oriented horizontally (scapular flap), vertically (parascapular flap), or both ways.
- The initial incision and dissection should start away from the triangular fossa (superiorly and laterally). The dissection should be subfascial to identify the teres major and minor muscles.
- Avoid transection of blood supply during dissection of the infraspinatus fascia from the medial skin island to the lateral scapular border. Also, avoid severing cutaneous branches close to the fascia of the infraspinatus fascia or compromising the circumflex scapular vessels while dissecting the skin from the teres major muscle attachments.
- Once the circumflex scapular vessel and the skin are identified, the lateral border of the scapula is exposed by directly incising the teres major and minor muscles to expose the periosteum overlying the scapula.
- Avoid avulsion of the circumflex scapular vessels during detachment of the teres major muscle.
- If the tip of the scapula is planned to be harvested, incomplete isolation of the angular branch at the level of the scapular tip leads to transection or injury during osteotomy. The angular artery has a variable origin; in about 50% of cases, it arises from the latissimus dorsi branch of the thoracodorsal artery.
- When planning the osteotomy, always maintain at least 1 cm of bone inferior to the glenoid fossa to avoid shoulder joint injury.

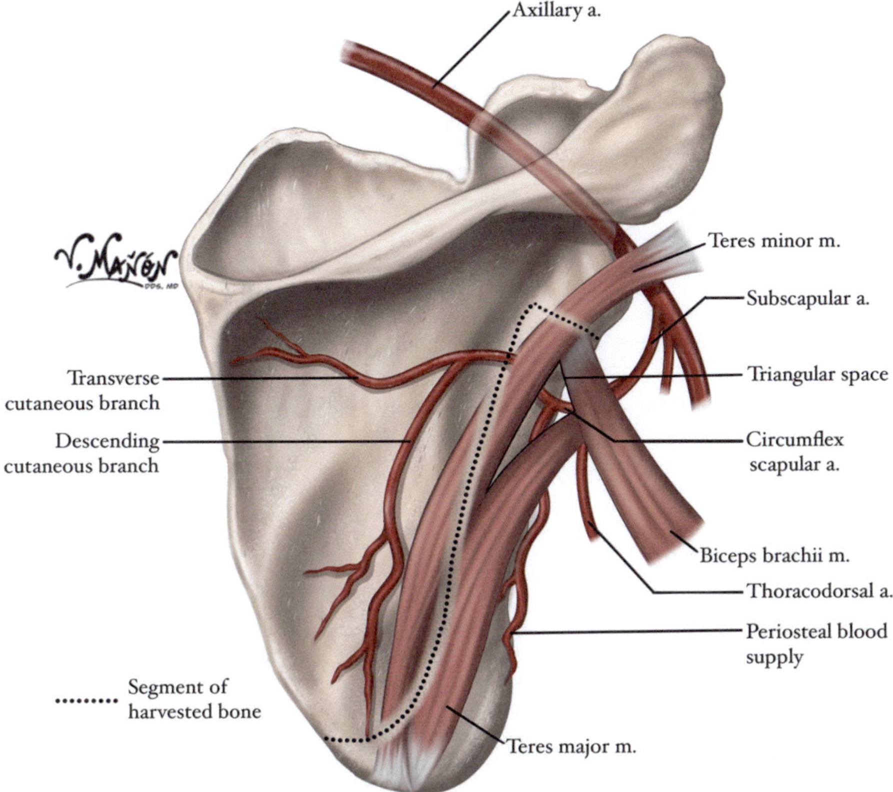

Fig. 36.1 The muscle and blood supply of the posterior axillary region and the scapula. The teres major, teres minor, and the long head of the triceps muscle bound the triangular space. The circumflex scapular artery (CSA) will divide into the transverse and descending cutaneous branches. The angular branch usually comes off the thoracodorsal artery

- Always leave a cuff of the subscapularis muscle on the bone to avoid injury to the periosteal blood supply to the flap.
- Reattach the teres major to the scapula by drilling holes into the bone and suturing the muscles. This will minimize the winging of the scapula postoperatively.
- Always prepare the recipient's vessels before starting the harvest of the scapula flap to minimize prolonged ischemia time.

Postoperative Consideration

- Shoulder morbidity is affected by deferred physical therapy, especially delaying shoulder strength and range of motion exercises in the ipsilateral harvested extremity. Sessions should start in the early postoperative period (within the first week) and continue after discharge.

Pearls

- Every flap should be tailored to the patient's specific needs.
- Always leave a cuff of the subscapularis muscle on the bone to avoid injury to the periosteal blood supply to the flap.

Pitfalls

- Be aware of the patient's position, as inadequate patient positioning limits exposure during the dissection of vascular structures in the axillary fossa.
- Avoid avulsion of the circumflex scapular vessels during detachment of the teres major muscle.

Further Readings

Urken ML, Bridger AG, Zur K, Genden E. The scapular osteofasciocutaneous flap a 12-year experience. Arch Otolaryngol Head Neck Surg. 2001;127(7):862–9.

Patel KB, Hubert T, Partridge A, et al. Assessment of shoulder function following scapular free flap. Head Neck. 2020;42(2):224–9. https://doi.org/10.1002/hed.25992.

Chundoo S, Naredla P, Thomas S. A brief clinical study: the use of a custom guide for scapula free flap harvest and mandibular reconstruction. J Craniofac Surg. 2022;33(7):2142–5. https://doi.org/10.1097/SCS.0000000000008739.

Choi N, Cho JK, Jang JY, Cho JK, Cho YS, Baek CH. Scapular tip free flap for head and neck reconstruction. Clin Exp Otorhinolaryngol. 2015;8(4):422. https://doi.org/10.3342/ceo.2015.8.4.422.

Vincent A, Sawhney R, Ducic Y. Perioperative care of free flap patients. Semin Plast Surg. 2019;33(1):5–12. https://doi.org/10.1055/s-0038-1676824.

Salgado C, Chim H, Schoenoff S, Mardini S. Postoperative care and monitoring of the reconstructed head and neck patient. Semin Plast Surg. 2010;24(3):281–7. https://doi.org/10.1055/s-0030-1263069.

Lese I, Biedermann R, Constantinescu M, Grobbelaar AO, Olariu R. Predicting risk factors that lead to free flap failure and vascular compromise: a single unit experience with 565 free tissue transfers. J Plast Reconstr Aesthet Surg. 2021;74(3):512–22. https://doi.org/10.1016/j.bjps.2020.08.126.

Nagai M, Dyalram D, Lubek JE. Failure of preoperative co-morbidity indices to predict the successful use of the composite scapula free flap for maxillofacial reconstruction in patients with significant medical co-morbidities. Int J Oral Maxillofac Surg. 2022;51(6):746–53. https://doi.org/10.1016/j.ijom.2021.10.009.

Park IH, Chung CH, Chang YJ, Kim JH. Clinical experiences with the scapular fascial free flap. Arch Plast Surg. 2016;43(5):438–45. https://doi.org/10.5999/aps.2016.43.5.438.

Schliephake H. Chapter 38: Common free vascularized flaps: the scapula. In: Maxillofacial surgery. 3rd ed. Amsterdam: Elsevier; 2017. p. 543–8.

Chapter 37
Practical Tips for Harvesting Latissimus Dorsi Free Flap

Brian Rethman, Salah Al Din Al Azri, James C. Melville, Andrew Huang, and Jonathan W. Shum

Abstract The latissimus dorsi flap (LDF) is a versatile soft tissue flap with a reliable vascular pedicle traveling in a consistent location along the ventral surface of the latissimus dorsi. It can be harvested as a muscle only, myocutaneous, split muscle, bilobed, osteomyocutaneous rib, and/or as part of a subscapular system chimeric flap. For example, the chimeric flap may include elements of scapula bone,

B. Rethman
Katz Department of Oral and Maxillofacial Surgery, The University of Texas Health Science Center at Houston, Houston's Health University, Houston, TX, USA

Oral and Maxillofacial Surgery, Bayne-Jones Army Community Hospital, Fort Johnson South, LA, USA

S. A. D. Al Azri
Katz Department of Oral and Maxillofacial Surgery, School of Dentistry, The University of Texas Health Science Center at Houston, Houston, TX, USA

J. C. Melville
Department of Oral and Maxillofacial Surgery, Oral, Head and Neck Oncology and Microvascular Reconstructive Surgery, University of Texas Health Science Center at Houston, Houston, TX, USA

UTHealth|The University of Texas Health Science Center at Houston Houston's Health University, Houston, TX, USA

A. Huang
Department of Otolaryngology-Head and Neck Surgery, Baylor College of Medicine, Houston, TX, USA

J. W. Shum (✉)
UTHealth|The University of Texas Health Science Center at Houston Houston's Health University, Houston, TX, USA

Department of Oral and Maxillofacial Surgery, Oral, Head and Neck Oncology and Microvascular Reconstructive Surgery, The University of Texas Health Science Center at Houston, Houston, TX, USA
e-mail: jonathan.shum@uth.tmc.edu

D. Amin, H. Marwan (eds.), *Pearls and Pitfalls in Oral and Maxillofacial Surgery*, https://doi.org/10.1007/978-3-031-47307-4_37

serratus anterior, and the latissimus dorsi. The pedicled myocutaneous latissimus dorsi flap has also been described as an alternative to the pectoralis major pedicled flap for head and neck reconstruction. Common indications for applying an LDF in the head and neck are reserved for defects with large surface area and volume loss, such as extensive neck and scalp defects. A maximum dimension of 20 × 40 cm may be harvested. The thoracodorsal perforator flap (TDAP) is a variation of the LDF that offers a thinner flap by splitting latissimus dorsi along the myocutaneous perforators without harvesting a significant portion of the muscle itself. The TDAP can be used for thinner, small- to medium-sized defects with a maximum dimension of 25 × 14 cm.

Although the LDF can be harvested as a pedicled or free tissue transfer, it is not a standard "workhorse" flap for head and neck patients due to the availability of the anterolateral thigh flap. The harvest can be limited by lateral decubitus or prone positioning. This can prevent a two-team approach, head and neck ablation, and reconstruction from working effectively simultaneously. The LDF or TDAP free flaps' vascular pedicle is based on the thoracodorsal artery and single vena comitans. The thoracodorsal artery is a continuation of the subscapular artery distal to the branch point of the circumflex scapular artery. The thoracodorsal artery immediately divides after perforation into the deep side of the latissimus into the lateral and medial branches. The vascular pedicle is consistent with less variability when compared to the ALT flap. The innervation of the latissimus dorsi muscle is from the thoracodorsal nerve, which arises from the posterior branch of the brachial plexus. It has multiple branches which run with the named vascular branches. The sensory nerve innervation arises from the ventral and dorsal rami of the thoracic spinal nerves. The purpose of this chapter is to review pearls and pitfalls for practical tips for harvesting latissimus dorsi free flap.

Practical Tips

Preoperative Consideration

- A thorough history and physical examination should be obtained. Significant concerns would include any previous history of trauma, surgery, or radiation to the donor site under consideration for harvest. A prior history of deep venous thromboembolism or any obvious deformities should also be noted.
- The vascular pedicle and perforators are consistent. No specific imaging is routinely required preoperatively.
- Consideration should be made to mark the lateral border of the latissimus dorsi with the patient standing up prior to entering the operating room.

Intraoperative Consideration

- The patient is positioned in lateral decubitus with the donor site upward and the shoulder joint abducted.
- The spider limb positioner can facilitate positioning of the upper extremity. The shoulder must be stabilized to prevent brachial plexus injury.
- Patient positioning routinely prevents a simultaneous two-team approach.
- Surgical landmarks include the posterior axillary crease, the tip of the scapula, and the lateral border of the latissimus dorsi muscle. If the lateral border was not marked with the patient standing, a line from the posterior axillary crease to the iliac crest halfway between the anterior and posterior iliac spines will approximate the border if it is difficult to palpate.
- A point 8 cm below the posterior axillary fold aligned parallel to the lateral border of the muscle, and 2 cm medial from the lateral border approximates the perforation point of the thoracodorsal neurovascular bundle into the muscle from the deep surface (Fig. 37.1).
- The skin paddle should be designed medial and parallel to the lateral border of the latissimus dorsi with a fusiform shape to aid in primary closure.
- After the lateral incision from the posterior axillary fold to the planned distal skin paddle is made, the first neurovascular bundle identified is the serratus anterior branch. This can be dissected proximally to the thoracodorsal bundle.
- The circumflex scapular neuromuscular bundle can be divided if a longer pedicle is needed. The pedicle can be taken to the subscapular artery if required.
- The flap can be harvested as a muscle-only flap, and a split-thickness skin graft can cover the muscle (Fig. 37.2).
- If a myocutaneous flap is harvested, the muscle flap should be slightly wider than the skin paddle to prevent undermining the vascular pedicle.
- Stay sutures between the skin and muscle around the flap boundaries should be placed to prevent shearing and damage to the perforators.

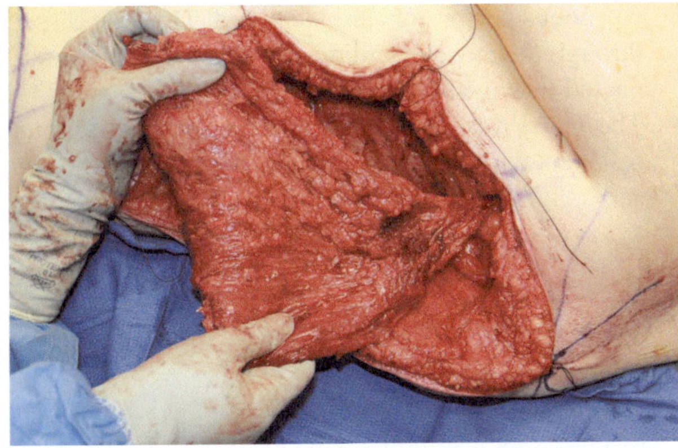

Fig. 37.1 Latissimus dorsi muscle-only flap is elevated

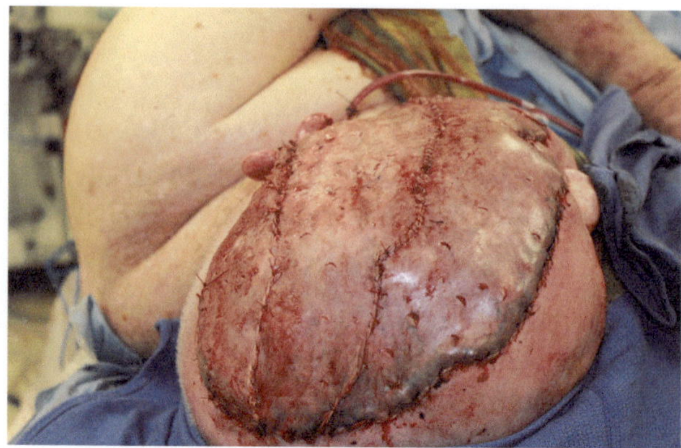

Fig. 37.2 The muscle-only latissimus dorsi is inset, and a split-thickness skin graft is placed

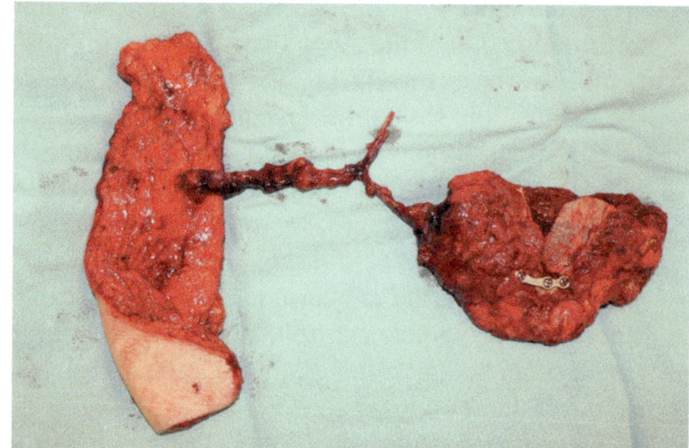

Fig. 37.3 Chimeric scapula bone-TDAP flap. The TDAP (left) is based on the lateral branch of the thoracodorsal artery, with a scapula tip based on the angular artery

- If the flap is 10 cm or less wide, it can generally be closed primarily. If the flap is larger, a skin graft may be required with a negative pressure dressing for 1 week.
- Two drains should be placed to prevent hematoma/seroma formation.
- For the TDAP variation, once the thoracodorsal neuromuscular pedicle is identified between the serratus anterior and the latissimus dorsi, the intramuscular cutaneous perforators are identified. They are dissected from deep to superficial through the muscle, and the latissimus is split longitudinally. The pedicle can be passed through after separation.
- The TDAP variation limits the amount of latissimus dorsi muscle taken with the fasciocutaneous portion and is a good choice if a significant flap bulk is unnecessary (Fig. 37.3).

Postoperative Consideration

- The patient may use the ipsilateral upper extremity in the immediate postoperative period but should avoid excessive movement for the first week.

- The gradual return of shoulder function and physical therapy can start after the first week. Strenuous exercise should be avoided for 6 weeks.
- The latissimus flap has a high rate of seroma formation. The drains should remain in place until there is less than 20 ml of fluid in 24 h.
- The patient may experience shoulder weakness with extension and adduction movements. Consideration should be made for other flaps in patients who use wheelchairs.

Pearls

- The vascular pedicle and perforators are consistent. No specific imaging is routinely required preoperatively.
- Consider marking the lateral border of the latissimus dorsi with the patient standing up before entering the operating room.
- Maintaining the orientation of the flap is vital to prevent torsion of the vascular pedicle.

Pitfalls

- It may be difficult to palpate the lateral border of the latissimus dorsi in an obese patient. The lateral border can be estimated by drawing a line from the posterior border of the axillary crease to the midline of the iliac crest.
- The serratus anterior neurovascular bundle is typically first identified and must not be mistaken for the thoracodorsal neurovascular bundle. To prevent this, do not divide the serratus anterior neurovascular bundle until the flap has been completely elevated.
- The muscle flap may be undermined obliquely, damaging the perforators or main thoracodorsal trunk. To prevent this, the muscle flap should be wider or parallel to the skin paddle.
- The bulky subcutaneous layer can cause shearing and damage the perforators during flap elevation. To prevent this, stay sutures are recommended.

Further Reading

International Federation of Facial Plastic Surgery Societies. Atlas of microvascular surgery: anatomy and operative techniques. Arch Facial Plast Surg. 2008;10(1):67.

Gold CK, Wong MS. Management of postradiation chest wall defects. In: Morita SY, Balch CM, Klimberg V, Pawlik TM, Posner MC, Tanabe KK, editors. Textbook of complex general surgical oncology. New York: McGraw Hill; 2018. https://accesssurgery.mhmedical.com/content.aspx?bookid=2209§ionid=168948130. Accessed 21 November 2022.

Ong HS, Ji T, Zhang CP. The pedicled latissimus dorsi myocutaneous flap in head and neck reconstruction. Oral Maxillofac Surg Clin North Am. 2014;26(3):427–34.

Slavin SA, Fox S. Latissimus dorsi myocutaneous flap. In: Guyuron B, Eriksson E, Persing JA, editors. Plastic surgery: indications and practice. Philadelphia: Saunders; 2009.

Gordon L, Bunche H, Alpert B. Free latissimus dorsi muscle flap with split-thickness skin graft cover: a report of 16 cases. Plast Reconstr Surg. 1982;70:173.

Fisher J, Bostwick J III, Powell RW. Latissimus dorsi blood supply after thoracodorsal vessel division: the serratus collateral. Plast Reconstr Surg. 1983;72:502.

Guerra AB, Metzinger SE, Lund KM, et al. The thoracodorsal artery perforator flap: clinical experience and anatomic study with emphasis on harvest techniques. Plast Reconstr Surg. 2004;114:32.

Hui KCW, Zhang F, Sutkin H, et al. Functional assessment of the shoulder following latissimus dorsi muscle donation in the handicapped. J Reconstr Microsurg. 1999;15:101.

Pennington D, Stern H, Lee K. Free flap reconstruction of large defects of the scalp and calvarium. Plast Reconstr Surg. 1989;83:655.

Part VI
Temporomandibular Surgery

Chapter 38
How to Perform Arthrocentesis

Jose Montero

Abstract Arthrocentesis is a well-known, evidence-based, minimally invasive procedure, described initially for severely limited mouth opening. It is a relatively simple procedure that should be part of any oral and maxillofacial surgeon skill set. Conservative and medical management of temporomandibular joint disorders (TMD) has been the first line of treatment for many decades. However, in the past few years, there has been a shift in the treatment algorithm. Multiple authors advocate that either shortening or omitting the traditional first line of treatment has shown to be beneficial and, in some cases, a more effective treatment modality for patients suffering from TMD. Understanding temporomandibular joint (TMJ) anatomy, instrumentation, and appropriate surgical techniques is key to successful outcomes in treating our patient population. Our profession also has a new tendency to introduce level I arthroscopy of the TMJ as part of the oral and maxillofacial surgery residency curriculum. The goal is to provide oral and maxillofacial surgery residents with the necessary armamentarium that would allow them to enhance the outcomes of arthrocentesis by being able to diagnose intra-articular pathology, perform guided intra-articular injections, and discuss specific findings and prognosis with patients, among other benefits. The purpose of this chapter is to review how to perform arthrocentesis. The arthroscopy procedure will be discussed in another chapter.

J. Montero (✉)
Baptist Hospital of Miami, Miami, FL, USA
e-mail: jmontero@miamioms.com

D. Amin, H. Marwan (eds.), *Pearls and Pitfalls in Oral and Maxillofacial Surgery*, https://doi.org/10.1007/978-3-031-47307-4_38

Practical Tips

Preoperative Consideration

Clinical Evaluation

1. Maximal interincisal opening (MIO) and range of motion

    (a) Check the velocity of opening
    (b) Deviation
    (c) Jaw protrusion and lateral excursion movement
    (d) Condylar subluxation

2. Joint noises

    (a) Opening clicks
    (b) Closing clicks
    (c) Crepitus
    (d) Grating sound

3. Joint and muscle pain

    (a) Check the lateral pole of the condyle by palpating the preauricular area.
    (b) Palpate masseter muscle and insertion of temporalis tendon at the coronoid process.
    (c) Palpate temple area for temporalis muscle assessment.

4. Joint loading maneuver (Mahan's sign)

    (a) A tongue blade broken in two and folded is placed in the premolar or molar area. *Direct loading* of the joint is opposite to the tongue blade. *Indirect loading* refers to the ipsilateral joint.

Radiographic Evaluation

Panoramic radiograph

- Obvious abnormal densities or opacities
- Mandibular ramus length
- Mandibular angle scalloping
- Missing teeth
- Teeth wear

TMJ cone-beam computed tomography scan (CBCT)

- Intra-articular space.
- The cortical bone and bone marrow of the condyles.
- Bone osteophytes.

- The posterior slope of the eminence.
- The author recommends sending the CBCT files to a maxillofacial radiologist to obtain a comprehensive report.

Open and closed T1–T2-weighted magnetic resonance imaging (MRI)

- Identify the condyle first.
- Locate the posterior slope of the eminence.
- Then look for the meniscus once the two previous structures have been identified.
- Look at the closed images and then the opened ones. If the reader cannot identify open and/or closed cuts, look at the teeth area to confirm.
- Displacement of the disk or not (in either open or close).
- Look for joint effusions.
- Read the report after MRI has been reviewed.
- Do not hesitate to call the radiologist for clarification.

Clinical Examination: Initial Consultation

- New patients that come to the clinic need to be approached rigorously to keep the consultation in the right direction. Having an orthopedic mindset during the consultation is recommended by the author.
- The goal is to categorize the patient into two broad groups in the first minutes of the consultation: temporomandibular joint disorders vs. orofacial pain. The latter is considered a separate entity. Therefore, it will not be addressed in this chapter.
- The systematic approach mentioned should start with basic questions and simple directions. History of the present illness should be obtained after the following is completed:
- Suggested directions and questions for the patient:

  - Open the mouth.
  - Close the mouth.
  - Move the mandible side to side.
  - Any pain or discomfort doing any of the above?
  - What did you have for breakfast this morning?
  - What happens when you chew something hard?

- If any of those actions and answers are normal, most likely, the patient will end the consultation in the orofacial pain category.
- Before starting the consultation, patients with TMD should be given a visual analog scale (VAS) form. Treatment decisions should be based on that VAS instead of advanced imaging findings. Very often, there will be patients with remarkable findings on MRIs and CBCTs who are asymptomatic with even normal joint function. The practitioner should be careful not to spend too much time reviewing first-time patients' records and concentrate more on clinical exams.

Intraoperative Consideration

- Palpation of the maximum concavity of the glenoid fossa with the tip of the thumb.
- Drawing the Holmlund-Hellsing line is recommended. Consider possible facial anatomical changes due to cosmetic surgery or previous trauma.
- The most acceptable measurements are:

  - 10–2 mm (first needle) and 20–10 mm (second needle)
  - 10–2 mm (first needle) and 7–2 mm (second needle)

- If done under IV light or moderate sedation, jaw protrusion should be considered when placing the first needle. Then, when placing the second most distal needle, the patient should be in occlusion.
- Recommended irrigation fluid: lactated Ringer (similar to human synovial fluid).
- Amount of fluids: equivalent to three 50 cc syringes (150 ml). Some authors advocate an irrigation fluid amount of up to 300 ml.
- Do not force fluids (either via cannula or needle). Sometimes the needle can be "stuck" in soft tissue or adhesions.
- Once arthrocentesis is completed, a total of 1 cc of hyaluronic acid (HA) or platelet-rich plasma (PRP) could be delivered after the procedure after removing one of the needles/portals.
- Patients should have an orthotic delivered immediately after the procedure.
- Physical therapy should be started by 24 h after the procedure.
- Physical therapy.

Stage	Goal	Exercises
I	Maintain mobility and strength	1. Limited active vertical opening, right and left excursion and protrusion 2. Isometrics in neutral
II	Increase range of motion	1. Active assisted exercises (guided by hand) to opening 2. Left and/or right side excursion 3. Protrusion
III	Smooth active range of motion without deviation or asymmetry	1. Feel for deviation in rotation, translation, and protrusion 2. Correct deviations in rotation, translation, and protrusion through isotonic resistance 3. Create smooth movement through isometrics 4. Create smooth motion with resistance throughout the range through active correction
IV	Progressively load	1. Opening and closing 2. Side excursion 3. Protrusion

Postoperative Consideration

- The patient should be seen at first week post-op.
- Physical therapy exercises should be reviewed.
- VAS form should be given to the patient and documented in the chart.
- Clinical pictures should be taken documenting MIO and occlusion.
- The patient should remain on a soft nonmechanical diet for 6 weeks and advance as tolerated.

Pearls

- Arthrocentesis can be implemented at any stage during TMD treatment.
- Protrude the jaw during the placement of the first needle. Then, when placing the second most distal needle, the patient should be in occlusion.
- Lactated Ringer is similar to human synovial fluid, and it is the recommended solution for irrigation.
- Use hyaluronic acid or PRP to supplement the procedure.

Pitfalls

- During the needle puncture, be aware of possible facial anatomical changes due to cosmetic surgery or previous trauma.
- Resistance during initial irrigation is common and indicates scarring and adhesion of the joint space.

Further Reading

Kaneyama K, Segami N, Nishimura M, Sato J, Fujimura K, Yoshimura H. The ideal lavage volume for removing bradykinin, interleukin-6 and protein from the temporomandibular joint by arthrocentesis. J Oral Maxillofac Surg. 2004;62(6):657–61.
McCain JP. Arthroscopy and arthrocentesis of the temporomandibular joint. In: Michael Miloro DM, editor. Peterson's principles of oral and maxillofacial surgery. Shelton: People's Medical Publishing House; 2011. p. 1069–122.

Chapter 39
Pearls and Pitfalls of Temporomandibular Joint Arthroscopy

Christopher K. B. Ward and Mohamed Abdel Hakim

Abstract Advanced TMJ arthroscopy is a technique-sensitive skill with a steep learning curve that requires dedication and repetition. Every step relies on the previous one, so errors compound technical difficulties. This chapter focuses on double puncture arthroscopy and should be reviewed regularly throughout learning this unique procedure, as some of the pearls and pitfalls are better understood with repetition. The purpose of this chapter is to review the pearls and pitfalls of temporomandibular joint arthroscopy.

Practical Tips

Preoperative Consideration

Patient Selection (for Beginners)

- Avoid patients with TMJ anatomy that is difficult to locate and palpate on clinical exam. For example, patients with increased facial adipose tissue from being overweight/obese can impair the palpation of anatomic landmarks and can alter the depth needed to access the joint, beyond the 25 mm safety rule (explained below).
- Avoid patients with limited neck range of motion. This will impact your ability to place the patient into an ideal position for the procedure.
- Avoid patients with a narrow joint space, making the first puncture challenging. Challenging punctures raise the risk of iatrogenic injuries.

C. K. B. Ward · M. A. Hakim (✉)
Oral and Maxillofacial Surgery and Hospital Dentistry, University of Michigan, Ann Arbor, MI, USA
e-mail: mohakim@med.umich.edu

D. Amin, H. Marwan (eds.), *Pearls and Pitfalls in Oral and Maxillofacial Surgery*, https://doi.org/10.1007/978-3-031-47307-4_39

Equipment Selection

- 0° arthroscopes are acceptable for diagnostic arthroscopy but not for operative arthroscopy because they cannot visualize the anterolateral aspect of the TMJ.
- A 30° arthroscope is recommended for advanced arthroscopy.

Intraoperative Consideration

Procedure Setup

- The head should be parallel to the floor to reduce the risk of ear injury (see technique tips below). If neck mobility is compromised, you may *airplane* the bed to achieve this position.
- There are **four** landmarks for a safe puncture:

  - **The maximum concavity of the glenoid fossa** should be palpated, and it is an important landmark for the entry point of the scope. Move the jaw forward, backward, and with a side-to-side motion (*with the condyle seated*) to palpate the relation of the condylar head to the maximum concavity. Mark this position with a dot, which will be called the fossa portal marking (Figs. 39.1 and 39.2). These movements confirm that you are palpating the glenoid fossa, not the eminence or the temporal fossa, as they allow you to palpate the **lateral pole of the condyle**. The lateral pole should align with the dot of the fossa portal and the maximum concavity of the glenoid fossa from an AP standpoint (Fig. 39.3).

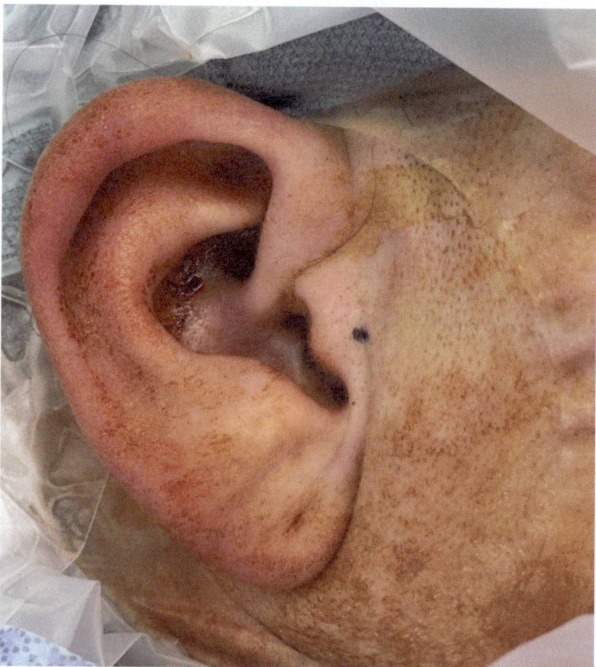

Fig. 39.1 The marking dot for the fossa portal. The marking dot is made anterior to the tragus and within the vicinity of the preauricular skin crease

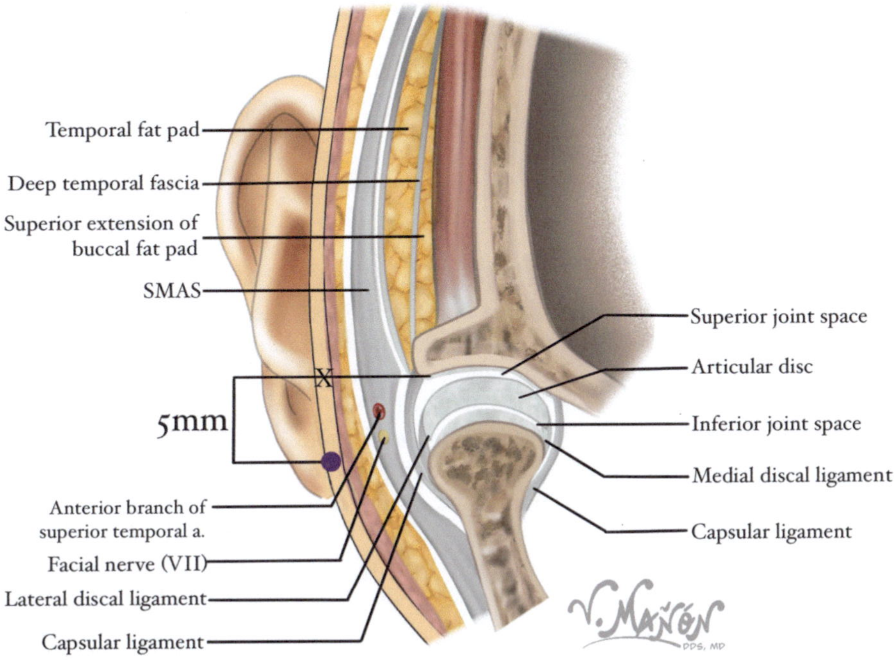

Fig. 39.2 The marking dot for the fossa portal (purple) should be 5 mm below where you palpate the maximum concavity of the glenoid fossa (**X**). This positions the scope more favorably into the superior joint space and avoids interference from the root of the zygomatic arch

Fig. 39.3 The marking dot for the fossa portal (purple) is in alignment with the condyle's lateral pole and the glenoid fossa's maximum concavity from a sagittal view

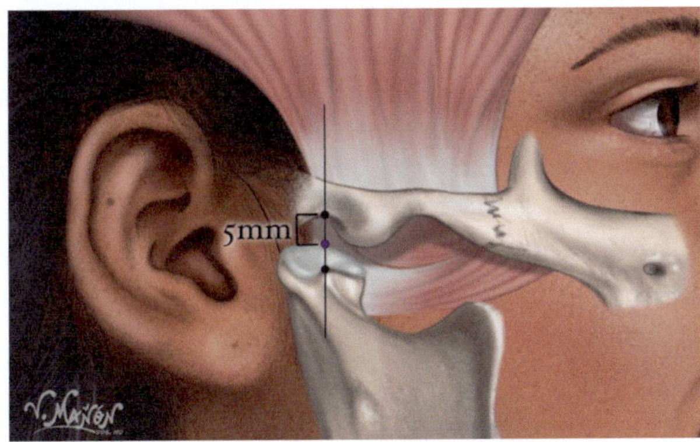

- This marking should be in front of the tragus and within proximity of the **preauricular skin crease** (Fig. 39.1). If you are too far posterior or anterior to the crease, repeat the first step.
- Lastly, examine the angulation of the **external auditory canal (EAC)** as it starts at the tragus and passes medially. An S-shaped EAC that courses anteriorly before passing medially is at a higher risk for injury.

- Pearl: The fossa portal marking dot should ideally be 5 mm below where you palpate the maximum concavity of the glenoid fossa. This positions the scope more favorably into the joint and avoids interference from the root of the zygomatic arch (Fig. 39.2).

Procedure

- Insufflation of the superior joint space

  - The insufflation puncture site is 5–10 mm inferior to the fossa portal mark. Use a 25-G needle and angle it 70–80° anteromedially and superiorly, targeting the back slope of the eminence. You should touch the bone when three-fourths of the needle is in (Fig. 39.4a–c).
  - Pitfall: An incorrect mediolateral angulation (too steep) will result in premature bony contact with the root of the zygomatic arch and failure to enter the joint. If this happens, withdraw the needle and increase your mediolateral angle closer to 80°.
  - Pitfall: Try not to move your thumb from the maximum concavity after joint insufflation to maintain this landmark (Fig. 39.4c). The distension from insufflation can distort your fossa portal marking made in the previous step.

- Trocar puncture and entry into the superior joint space

  - The side of the trocar should touch the tragus on entry for safe angulation and avoidance of EAC (Fig. 39.5b). Evaluating the EAC angulation can further guide the AP angulation of the trocar upon entry.
  - Pitfall: If the trocar is pointed too anteriorly on entry, the posterior slope of eminence will be scuffed. This is less consequential than an otologic injury.
  - The sharp tip of the trocar goes 5 mm beyond the cannula. Once you feel a "pop" from entry into the joint, switch to a pencil grip and gently spin to advance the cannula an additional 5 mm (Fig. 39.5c). The cannula will often deflect off the back slope of the eminence and enter the posterior recess.

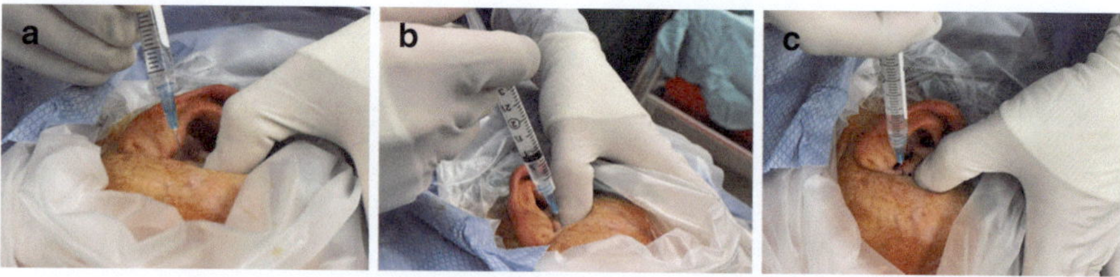

Fig. 39.4 A 25-G needle on a 3-cc syringe containing lactated Ringer's is angled 70–80° superiorly (**a**) and 70–80° anteromedially (**b**), targeting the back slope of the eminence. You should touch the bone when three-fourths of the needle is in (**c**). Try not to move your thumb from the maximum concavity after joint insufflation to maintain this landmark (**b, c**)

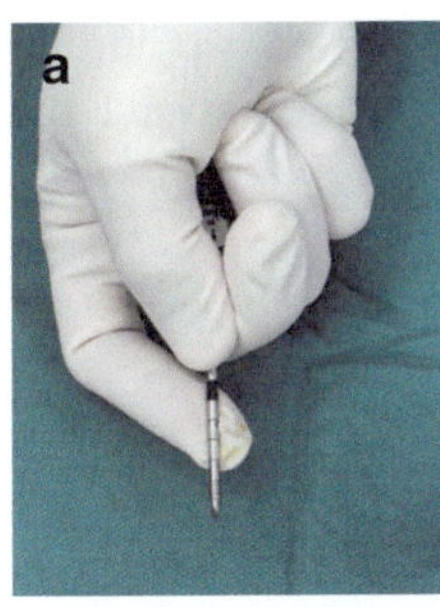
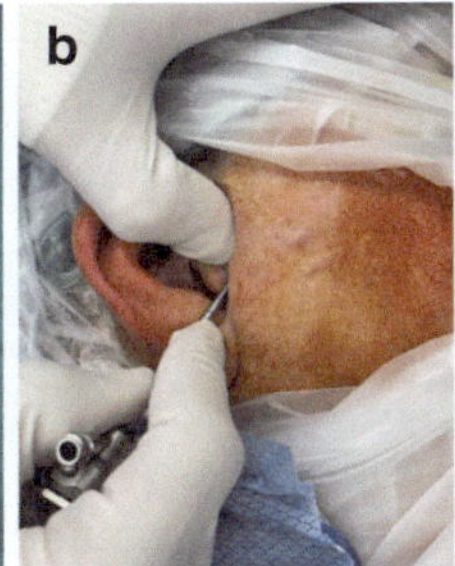
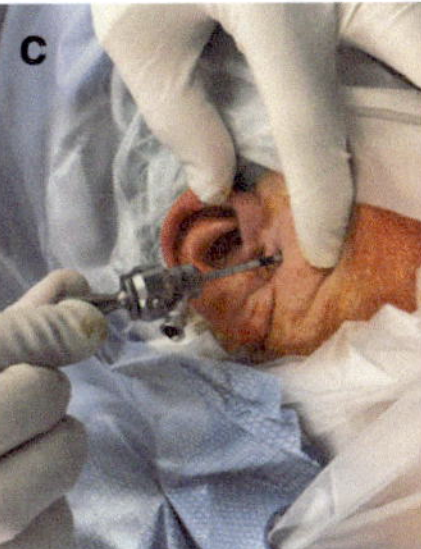
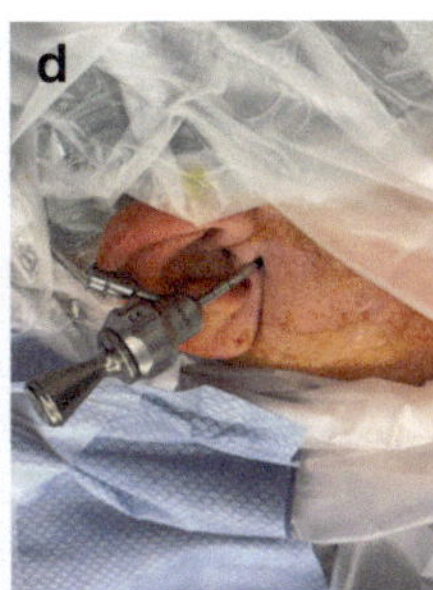

Fig. 39.5 Proper grip for holding the trocar for puncture into the joint capsule (**a**), the side of the trocar should touch the tragus on entry for safe angulation and avoidance of EAC (**b**) targeting the back slope of the articular eminence. Switch to a pencil grip and gently spin to advance the cannula an additional 5 mm (**c**), and then insert the sharp trocar and cannula to a maximum of **25 mm** (**d**)

Fig. 39.6 Puncturing the skin too cephalad will result in your scope pointing inferiorly. This will result in interference against the zygomatic arch/articular eminence when accessing the anterior recess

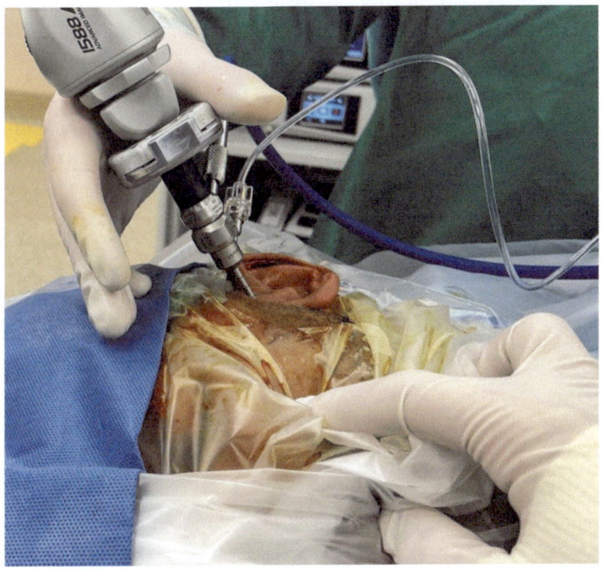

- If you puncture the skin too cephalad (refer to setup), your scope will point inferiorly, and you will struggle against the zygomatic arch/articular eminence (Fig. 39.6), especially when trying to access the anterior recess.
- Insert the sharp trocar and cannula to a maximum of 25 mm upon initial insertion (Fig. 39.5d).
- Pitfall: The middle of the superior joint space is, on average, 25 mm from the overlying skin, while the tympanic membrane is, on average, 35 mm from the tragus. Inserting the trocar deeper than 25 mm with the wrong angulation can result in perforation of the tympanic membrane, entry into the middle ear, damage to the auditory ossicles, and permanent hearing loss.

- – Pearl: In the event of poor AP angulation, where you inadvertently point too far posteriorly, the 25 mm rule will limit the injury to the EAC and save the patient from injury to the middle ear.

- Placement of a second cannula for operative arthroscopy

  - – Once a surgeon is comfortable with access and can consistently perform a diagnostic (level I) arthroscopy, placing a second cannula allows the surgeon to perform advanced arthroscopic procedures.
  - – To place a second cannula, the 30° arthroscope should be navigated into the anterior recess of the TMJ; you should visualize where the anterior slope of eminence meets the anterior synovial drape. A bubble can often be seen in this region along the anterolateral portion of the recess (Fig. 39.7).
  - – Pearl: Having your assistant seat the condyle posteriorly in a closed-mouth position will help present and open the anterior recess. Depressing the molars inferiorly in this position will help open the anterior recess further.
  - – Upon entering the most anterolateral portion of the joint, measure how deep the scope is, and measure the same distance on the skin for your second puncture to create an equilateral triangle (Figs. 39.8 and 39.9).
  - – Pearl: The most common distance from the first puncture site to the anterolateral recess is 25 mm. If your measurement is different, double-check your scope depth and location.
  - – Pearl: Seeing the lateral aspect of the joint capsule moving on your arthroscopic view when applying pressure to the selected second puncture site confirms the correct position. Use a 22-G needle to sound the path of the second puncture before switching to a trocar. The angulation and position of the 22-G needle should then be replicated with the trocar (Fig. 39.8a–f).

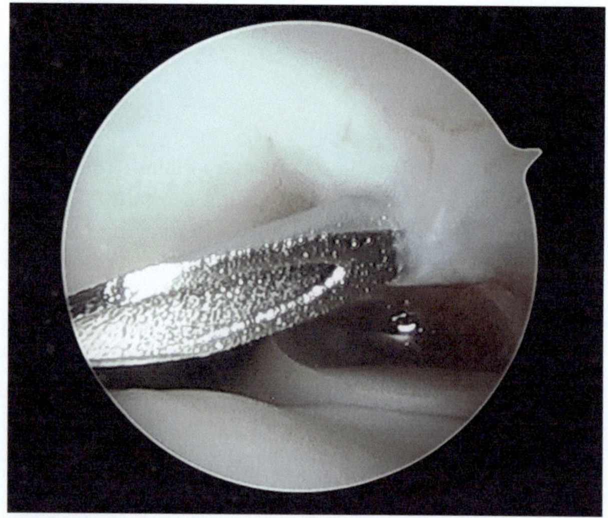

Fig. 39.7 The bubble is seen in the anterolateral region of the anterior recess. A 22-G needle is inserted into this region to confirm the path of the second puncture before switching to a sharp trocar to replicate the angle of insertion of the needle

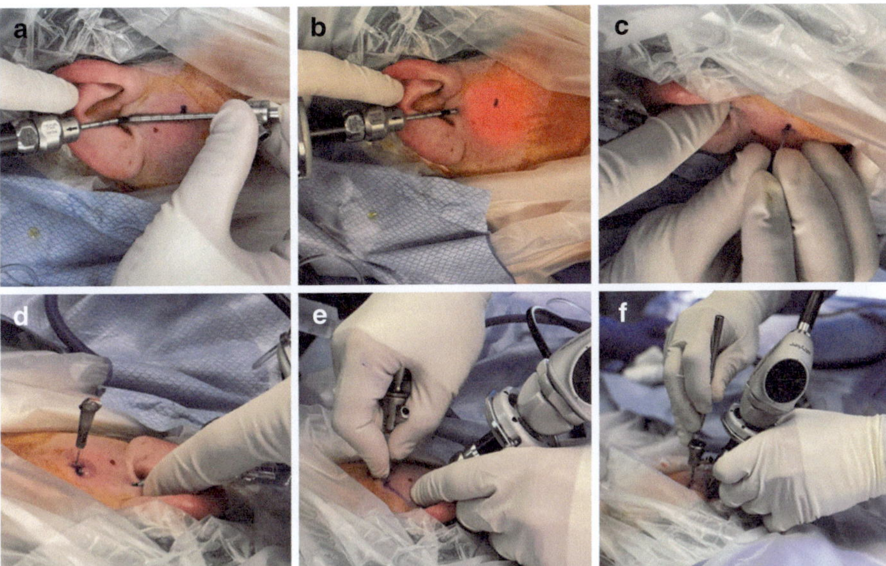

Fig. 39.8 Sequence for placement of a second cannula for operative arthroscopy. After navigating into the anterior recess, the measuring cannula marks the depth of the arthroscope on the external skin (**a**). This is most commonly measured at 25 mm, and a mark is made at this point for the second puncture. This mark can be verified by transillumination from the arthroscope (**b**). Use a 22-G needle to sound the path of the second puncture and visualize its entry into the anterior recess with the arthroscope before switching to a trocar (**c**, **d**). The angulation and position of the 22-G needle should then be replicated with the trocar to establish the secondary cannula port (**e**, **f**)

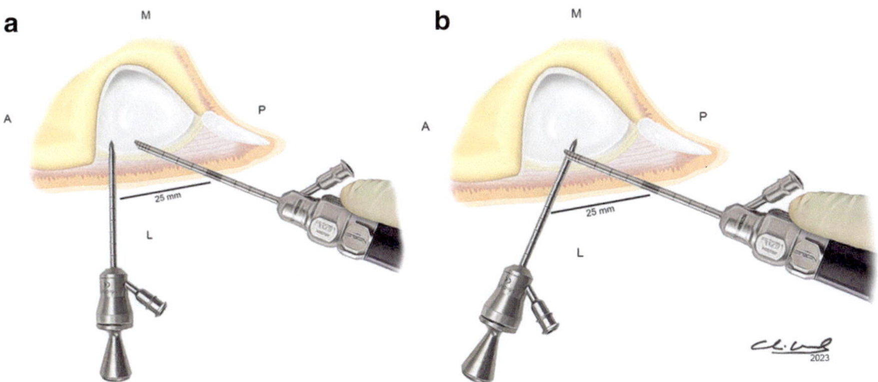

Fig. 39.9 Appropriate angulation of the second trocar into the anterior recess of the joint space. This is done by keeping 25 mm between the 30° arthroscope and the trocar and keeping the trocar in view during entry (**a**). Pointing too far posteriorly on the entry will result in not being able to see the operative cannula as it will be entering the joint space behind the view of the arthroscope (**b**)

- Pointing too far posteriorly during the second puncture could result in two issues:

  You will not see the operative cannula since it will be crossing behind the view of your scope.
  The first and second punctures are too close together, limiting your ability to operate in the anterior part of the joint.

- Pitfall: Multiple punctures in the joint capsule or excessive irrigation pressure can increase the risk of fluid extravasation, which increases postoperative swelling and discomfort if the extravasation is lateral or prolonged intubation if the extravasation is medial toward the lateral pharyngeal space.
- Pearl: In the event of lateral pharyngeal space extravasation, consider keeping the patient intubated for 1–2 h in an advanced care setting until the irrigant dissipates.
- Multiple attempts to puncture this region can lead to scuffing the anterior slope of the articular eminence.

Further Reading

Hakim MA, McCain JP, Ahn DY, Troulis MJ. Minimally invasive endoscopic oral and maxillofacial surgery. Oral Maxillofac Surg Clin North Am. 2019;31(4):561–7. https://doi.org/10.1016/j.coms.2019.07.001. Epub 2019 Aug 28.

McCain JP, Hossameldin RH. TMJ arthroscopy. In: Kademani D, Tiwana P, editors. Atlas of oral and maxillofacial surgery, vol. 2015. Philadelphia: Saunders; 2015. p. 1310–9.

Chapter 40
Pearl and Pitfalls of Total Joint Replacement of the Temporomandibular Joint

Patrick Wong, Courtney Evans, and Likith Reddy

Abstract Over the past few decades, alloplastic temporomandibular joint replacement (TJR) has proven to be a successful and predictable treatment modality for various temporomandibular joint (TMJ) pathologies. The primary goal of TMJ replacement (TJR) is to restore the form and function of the joint. The artificial joint can improve the range of motion and function of the jaw and is designed to last many years, providing long-term relief. But as with any surgical procedure, some potential risks and complications are associated with TMJ replacement surgery. There is the risk of bleeding, infection, nerve damage resulting in numbness and/or weakness in the jaw or face, and the potential for infection, loosening, or displacement of the artificial joint over time, requiring additional surgery to correct. Successful TJR surgery begins with proper patient selection and the preoperative workup. Although TJR can eliminate some patients' pain, the primary goal is restoring function; therefore, the surgeon must identify an actual articular pathology requiring joint replacement instead of simply treating TMJ pain.

Once the decision has been made to proceed with alloplastic TJR, a decision is made on whether a custom, patient-specific prosthesis or a mass-produced, stock prosthesis will be used. Presently, in the United States, there are two FDA-approved devices for TJR. The custom prosthesis is made by TMJ Concepts (Ventura, CA), and a stock prosthesis is available off the shelf and produced by Biomet-Lorenz Stock TJR (Parsippany, NJ). The indications for both prostheses are described below. TJR using custom prostheses is technically easier as the prosthesis components have been made specifically for the patient and are inherently easier to index. Furthermore, they can be used in a wider variety of patients. The disadvantage of custom joints compared to stock joints is that they are more costly and can take months to fabricate compared to their mass-produced, immediately available off-

P. Wong · C. Evans · L. Reddy (✉)
Oral and Maxillofacial Surgery, Texas A&M College of Dentistry, Dallas, TX, USA
e-mail: lreddy@tamu.edu

the-shelf counterparts. The purpose of this chapter is to review pearls and pitfalls in total joint replacement of the temporomandibular joint.

Practical Tips

Preoperative Considerations

Selection of Devices Custom vs. Stock

- Although recent evidence has shown that stock prostheses would fit in about 75% of patients requiring TJR, there are certain limitations to the stock prosthesis that would necessitate a custom prosthesis be fabricated.
- Common indications for custom TMJ prosthesis include:

  - Unusual or aberrant anatomy due to previous surgeries, trauma, congenital defects
  - Patients with craniofacial syndromes
  - Combined orthognathic surgery and planned mandibular advancements
  - Patients whose gap arthroplasty will exceed >35 mm

- Common indications for using stock TMJ prosthesis include:

  - Typical jaw anatomy
  - First TMJ replacement surgery

Intraoperative Considerations

- During the initial preauricular dissection, inadvertent entry into the external auditory meatus can occur if dissection is carried too far posteriorly. The dissection should proceed anteriorly to the tragal cartilage to reach the zygomatic arch and glenoid fossa.
- The initial incision may be endaural or preauricular based on the surgeon's preference; a small superior extension can help reduce unnecessary traction injury to the temporal branch of the facial nerve (CN VII).
- The main anatomic structure to negotiate during the preauricular approach is the frontal branch of the facial nerve (CN VII), as it courses anterosuperiorly along Pitanguy's line. Traction injury to the nerve due to excess retraction is a common cause of temporal branch weakness postoperatively. During the submandibular access, the marginal mandibular branch of the facial nerve (CN VII) can be in close approximation to the dissection as it travels anteriorly. In 19% of cases, the marginal mandibular branch will be found below the inferior border of the mandible in the region of the dissection. Care must be taken to avoid the nerve and have the nerve reflected carefully within the flap superiorly.

- Bleeding may occur at several points during the surgery. During the initial pre-auricular dissection, the superficial temporal vessels will be coursing parallel to the incision line. It is best to stay posterior to these vessels and cauterize/ligate them before they cause unnecessary bleeding and staining of the surgical field. A potential life-threatening bleeding may occur during the condylectomy portion of the procedure as the internal maxillary artery lies, on average, 5.1 mm medial to the medial extent of the sigmoid notch. This bleeding may be particularly difficult to stop due to poor visualization and retraction of the vessel.
- Prior to exposure of the zygomatic arch, there is commonly a small vessel traveling just over the arch; this vessel should be cauterized with bipolar or monopolar cautery before incision into the arch.
- It is often easier to perform the condylectomy in two steps, and the initial condylectomy usually does not leave a gap arthroplasty long enough to accommodate the minimum of 1.5 cm for the prosthetic device.
- After the initial condylectomy, a Dingman or Kocher bone clamp can be placed through the submandibular incision to direct the condylar stump superiorly and laterally to facilitate a second osteotomy in the most inferior aspect of the sigmoid notch. The lateral displacement will also direct the mandible away from the intermaxillary artery.
- Prior to entry into the oral cavity through the sterile Tegaderm, having a single surgeon drape the field off with sterile towels and place the patient into MMF can help reduce the risk of intraoral contamination of the prosthetic joints.
- In cases where the patient is edentulous or cannot reliably be placed into MMF, custom-fabricated surgical guides can be used to place predictive screw holes to help position the mandible in the desired position without the use of MMF.
- Poor fit of the prosthesis in TJR with a custom joint is usually due to inadequate dissection, as the device usually readily indexes into position.
- In the case of TJR with a stock prosthesis, some shaping of the glenoid fossa or buccal aspect of the ascending ramus may be required, which may be difficult for the novice surgeon.
- Frequently, the zygomatic arch and glenoid fossa must be shaped to be parallel to the Frankfort horizontal line. Furthermore, the surgeon must adequately remove any interferences on the medial aspect of the fossa component to avoid improper seating. Finally, in cases where the patient has a v-shaped mandible, the lateral ramus often needs to be reduced to prevent lateral flaring of the prosthesis.

Postoperative Considerations

- Postoperatively, patients should be initiated on early rehabilitation to facilitate early return to function; this can be accomplished with a TheraBite or tongue blade.

- Postoperatively, infection of the prosthesis is a dreaded complication. Sterile technique is imperative during the procedure. Operators should attempt to keep any contamination from the oral cavity to a minimum by covering the mouth with a sterile Tegaderm, except when the patient is wired into maxillomandibular fixation (MMF). The operator placing the patient into MMF should also replace the Tegaderm afterward and change their gloves to avoid joint contamination.
- Most cases of postoperative weakness to the marginal mandibular or temporal branches of the facial nerve (CN VII) are transient neuropraxia from retraction that will resolve with time.

Complications

- Periprosthetic joint infection: organisms that cause early (within 3 months after surgery) infections are introduced at the time of surgery, while late (3 months to 2 years after surgery) infections are more likely hematogenous in etiology. However, controlling sterility of the field and prosthesis, providing perioperative antibiotics and improving patient nutrition, controlling systemic disease, and smoking cessation can minimize the likelihood of infection.
- Heterotopic bone formation: Bone formation around the TMJ prosthesis where the native bone does not normally exist. This can result in pain and limit function. Surgical removal of bone is necessary to regain mobility in combination with autogenous fat grafting to prevent a recurrence.
- Dislocation: Anterior condylar component dislocation is more common in patients with unilateral or bilateral coronoidectomy. Posterior condylar component dislocation is typically seen when TMJ prosthesis does not utilize a posterior stop in combination with orthognathic surgery. Immediate dislocation is managed with manual reduction and light intermaxillary elastic traction placement. Late dislocation may require surgical intervention should manual reduction be inadequate.
- Persistent or worsening pain: both intrinsic (nociception from somatic or visceral tissue) and extrinsic (non-nociceptive pain) pain are associated with TMJ prosthesis. The surgeon must appropriately diagnose and manage properly.
- Material hypersensitivity: can likely be avoided with adequate medical history and allergy testing. Custom prostheses can be fabricated with all titanium metal components with prior FDA approval.

Pearls

1. Temporomandibular joint replacement (TJR) can predictably restore function in even severely debilitated patients; however, pain may persist, especially in patients with centralized pain mechanisms.

2. Both stock and custom TJR prostheses can be used; however, the surgeon must consider the indications for both options and tailor the choice based on the specific patient.
3. A two-stage condylectomy can safely ensure the surgeon has removed enough of the proximal mandible to fit the prosthesis and avoid excessive bleeding.

Pitfalls

1. Excess retraction forces can cause transient or permanent weakness to the facial nerve branches encountered in the preauricular and submandibular dissections. Extension of incisions can help avoid undue retraction forces.
2. Significant bleeding from the internal maxillary artery can be encountered during the condylectomy or coronoidectomy if sharp instruments are placed too far from the mandible.
3. Contamination of the joint with flora from the oral cavity should be minimized. The mouth should be covered with a sterile Tegaderm during the entire procedure except for when the surgeon places the patient into maxillomandibular fixation (MMF).

Further Reading

Abramowicz S, et al. Adaptability of Stock TMJ Prosthesis to Joints That Were Previously Treated with Custom Joint Prosthesis. International Journal of Oral and Maxillofacial Surgery. 2011;41(4):518–20. Web.

Brown ZL, Sarrami S, Perez DE. Will They Fit? Determinants of the Adaptability of Stock TMJ Prosthesis Where Custom TMJ Prosthesis Were Utilized. International Journal of Oral and Maxillofacial Surgery. 2021;50(2):220–26. Web.

Hakan O, et al. Maxillary Artery : Anatomical Landmarks and Relationship with the Mandibular Subcondyle. Plastic and Reconstructive Surgery (1963). 2007;120(7):1865–70. Web.

Harper DE, Schrepf A, Clauw DJ. Pain Mechanisms and Centralized Pain in Temporomandibular Disorders. Journal of Dental Research. 2016;95(10):1102–1108. https://doi.org/10.1177/0022034516657070.

Louis GM. Temporomandibular Joint Total Joint Replacement – TMJ TJR A Comprehensive Reference for Researchers, Materials Scientists, and Surgeons. Ed. Louis G. Mercuri. 1st ed. 2016. Cham: Springer International Publishing. 2016. Web.

Reed OD, Grabb WC. Surgical anatomy of the mandibular ramus of the facial nerve based on the dissection of 100 facial halves. Plastic and Reconstructive Surgery (1963). 1962;29(3):266–72. Web.

Siegmund BJ, et al. Reconstruction of the temporomandibular joint: a comparison between prefabricated and customized alloplastic prosthetic total joint systems. International Journal of Oral and Maxillofacial Surgery. 2019;48(8):1066–71. Web.

Chapter 41
Pearls and Pitfalls in Botox Injections for TMD

Jose Montero and Jorge Beltran

Abstract OnabotulinumtoxinA (Botox®) corresponds to a neurotoxin protein secreted by the bacterium *Clostridium Botulinum*. Its mechanism corresponds to blocking the release of acetylcholine from presynaptic motor nerve endings, resulting in the relaxation of muscles and the relief of neurogenic pain. It has an analgesic effect at the central level, although it is still controversial in the literature. Botox® affects the nociceptive mechanism by preventing the release of inflammatory mediators such as glutamate and substance P. Ultimately, its analgesic action also includes an effect on the postganglionic sympathetic ending, inhibiting the release of norepinephrine and ATP, two stimulating neurotransmitters of muscle nociceptors.

The application of botulinum toxin in its subtypes A and B is widely used in the management of the muscular component of temporomandibular disorders as a second line of treatment or as a coadjuvant strategy to reduce joint loading from masticatory muscles and to reduce intramuscular pain associated with parafunctional habits (e.g., clenching, teeth grinding). Botox® therapy is often combined with traditional medical/conservative management such as orthotic therapy, NSAIDS, muscle relaxants, diet restrictions, patient education, physical therapy, etc.

A relevant element to consider when using Botox® is the correct indication. To do this, we must consider some diagnoses and conditions to be ruled out, which can confuse the clinician at the time of patient evaluation and lead to the use of this therapy incorrectly and with uncertain results.

Among these, we have:

- Postherpetic neuralgia.
- Postherpetic trigeminal neuralgia.
- Painful anesthesia.
- Persistent dentoalveolar pain.

J. Montero (✉)
Jackson Memorial Hospital/University of Miami, Miami, FL, USA

J. Beltran
Department of Oral and Maxillofacial Surgery, School of Dentistry, University of Concepción, Concepción, Chile

© The Author(s), under exclusive license to Springer Nature Switzerland AG 2024
D. Amin, H. Marwan (eds.), *Pearls and Pitfalls in Oral and Maxillofacial Surgery*, https://doi.org/10.1007/978-3-031-47307-4_41

- Giant cell arteritis.
- Post-traumatic pain.
- Chronic migraine.
- Pain associated with cancer.
- Intra-articular pain (TMJ).
- Burning mouth syndrome.
- Persistent idiopathic facial pain.
- Neuralgia trigeminal.
- Glossopharyngeal neuralgia.

Preoperative Evaluation

It is important to assess the general masticatory muscle architecture prior to considering Botox® application. Hypertrophic masseter and temporalis muscles are usually reasonably easy to identify (Fig. 41.1). Muscle firmness and volume should also be documented during the clinical exams. Lastly, preoperative radiographic evaluation can help identify clenching or teeth grinding signs by looking at the mandibular angles. A scalloping pattern at the mandibular angles secondary to excessive masseter strength is often noticed in clencher and grinder patients (Fig. 41.2).

Technique and Doses

The most common injection sites, according to the literature, are:

1. Temporal and masseter muscles.
2. Lateral pterygoid muscle.
3. Intra-articular TMJ injection.

Fig. 41.1 Masseter hypertrophy

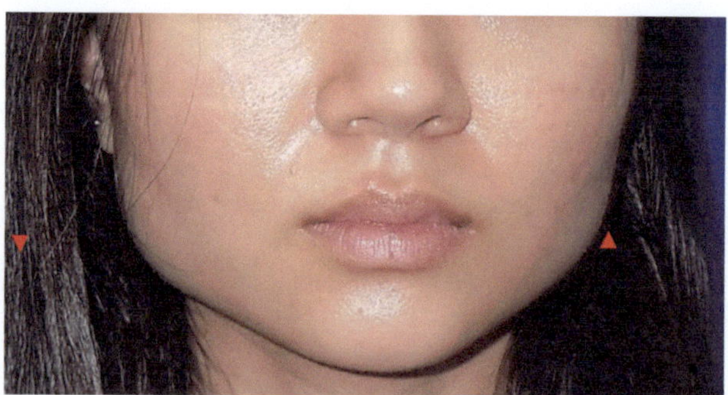

Fig. 41.2 Mandibular angle scalloping

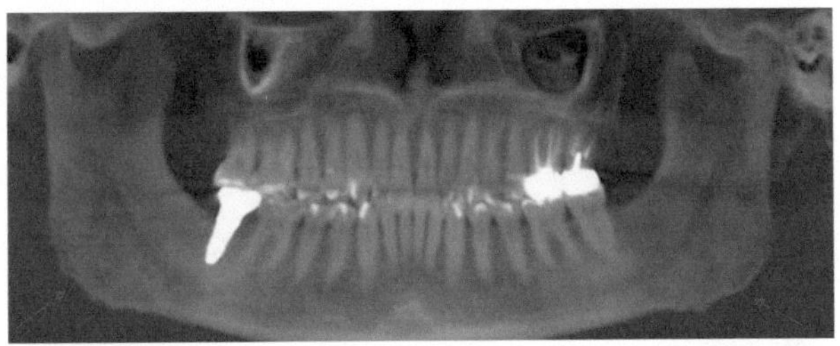

Regarding the dose, it is important to note that there is no consensus regarding the number of units to be infiltrated in each muscle. Another element to consider is that the presentations and dilution methods, as well as the potency per unit of a solution, are different according to the manufacturer, so the clinician must necessarily become familiar with each presentation of botulinum toxin prior to its administration in the patient. Brands authorized by the U.S. Food and Drug Administration (FDA) include Botox® (onabotulinumtoxinA), Dysport® (abobotulinumtoxinA), Xeomin® (incobotulinumtoxinA), and Myobloc® (rimabotulinumtoxinB).

The variety of commercial options make it difficult to find a universally adopted dosage protocol based on effects obtained by using botulinum toxin, so it is advisable to standardize the brand of drug to be used. On the other hand, it is agreed that the desired effect of muscle relaxation and analgesia is associated with the amount and concentration of botulinum toxin used. Most studies show promising results in relieving painful symptoms and muscle relaxation using between 20 and 40 U on each muscle as well as multiple points of injection (Table 41.1). It is estimated that the lethal dose goes between 2700 and 3000 IU, which is quite far from what is indicated in managing temporomandibular disorders. Finally, a periodicity of control is recommended at 3 and 12 weeks.

Infiltration in Temporal and Masseter Muscles

The safe zone for intramuscular infiltration of the masseter is defined by a line joining the tragus and the labial commissure (Fig. 41.3), while the anterior and posterior boundary of this zone is determined by the respective edges of the masseter. The injection of three to five points near the lower insertion of the masseter is described in the literature.

The patient is observed for 30 min after injection in case of an adverse reaction, which is rare.

The most common doses of Botox® range from 25 to 50 IU from each masseter muscle, according to pain severity and muscle volume. The authors recommend 25 units as a minimum dose for the average patient. Injections of Botox in the temporalis muscle area usually maintain in the anterior aspect of the muscle anatomy. Four to five points are selected. Twenty-five units of Botox® is usually sufficient to achieve a therapeutic effect (Fig. 41.4).

Table 41.1 Amount of units and locations

Author	Dosage used	Number of injection points in each muscle	Number of patients	Result
Justo M. Alcolea et al. (2019)	30_95 u in each patient 7–5-19 U by injection	Three points (masseter)	25	Success
Luca Guarda-Nardini y cols. (2014)	30 U masseter 20 U temporalis	Four points (masseter) Three points (temporalis)	20	Success
Hessa Al-Wayli et al. (2017)	20 S	Three points (masseter)	50	Success
Long-dan Zhang y cols. (2016)	25 S	Three points (masseter)	30	Success
Young Joo Shim y cols. (2020)	25 U masseter 25 U temporalis	Two points	23	Success
William G. Ondo et al. (2018)	60 U masseter 40 U temporalis	Two points (masseters) Three points (temporalis)	23	Success
Fatih Asutay et al. (2017)	20 U masseter	Four points (masseter)	25	Success

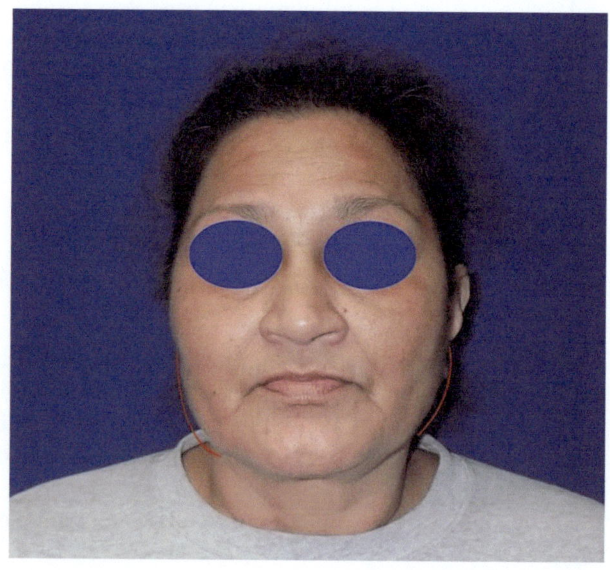

Fig. 41.3 Masseter muscle suggested injection points

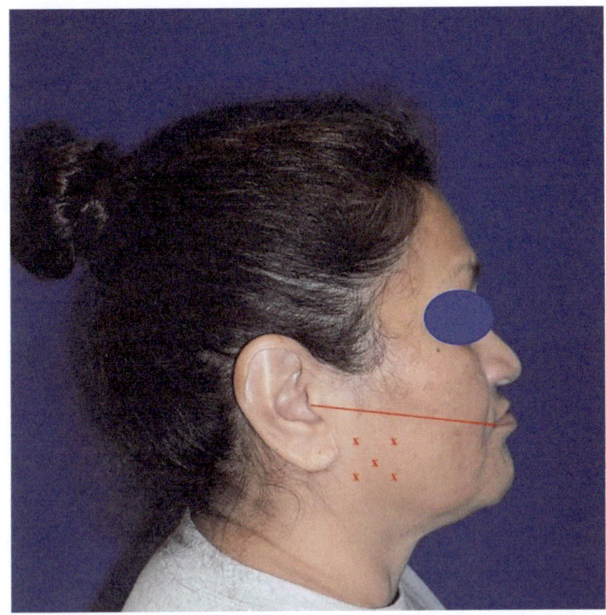

Fig. 41.4 Temporalis muscle suggested injection points

Technique: (Botox®)

- Reconstitute following manufacture instructions:

  100 unit vial: Dilute with 2.50 mL of preservative-free 0.9% sodium chloride, USP only.

  50 unit vial: Dilute with 1.25 mL of preservative-free 0.9% sodium chloride, USP only.

  Resulting dose for both dilutions: 4 units per 0.1 mL.

- Use a TB/insulin syringe with a 30 G needle.
- Prep the area with an alcohol pad.
- Palpate the anatomy of the muscle looking for tender/painful points. When found, proceed to deposit 0.1 mL in the selected area. Asking the patient to clench prior to injection helps to have a better clinical impression of the muscle shape and boundaries. The patient can relax the muscles after the selected area has been identified. Aspirate, if possible, prior to injection.
- Apply pressure if it is noticed that a small capillary vessel has been encountered.
- Provide an ice pack to the patient after completing the session.

Infiltration in Lateral Pterygoid Muscle

Based on the pathophysiological mechanisms that generate TMJ clicks and their probable relationship, an increase in the tone of the lateral pterygoid muscle and its influence on the disc position when using botulinum toxin can lead to reducing the symptoms and signs derived from the such condition; this considering its muscle relaxation effect.

Technique

After reconstitution (see previous muscle group).

Intraoral

The patient is placed supine, with a slight back tilt of the head and maximum mouth opening. From the contralateral side, at an angle of 45° to the tuberosity, is directed to the condyle neck, to the insertion area of the lateral pterygoid.

Arthroscopically

During TMJ arthroscopy, the fullness of the lateral pterygoid muscle can be identified in the most anterior-medial aspect of the superior joint space. This location is described arthroscopically as the "pterygoid shadow." See (Fig. 41.5). As it can be

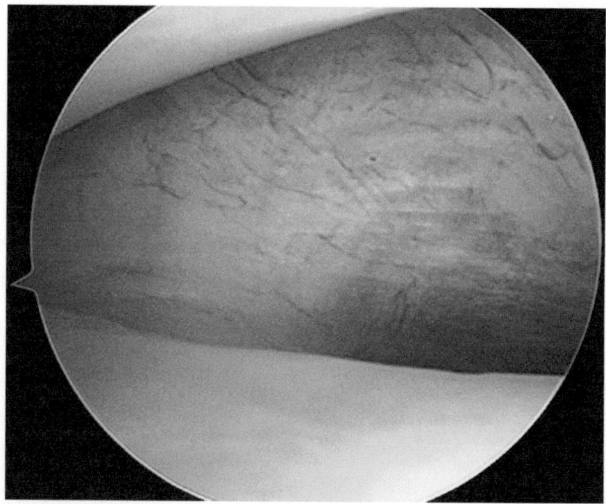

Fig. 41.5 Pterygoid shadow

appreciated, Botox® can be easily directed into the muscle once it is visualized arthroscopically. A 20 G or 22 G spinal needle can be used.

Intra-Articular Infiltration

has been described in the literature, and its main objective is reducing pain due to its antinociceptive effect, inhibiting inflammatory mediators, and releasing neuropeptides from joint nociceptors, thereby decreasing joint pain and neurogenic inflammation. There are not many reports of results and techniques. The authors do not consider intra-articular injection a great advantage, considering the well-known and documented benefits of other medications used in intra-articular infiltration (i.e., sodium hyaluronate, steroids, plasma-derived products, etc.).

Good results have been described with the use of doses of 30 U in each joint, with a decrease in pain for 3 months; doses of 20 IU were insufficient for management, and higher doses (40–50 U) have not been shown to have better results.

Batifol et al. describe the technique of intra-articular injection of Botox® as follows:

- Contralateral head rotation.
- Undiluted 1% subcutaneous local anesthesia in TMJ area.
- Using the indicated dilution, 30 IU is infiltrated into each joint.
- The anatomical reference points are the posterior edge of the condyle and the ramus and the lower edge of the zygomatic arch to obtain 30 IU (Botox®), which can be better palpated when asking the patient to open the mouth.
- Using the indicated dilution, 30 IU is infiltrated into each joint using a 23 G needle of 0.6 mm in diameter and 25 mm in length, which is introduced into the posterosuperior border of the condyle in the joint space.

Complications

When injecting Botox→, we must bear in mind that its local and systemic distribution depends on the following factors:

(a) Propagation: It is the physical movement of the toxin and is subject to variables related to the injection technique, volume, and size of the needle.
(b) Diffusion: Where the soluble molecule is dispersed by passive transport beyond its injection site, calculated for botulinum toxin at approximately 1 cm.
(c) Migration: By axonal-neuronal transport or hematogenous pathway.
(d) Volume and dilution.

The literature reports a low incidence of side effects after treatment. All of them were transient and of short duration in time—to mention in descending order:

- Effects on chewing such as sensitivity, fatigue, and difficulty.
- Unwanted aesthetic change (lower lip, eyelid).
- Pain at injection site.
- Ecchymosis edema and speech difficulty.

Further Reading

Sari BC, Develi T. The effect of intraarticular botulinum toxin-A injection on symptoms of temporomandibular joint disorder. J Stomatol Oral Maxillofac Surg. 2022;123:e316–20.

Lora VR, Clemente-Napimoga JT, Abdalla HB, Macedo CG, Canales GT, Barbosa CM. Botulinum toxin type A reduces inflammatory hypernociception induced by arthritis in the temporomadibular joint of rats. Toxicon. 2017;129:52–7.

Drinovac Vlah V, Filipović B, Bach-Rojecky L, Lacković Z. Role of central versus peripheral opioid system in antinociceptive and anti-inflammatory effect of botulinum toxin type A in trigeminal region. Eur J Pain. 2018;22:583–91.

Matak I. Involvement of substance P in the antinociceptive effect of botulinum toxin type A: evidence from knockout mice. Neuroscience. 2017;358:137–45.

Batifol D, Huart A, Finiels PJ, Nagot N, Jammet P. Effect of intra-articular botulinum toxin injections on temporo-mandibular joint pain. J Stomatol Oral Maxillofac Surg. 2018;119(4):319–24.

Zakrzewska JM. Differential diagnosis of facial pain and guidelines for management. Br J Anaesth. 2013;111(1):95–104.

Schiffman E, Ohrbach R, Truelove E, Look J, Anderson G, Goulet JP, et al. Diagnostic criteria for temporomandibular disorders (DC/TMD) for clinical and research applications: recommendations of the international RDC/TMD consortium network and orofacial pain special interest group. J Oral Facial Pain Headache. 2014;28(1):6–27.

Ernberg M. Efficacy of botulinum toxin type A for treatment of persistent myofascial TMD pain: a randomized, controlled, double-blind multicenter study. Pain. 2011;152:1988–96.

Thambar. Botulinum toxin in the management of temporomandibular disorders: a systematic review. Br J Oral Maxillofac Surg. 2020;58:508–19.

Patel J, Cardoso J, Mehta S. A systematic review of botulinum toxin in the management of patients with temporomandibular disorders and bruxism. Br Dent J. 2019;226:667–72.

Schwartz M. Treatment of temporomandibular disorders with botulinum toxin. Clin J Pain. 2002;18(6):198–203.

Kim SY. Treatment of non-odontogenic orofacial pain using botulinum toxin-A: a retrospective case series study. Maxillofac Plast Reconstr Surg. 2018;40:21.

Mor N. Temporomandibular myofascial pain treated with botulinum toxin injection. Toxins (Basel). 2015;7(8):2791–800.

Clark GT. The management of oromandibular motor disorders and facial spasms with injections of botulinum toxin. Phys Med Rehabil Clin N Am. 2003;14(4):727–48.

Alvarez-Pinzon N. Botulinum toxin for the treatment of temporomandibular disorders. Int J Odontostomat. 2018;12(2):103–9.

Ramirez-Castaneda J. Diffusion, spread, and migration of botulinum toxin. Mov Disord. 2013;28(13):1775–83.

Katz H. Botulinum toxins in dentistry—the new paradigm for masticatory muscle hypertonicity. Dent J. 2005;27(1):7–12.

Alcolea JM. Bruxism treatment with botulinum toxin type A. Prospective clinical study. Cir Plást Iberolatinoam. 2019;45(4):435–48.

Ondo WG. Onabotulinum toxin-A injections for sleep bruxism. Neurology. 2018;90(7):e559–64.

Guarda-Nardini L. Efficacy of botulinum toxin in treating myofascial pain in bruxers: a controlled placebo pilot study. Cranio. 2008;26(2):126–35.

Al-Wayli H. Treatment of chronic pain associated with nocturnal bruxism with botulinum toxin. A prospective and randomized clinical study. Journal of clinical and experimental. Dentistry. 2017;9(1):e112–7.

Shim YJ. Botulinum toxin therapy for managing sleep bruxism: a randomized and placebo—controlled trial. Toxins (Basel). 2020;12(3):168.

Part VII
Facial Cosmetic Surgery

Chapter 42
Injectable Soft Tissue Fillers and Their Use in Facial Rejuvenation

Daria Hamrah and Brayann Aleman

Abstract Minimally invasive and nonsurgical procedures for facial rejuvenation have increased exponentially in the last decade. The main reasons for the above are the consumer's demand for reduced downtime and accessibility of cosmetic treatments, as well as the increased awareness with emphasis on self-improvement. That is why in particular dermal fillers and neuromodulators have been increasingly performed not just by surgeons but also physicians across all specialties as well as mid-level practitioners at medical spas. This is not surprising as dermal fillers have become the gateway treatment in aesthetic medicine and have become a household name in our society globally.

Keeping up to date with the accelerated evolution of injectables is challenging for many practitioners and demands continuous education and knowledge update.

With the increasing popularity of social media, the above trend has increased exponentially as the "selfie culture" has made us more aware and observant of our facial features than ever before. This coupled with the race to compete with the aesthetic norms and constant comparison with our peers and beauty idols has created what is today known as "Zoom dysmorphia." The latter, classically known as body dysmorphic syndrome, has been reported in the literature to comprise roughly 7–10% of patients walking into an aesthetic practice.

Today, dermal filler treatments have increased by 174%, with an average of 3,410,730 fillers injected. This is despite the decreased access to cosmetic procedures from 2019 to 2020 due to the COVID-19 pandemic (Plastic Surgery Statistics Report, 2020).

Despite the above trend, there has been a paradigm shift in the way we utilize facial fillers in aesthetic medicine today. Traditionally, fillers were utilized to coun-

D. Hamrah (✉) · B. Aleman
NOVA SurgiCare, PC, McLean, VA, USA
e-mail: drhamrah@novasurgicare.com
http://www.novasurgicare.com

© The Author(s), under exclusive license to Springer Nature Switzerland AG 2024
D. Amin, H. Marwan (eds.), *Pearls and Pitfalls in Oral and Maxillofacial Surgery*, https://doi.org/10.1007/978-3-031-47307-4_42

ter the gravitational effects of the aging process, which is initiated by the increased laxity of the dermal as well as the deeper SMAS (superficial musculoaponeurotic system). This occurs because of the downregulation of collagen and elastin production of our soft tissues in combination with bone atrophy, and the net result is ptosis and transposition of the facial soft tissues.

In recent years, we have learned that this is not possible without over-volumization and distortion of the facial features, which has created a rather unaesthetic appearance and proper interference with the mobility of the facial soft tissues during animation.

As a result, it has changed our present view and approach in the utilization of dermal fillers in facial rejuvenation and is now mainly recommended for the correction of absolute deficits, hollowness, and the enhancement of wanted facial features.

The specialized training of oral and maxillofacial surgeons gives us the advantage of a comprehensive understanding of facial anatomy and aesthetics.

This is important as only the proper diagnosis can lead to the proper choice of any therapeutic treatment.

In-depth knowledge of facial anatomy and physiology is also important since, by definition, any injection into the human body is considered an invasive procedure and can lead to potential adverse effects like tissue necrosis, emboli, blindness as a result of intravascular injection, or occlusion.

In addition, the proper management of patient expectations warrants precise physician-patient communication, patient counseling, and informed consent that includes the knowledge of and ability to manage possible complications and adverse effects associated with injectables.

History

Facial soft tissue fillers were first described in 1893 by Dr. Franz Neuber, who utilized free fat autograft to correct facial soft tissue defects. Later, liquid silicone was used to correct and enhance body contours in the 1940s.

In the 1980s, bovine xenograft dermal collagen was approved by the FDA as a dermal filler. Although it had a high success rate, it came with the caveat of a high resorption rate and the complex pre-treatment double skin test requirement to examine possible allergic reactions.

The true evolution of today's paradigm in dermal fillers started in 2003 with the introduction of hyaluronic acid dermal fillers. Hyaluronic acid is a glycosaminoglycan disaccharide that can be found in human tissue. Since it is extracted from bacterial fermentation, it completely avoids the need for allergy skin tests because of its lack of proteins. This made it safer and more user-friendly, which has resulted in its dominance as the gateway drug in facial aesthetic medicine.

General Classification of Dermal Fillers

Dermal fillers can be categorized by their biological component, biodegradability, biological behavior, and clinical applications. Table 42.1 summarizes the present existent dermal fillers.

Rheology and Biological Considerations of Dermal Fillers

- Rheology is the science that studies the consistency, compression, and elasticity properties of liquids and gels.
- G prime: Refers to the viscoelasticity properties of the filler. The higher the force required to deform the object, the higher its elasticity. In summary, the higher the G prime, the more filler will be able to volumize because it will resist the counterforces and tension of the surrounding tissues. If the objective is to smooth and blend contours, a low G prime filler will be more appropriate.
- Hydrophilic property: Is the degree of affinity for water. The higher the concentration of HA, the greater the hydrophilic attraction.
- Cross-linking: Is the percentage of cross-linker molecules for every 100 units of HA. Cross-linking is designed to reduce the oxidative and enzymatic resorption of the filler, thereby increasing its longevity. In addition, it improves the viscoelastic (G prime) properties of the filler.

Table 42.1 Characteristics of current existent dermal fillers

Category	Substances	Common brand names	Origin
Permanent	Fat	N/A	Autologous
Biodegradable	Bovine collagen	Zyderm I, Zyderm II, and Zyplast	Xenogenic
Biodegradable	Human tissue collagen matrix	Dermalogen, Dermaplant	Allogenic
Biodegradable	Acellular human dermal matrix	Alloderm	Allogenic
Biodegradable	PLLA	Sculptra	Synthetic
Biodegradable	Hyaluronic acid	Captique, Esthélis, Elevess, Hylaform, Juvederm, Perlane, Prevelle, Puragen, Restylane	Bacterial fermentation
Nonbiodegradable	Polyalkylimide	Aquamid	Synthetic
Nonbiodegradable	Calcium hydroxylapatite	Radiesse	Synthetic
Nonbiodegradable	Polymethyl-methacrylate microspheres	Artefill, Bellafill	Synthetic

- Longevity: It is important to differentiate filler clinical tissue effect duration from biological filler longevity. Interestingly, even when the manufacturer determined an average filler clinical duration, the clinical effect varies depending on the material utilized and its rheological properties, the anatomic area injected, the technique utilized, and the volume infiltrated.
- Reversibility: Presently, only hyaluronic acid-based fillers are reversible. The injection of hyaluronidase can dissolve the naturally existent hyaluronic acid within the tissues and may be associated with skin laxity and loss of support subsequently.

Patient Evaluation

Dermal filler indications

1. Mild developmental skeletal or soft tissue deficiencies.
2. Soft tissue atrophy and camouflage of mild changes due to aging.
3. Minor contour enhancement.
4. Static wrinkles.
5. Trauma-related hypoplasia (soft tissue defects).
6. Dermal scars (atrophic scars, acne scars, viral scars).
7. Disease-related soft tissue atrophy (HIV/AIDS).
8. Congenital diseases (Parry-Romberg syndrome, hemifacial microsomia, Goldenhar syndrome, and rheumatoid conditions affecting lower jaw growth, unilateral condylar hyperplasia).

Dermal filler contraindications

1. Hypersensitivity.
2. Active infection of the injection site.
3. Active inflammation in the treating area.
4. Unrealistic patient expectations.
5. Immunosuppressed patient.
6. Pregnancy, breastfeeding.

Patient Evaluation

It is the surgeon's responsibility to diagnose, educate, and guide the patient through different treatment options that are result based and match the patient's expectations.

Also, a detailed and targeted history of previous facial filler injections including specific location of the face, volume, and type of filler is essential.

The questionnaire should include:

1. Medical conditions.

    (a) Bleeding disorders.
    (b) Viral infections.
    (c) Psychiatric disorders.
    (d) Autoimmune disease.
    (e) Immunosuppression.
    (f) Dermatologic conditions.

2. Allergies and type of reaction.

    (a) Environmental.
    (b) Food.
    (c) Medications.
    (d) Other substances.

3. Medications.

    (a) Anticoagulants.
    (b) Supplementation.

4. Surgical interventions.
5. Prior anesthetic events/complications.
6. Vaccination status.

    (a) COVID vaccination.
    (b) Viral vaccination.

7. Mental health status.
8. Motivation and expectations for treatment.
9. Past cosmetic surgical or nonsurgical treatments.

A systematic physical evaluation of the muscular-cutaneous complex, deep and superficial fat compartments, facial skeleton, and degree of aging changes will dictate the choice of the ideal treatment. Further, they should be custom-tailored to the patient's gender, age, and specific expectations discussed in the consultation process.

Preoperative Photograph

Proper standardized high-quality clinical photographs should be taken utilizing high-definition cameras and proper studio lighting. In general, smartphone cameras should be avoided due to fish-eye effect of the lens and the distortion of facial proportions produced by the lack of optical zoom and distance from the lens to the object.

In general, clinical photography serves as:

1. Diagnostic tool.
2. Communication tool between surgeon and patient.
3. Evidence of postoperative changes and improvements.
4. Study tool for the surgeon for self-critical assessment.
5. Medicolegal evidence.
6. Possible postproduction tool for marketing and education.

Treatment Plan and Filler Selection

See Table 42.3.

Injection techniques:

1. Linear threading.
2. Serial puncture.
3. Cross-hatching.
4. Tower technique.
5. Fanning.

Indication	Depth	Angle
Fine rhytids	Papillary dermis	10–30°
Moderate rhytids	Reticular dermis	30–45°
Deep rhytids and volume	Fat, subperiosteal	45–90°

Post-Procedure Considerations

General recommendations are:

Immediate:

1. Avoid palpation and massage of the area.
2. No cosmetic products for at least 24 h.
3. Avoid NSAIDs and anticoagulants for 24 h.
4. Avoid skin treatments (laser, radiofrequency, micro-needling, peels, etc.).
5. Avoid sun exposure; apply sunblock after 24 h.
6. Antiviral therapy 3 days before and 3 days after in case of history of herpesvirus.

Complications

Overtreatment

- Understand the patient's expectations and guide the patient on possible outcomes and treatment plan.
- Perception shifting, either from the patient, practitioner, or both, may lead to unaesthetic outcomes.
- Perform soft tissue augmentation conservatively with small doses and gradually.
- Conservative treatment allows the practitioner to reevaluate the contours after the post-op swelling resolves and retreats if necessary.

Pain

- Most HA filler contains lidocaine within their formulation, diminishing discomfort and injection pain.
- Local anesthesia in presentations such as creams, ointments, and gels can be utilized to increase patient comfort. Icing also decreased pain perception.
- Regional facial blocks and a minimal amount of local anesthetic are recommended to decrease soft tissue distortion.

Bruising and Swelling

- Postinjection bruising and swelling are self-limiting and resolve without complications. Warm compresses and medications such as arnica may help to accelerate bruising resolution.

Tyndall Effect

- The Tyndall effect is defined by the scattering of a light beam when it passes through a colloidal medium.
- This phenomenon is usually observed where the skin thickness is thin. When the filler is injected, it distends the skin, allowing the daylight to penetrate through the thin skin and revealing the translucent material injected.
- Adequate depth of injection into deeper layers avoids this complication. The treatment consists of massaging, hyaluronidase injections, or direct excision.

Migration

- Injection of large volumes, inadequate filler selection, excessive injection force, repeated injections on an anatomic site, excessive postinjection massage, poor injection technique, and muscle activity are factors associated with this phenomenon.

Allergic Reactions

- Rare complication. Signs and symptoms of hypersensitivity include local urticaria, swelling, and angioedema. The treatment comprises antihistaminic medications, steroids, hyaluronidase injections, and direct excision.

Skin Necrosis

According to different studies, the incidence of vascular occlusion is 3–9 in 10,000 injections. The areas of higher risk of vascular complications are the nose and nasolabial fold (52%), forehead and eyebrows (12.1%), glabella (8.2%), lower eyelid and tear trough (7.1%), cheeks (7.1%), lips (6.2%), temporal region (16%), perioral (2.7%), and lastly the chin (2.5%).

Signs of vascular compromise:

1. Ischemia.
2. Numbness.
3. Pain.
4. Blanching.
5. Mottling.
6. Blistering.

Different protocols have been published:

1. Diagnose and treat within 90 min.
2. Warm compress and massage 5–10 min every 30–60 min (avoid burning the skin).
3. Hyaluronidase injections (500–1500 IU and repeat every 24 h as needed).
4. Aspirin two pills of 325 mg daily for 1 week.
5. Nitroglycerin pastes every 8 h daily until improvement.
6. Hyperbaric oxygen.
7. Daily follow-up.
8. Routine wound care (daily dressings, antibiotic ointment).
9. Adequate wound and patient hydration.
10. Wound debridement as needed.

Recommendations before any injections include:

1. Injection of <0.1 ccs per injection.
2. Retrograde injection.
3. Aspiration.
4. Low injection pressure.
5. Use of cannulas.
6. Knowledge of the anatomic area.
7. Possible use of lidocaine with epinephrine.

Blindness

The areas with a higher risk are the glabellar complex, nose, nasolabial fold, forehead, and temple, respectively.

Recommended management:
- Abort the procedure immediately.
- Hyaluronidase injection (retrobulbar) 300–600 units (27–30-gauge 1.5-in. needle).
- Aspirin 325 mg two tabs chewed.
- Hot pads.
- Nitropaste gel.
- Ocular massage.
- Emergency room transportation.
- Ophthalmology consultation within 90 min (retina specialist).
- Continuous assessment to rule out a cerebrovascular accident.

Preventive measurements:

1. Injection of <0.1 ccs per injection.
2. Retrograde injection.
3. Aspiration.
4. Low injection pressure.
5. Use of cannulas.
6. Knowledge of the anatomic area.
7. Possible use of lidocaine with epinephrine.

Lymphatic Disruption

Due to the volumetric expansion of the tissues postinjection, fillers may cause partial or total occlusion of the lymphatic systems by collapsing the lymphatic channels.

Risk factors for persistent edema are:

1. Females.
2. A previous surgical procedure in the affected area.
3. Repeated filler injections in a specific anatomic area.
4. History of allergies.
5. History of eyelid edema or festooning.
6. Fillers with high HA content (higher water affinity).
7. Large volumes of filler injected.
8. Age (50–60 years old).

Treatment includes hyaluronidase injections in the case of HA fillers to dissolve the agent, direct excision, and radiofrequency therapy. Ultrasound can be utilized to locate the exact location of the fillers within the tissues.

Pearls (Table 42.2)

1. Understanding facial anatomy and physiology of the facial musculature and spaces is essential to achieving optimal results.

Table 42.2 Hyaluronic acid fillers and rheological properties

Product	HA concentration (mg/mL)	% Cross-linked
Restylane	20	1.20%
Restylane Lyft	20	1.20%
Restylane Silk	20	1.20%
Restylane Kysse	20	7%
Restylane Contour	20	7%
Restylane Defyne	20	8%
RHA 2	23	3%
RHA 3	23	3.50%
RHA 4	23	4%
Juvederm Ultra	24	6%
Juvederm Ultra Plus	24	8%
Juvederm Voluma	20	Highly (proprietary)
Juvederm Volbella	15	Highly (proprietary)
Juvederm Vollure	17.5	Highly (proprietary)
Revanesse Versa	25	7%
Belotero	22.5	Cannot be measured

2. Utilize cannulas to mitigate the risk of accidental intra-vascular injections and resultant vascular occlusion that can lead to tissue necrosis, blindness, or emboli.
3. In general, avoid large volume injections to a particular area in order to avoid extreme tissue expansion that can lead to soft tissue thinning and rhytidosis that is difficult to treat.
4. Frequent aspiration and injection of small conservative doses in a retrograde manner with low injection pressure are essential in avoiding inadvertent intra-vascular injections.
5. Have an emergency plan ready for all possible complications prior to injecting.

Pitfalls (Tables 42.2, 42.3)

1. Injection of filler in areas with constant dynamic muscular activity will cause filler migration and have the opposite effect on the desired outcome.
2. Incorrect product selection, poor injection technique, and use of needles without aspiration significantly increase the risk of intra-vascular injection and resultant vascular occlusion.
3. Proper patient selection is key to success. Dermal fillers are not a replacement for surgery. They cannot defy gravity and, therefore, cannot "lift" the tissues. This is rather an illusion caused by inflation and expansion of the soft tissues. Understanding resultant volume changes is essential in predicting a positive aesthetic outcome and meeting the patient's expectations.

Table 42.3 Filler selection according to the anatomic area

Location	Filler
Brow augmentation	Restylane-L Belotero balance
Tear through and A-frame deformity	Restylane-L Belotero balance
Malar augmentation	Restylane Lyft Restylane contour, RHA-4, Juvederm Voluma
Lip augmentation	Restylane Kysse Restylane Refyne Versa lips Juvederm Ultra
Nasolabial folds	Juvederm Ultra Juvederm Ultra Plus Juvederm Vollure Restylane Refyne Restylane Defyne RHA-3
Fine lines	RHA-2 Belotero Balance
Nonsurgical rhinoplasty	Restylane Lyft Restylane-L

Further Reading

Hamrah D, Watson SW. Injectable soft tissue fillers and their use in facial rejuvenation, vol. 16.

Tezel A, Fredrickson GH. The science of hyaluronic acid dermal fillers. J Cosmet Laser Ther. 2008;10(1):35–42. https://doi.org/10.1080/14764170701774901.

Hyaluronan: structure and physical properties. https://www.glycoforum.gr.jp/article/01A2.html. Accessed 8 Oct 2022.

Master M. Hyaluronic acid filler longevity and localization: magnetic resonance imaging evidence. Plast Reconstr Surg. 2021;147:50e–3E. https://doi.org/10.1097/PRS.0000000000007429.

Master M, Roberts S. Long-term MRI follow-up of hyaluronic acid dermal filler. Plast Reconstr Surg Glob Open. 2022;10(4):E4252. https://doi.org/10.1097/GOX.0000000000004252.

Wang H, Guan J, Zhang X, et al. Effect of cold application on pain and bruising in patients with subcutaneous injection of low-molecular-weight heparin: a meta-analysis. Clin Appl Thromb Hemost. 2020;26:1076029620905349. https://doi.org/10.1177/1076029620905349.

Algafly AA, George KP. The effect of cryotherapy on nerve conduction velocity, pain threshold and pain tolerance. Br J Sports Med. 2007;41(6):365–9. https://doi.org/10.1136/BJSM.2006.031237.

Kuzu N, Ucar H. The effect of cold on the occurrence of bruising, haematoma and pain at the injection site in subcutaneous low molecular weight heparin. Int J Nurs Stud. 2001;38(1):51–9. https://doi.org/10.1016/S0020-7489(00)00061-4.

Smith KC, Comite SL, Storwick GS. Ice minimizes discomfort associated with injection of botulinum toxin type a for the treatment of palmar and plantar hyperhidrosis. Dermatol Surg. 2007;33(SUPPL. 1):S88. https://doi.org/10.1111/j.1524-4725.2006.32337.x.

Kuwahara H, Ogawa R. Using a vibration device to ease pain during facial needling and injection. Eplasty. 2016;16:e9. Accessed 15 Oct 2022.

Mally P, Czyz CN, Chan NJ, Wulc AE. Vibration anesthesia for the reduction of pain with facial dermal filler injections. Aesthetic Plast Surg. 2014;38(2):413–8. https://doi.org/10.1007/s00266-013-0264-4.

Sharma P, Czyz CN, Wulc AE. Investigating the efficacy of vibration anesthesia to reduce pain from cosmetic botulinum toxin injections. Aesthet Surg J. 2011;31(8):966–71. https://doi.org/10.1177/1090820X11422809.

King M. Management of tyndall effect. J Clin Aesthet Dermatol. 2016;9(11):E6. Accessed 16 Oct 2022.

Delorenzi C. Complications of injectable fillers, part I. Aesthet Surg J. 2013;33(4):561–75. https://doi.org/10.1177/1090820X13484492.

Povolotskiy R, Oleck NC, Hatzis CM, Paskhover B. Adverse events associated with aesthetic dermal fillers: a 10-year retrospective study of FDA data. Am J Cosmet Surg. 2018;35(3):143–51. https://doi.org/10.1177/0748806818757123.

Halepas S, Peters SM, Goldsmith JL, Ferneini EM. Vascular compromise after soft tissue facial fillers: case report and review of current treatment protocols. J Oral Maxillofac Surg. 2020;78(3):440–5. https://doi.org/10.1016/j.joms.2019.10.008.

Vascular compromise from soft tissue augmentation: experience with 12 cases and recommendations for optimal outcomes—PubMed. https://pubmed.ncbi.nlm.nih.gov/25276276/. Accessed 18 Oct 2022.

Hwang CJ. Periorbital injectables: Understanding and avoiding complications. J Cutan Aesthet Surg. 2016;9:73–9. https://doi.org/10.4103/0974-2077.184049.

Oranges CM, Brucato D, Schaefer DJ, Kalbermatten DF, Harder Y. Complications of nonpermanent facial fillers: a systematic review. Plast Reconstr Surg Glob Open. 2021;9(10):e3851. https://doi.org/10.1097/gox.0000000000003851.

Cohen JL, Biesman BS, Dayan SH, et al. Treatment of hyaluronic acid filler-induced impending necrosis with hyaluronidase: consensus recommendations. Aesthet Surg J. 2015;35(7):844–9. https://doi.org/10.1093/ASJ/SJV018.

van Loghem JAJ, Humzah D, Kerscher M. Cannula versus sharp needle for placement of soft tissue fillers: an observational cadaver study. Aesthet Surg J. 2017;38(1):73–88. https://doi.org/10.1093/asj/sjw220.

Iwayama T, Hashikawa K, Osaki T, Yamashiro K, Horita N, Fukumoto T. Ultrasonography-guided cannula method for hyaluronic acid filler injection with evaluation using laser speckle flowgraphy. Plast Reconstr Surg Glob Open. 2018;6(4):e1776. https://doi.org/10.1097/GOX.0000000000001776.

Alam M, Kakar R, Dover JS, et al. Rates of vascular occlusion associated with using needles vs cannulas for filler injection. JAMA Dermatol. 2021;157(2):174–80. https://doi.org/10.1001/jamadermatol.2020.5102.

Pavicic T, Webb KL, Frank K, Gotkin RH, Tamura B, Cotofana S. Arterial wall penetration forces in needles versus cannulas. Plast Reconstr Surg. 2019;143(3):504E–12E. https://doi.org/10.1097/PRS.0000000000005321.

Chatrath V, Banerjee PS, Goodman GJ, Rahman E. Soft-tissue filler-associated blindness: a systematic review of case reports and case series. Plast Reconstr Surg Glob Open. 2019;7(4):e2173. https://doi.org/10.1097/GOX.0000000000002173.

Kim YK, Jung C, Woo SJ, Park KH. Cerebral angiographic findings of cosmetic facial filler-related ophthalmic and retinal artery occlusion. J Korean Med Sci. 2015;30(12):1847–55. https://doi.org/10.3346/JKMS.2015.30.12.1847.

Fundus artery occlusion caused by cosmetic facial injections—PubMed. https://pubmed.ncbi.nlm.nih.gov/24762584/. Accessed 18 Oct 2022.

LETTERS AND COMMUNICATIONS restoration of visual loss with retrobulbar hyaluronidase injection after hyaluronic acid filler. Published online 2017.

Paap MK, Milman T, Ugradar S, Silkiss RZ. Assessing Retrobulbar hyaluronidase as a treatment for filler-induced blindness in a cadaver model. Plast Reconstr Surg. 2019;144(2):315–20. https://doi.org/10.1097/PRS.0000000000005806.

Chapter 2. The lymphatic anatomy of the lower eyelid and the malar region of the face. In: Facial volumization. Published online 2017. https://doi.org/10.1055/B-0037-146353.

Decates TS, Kruijt Spanjer EC, Saini R, Velthuis PJ, Niessen FM. Unilateral facial edema after filler injection of the lower eyelid. Dermatol Ther. 2020;33(4):e13539. https://doi.org/10.1111/dth.13539.

Griepentrog GJ, Lucarelli MJ, Burkat CN, Lemke BN, Rose JG. Periorbital edema following hyaluronic acid gel injection: a retrospective review. Am J Cosmet Surg. 2011;28:251–4.

Plastic surgery procedural statistics from the American Society of Plastic Surgeons 2020.

Chapter 43
Facial Laser Skin Resurfacing in Facial Cosmetic Surgery

Daria Hamrah and Brayann Aleman

Abstract In the past several decades, technological advances have become an essential part of cosmetic treatments in aesthetic and rejuvenative medicine. Photorejuvenation is defined as the treatment of photoaged skin utilizing laser or light-based technologies. While laser procedures can be done independently, the combination of laser procedures in conjunction with nonsurgical or surgical treatments synergistically enhances comprehensive facial rejuvenation outcomes. This chapter will limit our discussion to facial skin resurfacing treatments, the biology of skin aging, the scientific basis of phototherapy, patient evaluation, treatment, and management of complications.

Introduction to Lasers

Laser is an acronym that originated from light amplification by stimulated emission of radiation.

A chromophore is an endogenous light-absorbing chemical, an atom or group whose presence is responsible for color. The primary skin chromophores are:

1. Oxyhemoglobin (vascular lesions).
2. Melanin (pigmented lesions).
3. Water (collagen stimulation).

The laser medium is a substance that emits a particular light wavelength when stimulated by an external energy source.

D. Hamrah (✉) · B. Aleman
NOVA Surgicare PC, McLean, VA, USA
e-mail: drhamrah@novasurgicare.com; www.novasurgicare.com

© The Author(s), under exclusive license to Springer Nature Switzerland AG 2024
D. Amin, H. Marwan (eds.), *Pearls and Pitfalls in Oral and Maxillofacial Surgery*, https://doi.org/10.1007/978-3-031-47307-4_43

Laser mediums:

1. Solid (alexandrite, ruby, neodymium-doped yttrium aluminum garnet).
2. Liquid (dyes).
3. Gas (carbon dioxide).

Laser Physics and Principles

Absorption: When a laser is directed against the skin, it can be absorbed (the most essential and desired effect), reflected, scattered, or transmitted.

Wavelength (nm): The distance between the peak of each wave at a specific time. The longer the wavelength, the deepest the laser penetration. Each chromophore has a specific wavelength depending on the medium utilized.

Fluence (J/cm^2) or density: The energy delivered per unit area. The higher the fluence, the higher the thermal injury to the peripheral tissue.

Pulse width or pulse duration (picoseconds): Time the laser beams contact the skin. The longer the pulse duration, the deeper the laser beam will penetrate.

Spot size (mm): It is the diameter of the laser beam on the skin surface. Small spot sizes have greater scattering and less penetration.

Repetition rate (Hz): It is defined as the number of pulses per second. High Hz allows the treatment of large surface areas in a short period. Low Hz is used to treat small lesions or areas.

Power or irradiance (W/cm^2): The frequency of the energy emitted from the laser.

Spot density: Determines the percentage of skin treated per pulse. High density is directly proportional to treatment intensity, healing time, and skin resurfacing improvement.

Variable pulse sequencing: The delay between pulses allows skin relaxation and thermal dissipation between pulses (relaxation time).

Thermal relaxation time: Time for 50% heat dissipation into the surrounding tissue. The pulse width should heat the desired chromophore with limited peripheral heat transmission and tissue damage.

Selective photothermolysis: This is the treatment of a specific chromophore with a chromophore-specific wavelength with a precise amount of energy (fluence) required to damage its target tissue for a specific time (pulse length) with minimal thermal damage to the peripheral tissues (thermal relaxation time).

Laser Treatment Indications

1. Red vascular lesions.
2. Dyschromia.

3. Mild to moderate rhytids.
4. Tattoo removal.
5. Hair removal.
6. Skin resurfacing.

Laser Treatment Contraindications

1. Active skin infection and acne.
2. Dermatoses.
3. Keloidal and poor healing/scarring (genetic, medication-induced).
4. Livedo reticularis.
5. Sun exposure and self-tanning treatments within 4 weeks before the treatment.
6. Uncontrolled medical conditions.
7. Photosensitive disorder.
8. Patient under photosensitizing medications (i.e., tetracycline).
9. Collagen and vascular disease secondary to steroid or autoimmune disorders.
10. History of radiation therapy to the intended treating area.
11. Patients with psychological and social disturbances (BDD) and unrealistic expectations.
12. Topical retinoid within 1 week before treatment.
13. History of extensive electrolysis to face.
14. Recent skin resurfacing, either laser, chemical, or physical.
15. Pregnancy.
16. Fitzpatrick V–VI.

Fractional Vs. Nonfractional Devices

Fractional devices deliver energy in microthermal zones distributed in a grid-like pattern. Selective basal layer preservation allows faster epidermal regeneration.

Nonfractional laser devices deliver energy to the entire surface without interruption.

Ablative Vs. Nonablative

Nonablative Devices

Controlled temperature elevation (up to 100 °C) *without* tissue removal or vaporization. The tissue is also coagulated, leaving an intact stratum corneum.

Ablative Devices

Work by controlled skin temperature elevation (up to 100 °C) *with* tissue vaporization, removing epithermal and dermal tissues and leaving an open wound.

Patient Evaluation

Physical Examination

1. General complete physical examination.
2. Fitzpatrick scale (melanin content and UV sensitivity).
3. Glogau classification of photoaging.
4. Skin lesions.

Preoperative Instructions and Skin Preparation

The purpose of skin preparation is to ensure proper healing ability of the skin posttreatment as well as avoidance of possible laser complications. The following protocol is recommended:

Four weeks before the treatment:

1. Preoperative photographs.
2. Mineral-based sunscreen, SPF >30 (containing zinc oxide or titanium oxide).
3. Retinoids (promote epidermal healing and accelerate epithermal cell turnover).
4. Hydroquinone 4–8% (reduction of melanin production by inhibition of tyrosinase, selective damage to melanocytes and melanosomes).
5. Topical vitamin C (antioxidant which decreases epidermal oxidation and promotes collagen formation).

Two weeks before the treatment:

1. Antiviral and antibiotic prophylactic medications:

    (a) Acyclovir 400 mg PO every 12 h starting 3 days preoperatively and continuing for 5 days postoperatively to decrease the risk of post-operative herpes virus infections.

    (b) Cephalexin 500 mg PO three times per day for 5 days postoperatively.

2. Review and provide all preoperative and postoperative instructions, medications, and skin care regimens.
3. Discontinue anticoagulants and any supplements.

Intraoperative Laser Treatment (Tables 43.1 and 43.2)

1. Follow laser safety guidelines.
2. Remove jewelry, contact lenses, makeup, and skin care products.
3. Position the patient in a supine position.
4. Clean skin with alcohol.
5. Anesthesia and analgesia (topical, sedation, general anesthesia).
6. Remove all traces of topical anesthesia, wipe the skin with alcohol, and let it dry.
7. Eye protection (metallic lenses or metallic corneal shields) .
8. Hold the laser handpiece perpendicular to the treating surface (90°).
9. Perform systematic passes with appropriate laser settings based on skin type, condition, and treatment goal.
10. Continuous skin response evaluation to avoid unwanted laser effects.
11. Blend by feathering the transition lines between treated and untreated surfaces.
12. Do not debride (higher risk of scarring); leave eschar over skin.

Unwanted laser effects:

1. Wide surface bleeding.
2. Blistering.
3. Severe whitening to severe graying.

Wanted laser effects on tissue:

1. White spots and erythema.
2. Sebum vaporization.
3. Darkening of pigmented lesions.
4. Pinpoint bleeding (Er:YAG).

Table 43.1 Laser settings and depth of treatment

Laser settings	Superficial skin treatments	Deep skin treatments
Wavelength	Short	Long
Pulse width	Short	Long
Spot size	Small	Large
Fluence	Low	High

Table 43.2 Parameter selection according to patient characteristics

Laser settings	Fitzpatrick I–III and facial areas	Fitzpatrick IV–VI and nonfacial areas
Wavelength	Short	Long
Pulse width	Short	Long
Spot size	Small	Large
Fluence	High	Low

Immediate Aftertreatment

1. Skin cooling for 30 min.
2. Occlusive ointments like petrolatum or Vaseline (nonantibiotic, fragrance-free, colorant-free).
3. Avoid UV exposure.
4. Review all postoperative medications and skin care products with the patient and caregiver.

Postoperative Follow-Up Visits

Day one: General evaluation and postoperative recommendation reinforcement.

One and two weeks: Assess skin healing, reinforce postoperative recommendations, and patient and relative's psychological reinforcement. After 2 weeks, if the skin has epithelized completely, one may restart retinol and hydroquinone as tolerated.

One, three, and six months: Photographic objective comparison with preoperative photos, reinforcing skin care measurements, adjunctive skin treatments like regular facials, and patient-specific skin care regimen for maintenance.

One year: Photographic objective comparison with preoperative photos, reinforcing skincare regimen. and adjunctive skin treatments. Retreat if desired or necessary.

Postoperative Instructions and Skin Care Regimen

Day one until epithelialization:

1. Apply moisturizer ointment as needed. The skin should be hydrated at all times.

   Day two until epithelization:

1. Wash your face six times daily with mineral water or diluted acetic acid.
2. Apply the moisturizer ointment as needed during the day. Avoid dehydration.

   Day four and above:

1. Apply moisturizer ointment as needed.
2. Mineral-based sunscreen SPF 30+ every 2 h once the epidermal scab has peeled off. Avoid manual debridement of the scab to avoid scarring.
3. Use an antioxidant gentle cleanser three times daily to cleanse the skin once the scab is gone.

Complications

1. *Pain:* Persistent pain or severe pain should be evaluated for possible infection.
2. *Erythema:* Persistent erythema (>4 weeks) is treated with topical steroids or vascular lasers.
3. *Dermatitis:* Accompanied by pruritus, associated with topical antibiotics (Bacitracin, triple antibiotic ointments), vitamin E, and herbal supplementation.

   (a) *Treatment*: Discontinue topical, herbal, and supplements. Topical steroids, cold compresses, and oral antihistamine medication.

4. *Dyschromias:*

   (a) *Hypopigmentation*: Delayed presentation (6–12 months post-op) may be permanent.

      • *Treatment*: excimer laser, narrowband UVB treatment, ambient light sunlight, and cosmetic makeup.

   (b) *Postinflammatory pigmentation (PHI)*: Associated with postoperative sun exposure, poor patient compliance, and predisposition to PIH.

      • *Treatment (supportive):* mineral-based sunscreen (SPF >30), retinol hydroquinone 4%, cholic acid, and superficial treatments.

5. *Infection:* The provider should have a low tolerance and culture the wound and initiate empiric treatment and definitive treatment once infection culture results are obtained.

   (a) *Bacterial*: Streptococcus (group A Streptococcus), Staphylococcus (*S. aureus*, MRSA [uncommon]), and *Pseudomonas aeruginosa.*

      • *Treatment*:

         Doxycycline 100 mg PO every 12 h.
         Clindamycin 300 mg PO every 6 h.
         Sulfamethoxazole/trimethoprim 800 mg/ 160mg PO every every 12 hours.

   (b) *Viral*: Most frequently reactivation of HSV, tingling, burning, discharge, and vesicle formation.

      • *Treatment:*

         Acyclovir 800 mg PO five times per day.
         Valacyclovir 500–1000 mg PO every 8 h.
         Famciclovir 500 mg PO every 8 h.

   (c) *Fungal*: Difficult to diagnose, resemble acne, pain, purulence, erythema, pruritus, and crusting.

- *Treatment*: Discontinue ointment, fluconazole 100 mg PO daily, and definitive treatment based on cultures.

6. *Burn:* Overaggressive treatment parameters.

   (a) *Treatment*: ice pack, occlusive dressings, and ointments that allow proper healing and close re-evaluation.

7. *Scarring:* Overaggressive treatment parameters, infection, poor patient compliance, and predisposition.

   (a) *Treatment*: topical corticosteroid treatment, 5FU injections, and triamcinolone acetonide 10 mg/ml injections (1–2 mg) every 4–6 weeks.

8. *Damage to adjacent structures.*

Conclusion

Skin laser resurfacing is an integral treatment modality of comprehensive facial rejuvenation and cosmetic treatment. To achieve positive outcomes and avoid complications, proper patient selection, skin preparation, laser parameters as well as proper postoperative care, and close follow-up are critical. Patient compliance is the most challenging and unpredictable variable in these treatments due to the need for meticulous home care. Understanding the science and technology associated with laser treatments is a paradigm for successful treatment outcomes.

Pearls

1. Targeted preoperative skin preparation and postoperative skincare are important treatment steps to achieve optimal results and avoid postoperative inflammatory hyperpigmentation and wound healing problems. Further, a pre- and perioperative empiric antiviral and antibiotic regimen is recommended to avoid possible infections during the recovery phase.
2. Ablative laser treatments are more effective for treating deeper rhytidosis, acne scarring, and other deep skin imperfections. However, they should be used with caution in patients with darker skin tones (FP III–V) due to the risk of pigmentation changes.
3. Nonablative lasers are less invasive as they only treat skin surface partially based on the density chosen and, therefore, safer for patients with darker skin types. As a result, they may require multiple treatments for optimal results.
4. Laser therapy is not a one-size-fits-all approach. A customized treatment plan should be created for each patient, based on skin type and condition, utilizing the proper laser according to individualized settings.

Pitfalls

1. Uneven results: Lasers should be regularly maintained and calibrated. Failure to do so may result in uneven skin color, tone, and texture and, in some cases, severe skin damage and burns.
2. Hypopigmentation or hyperpigmentation: Depending on the type of laser used and the patient's skin type, the laser may cause changes skin dyschromias. Hypopigmentation or loss of skin color and hyperpigmentation or darkening of skin color are potential complications. This is why it is crucial to match the laser type and intensity to the patient's skin type and condition. Typically testing a conspicuous area is recommended prior to any treatment.
3. Prolonged erythema: Post-laser skin may appear erythematous and sensitive for several weeks and, in some cases, even for several months. The proper postoperative skin care, as well as management of the patient's expectations, is essential as part of comprehensive patient management.
4. Lasers are to be avoided in patients prone to excessive scarring or keloids.

Further Reading

Houreld NN. The use of lasers and light sources in skin rejuvenation. Clin Dermatol. 2019;37(4):358–64. https://doi.org/10.1016/J.CLINDERMATOL.2019.04.008.

Small R. A practical guide to laser procedures. p. 282. https://www.wolterskluwer.com/en/solutions/ovid/practical-guide-to-laser-procedures-a-9237. Accessed 25 Nov 2022.

Chakravarthi M, Shilpakar R, KrupaDS S. Carbon dioxide laser guidelines. J Cutan Aesthet Surg. 2009;2(2):72. https://doi.org/10.4103/0974-2077.58519.

Preissig J, Hamilton K, Markus R. Current laser resurfacing technologies: a review that delves beneath the surface. Semin Plast Surg. 2012;26(3):109. https://doi.org/10.1055/S-0032-1329413.

Kaushik SB, Alexis AF. Nonablative fractional laser resurfacing in skin of color: evidence-based review. J Clin Aesthet Dermatol. 2017;10(6):51. Accessed 25 Nov 2022.

Roy D, Sadick NS. Ablative facial resurfacing. Ophthalmol Clin North Am. 2005;18(2):259–70. https://doi.org/10.1016/j.ohc.2005.03.005.

Boehm KS, Avashia YJ, Savetsky IL, Rohrich RJ. Laser resurfacing: safety and technique. Plast Reconstr Surg Glob Open. 2020;8(4):e2796. https://doi.org/10.1097/GOX.0000000000002796.

Zubair R, Sliney D. ASLMS laser safety guide in dermatology and plastic surgery. American Society for Laser Medicine and Surgery. 2021. [Internet]. Available from: https://www.aslms.org/docs/default-source/for-professionals/mentorship-program/alsms-laser-safety-guide-final.pdf?sfvrsn=1f1f43b_5.

Lolis M, Dunbar SW, Goldberg DJ, Hansen TJ, MacFarlane DF. Patient safety in procedural dermatology: part II. Safety related to cosmetic procedures. J Am Acad Dermatol. 2015;73(1):15–24. https://doi.org/10.1016/J.JAAD.2014.11.036.

Metelitsa AI, Alster TS. Fractionated laser skin resurfacing treatment complications: a review. Dermatol Surg. 2010;36(3):299–306. https://doi.org/10.1111/J.1524-4725.2009.01434.X.

Niamtu J. Cosmetic facial surgery. New York: Elsevier; 2018. https://doi.org/10.1016/B978-0-323-39393-5.00017-0.

Wright EJ, Struck SK. Facelift combined with simultaneous fractional laser resurfacing: outcomes and complications. J Plast Reconstr Aesthet Surg. 2015;68(10):1332–7. https://doi.org/10.1016/J.BJPS.2015.06.001.

Ramsdell W. Fractional CO2 laser resurfacing complications. Semin Plast Surg. 2012;26(3):137. https://doi.org/10.1055/S-0032-1329415.

Prohaska J, Hohman MH. Laser complications. In: Complications in anesthesia; 2022. p. 567–9. https://doi.org/10.1016/B978-1-4160-2215-2.50144-7.

Griffin AC. Laser resurfacing procedures in dark-skinned patients. Aesthet Surg J. 2005;25(6):625–7. https://doi.org/10.1016/J.ASJ.2005.09.019.

Gilbert S, McBurney E. Use of valacyclovir for herpes simplex virus-1 (HSV-1) prophylaxis after facial resurfacing: a randomized clinical trial of dosing regimens. Dermatol Surg. 2000;26(1):50–4. https://doi.org/10.1046/J.1524-4725.2000.99166.X.

Vanaman M, Fabi SG, Carruthers J. Complications in the cosmetic dermatology patient: a review and our experience (part 2). Dermatol Surg. 2016;42(1):12–20. https://doi.org/10.1097/01.DSS.0000479796.34703.94.

Barkana Y, Belkin M. Laser eye injuries. Surv Ophthalmol. 2000;44(6):459–78. https://doi.org/10.1016/S0039-6257(00)00112-0.

Chapter 44
How to Perform Blepharoplasty

Marawan El Naboulsy, Faisal A. Quereshy, and Victoria A. Mañón

Abstract Blepharoplasty is one of the most performed cosmetic procedures in the world. This is attributed to its profound impact on the brow and cheek rejuvenation. Blepharoplasty augments the upper and lower eyelids to treat dermatochalasis and loose or redundant eyelid skin. The keys to safe and predictable surgical outcomes include a diligent medical history review, comprehensive facial examination, and thoughtful preoperative planning. Physical examination should consider brow, eyelid, and cheek projection. This narrative aims to address common pitfalls to avoid complications. The purpose of this chapter is to review pearls and pitfalls in blepharoplasty.

Practical Tips

Preoperative Consideration

- A succinct discussion of possible complications, post-op course, and management of patient expectations.
- Identification of existing facial asymmetries and review of pre-op photos with patients.
- Pre-op demonstration of approximate post-op results by pinching the skin to simulate outcomes.
- Misdiagnosing excessive brow skin for eyelid skin, resulting in suboptimal results and dissatisfied patients.

M. El Naboulsy · F. A. Quereshy (✉)
Department of Oral and Maxillofacial Surgery, Case Western Reserve University, Cleveland, OH, USA
e-mail: mxe223@case.edu; faq@case.edu

V. A. Mañón
Department of Oral and Maxillofacial Surgery, University of Texas Health at Houston, Houston, TX, USA
e-mail: Victoria.a.manon@uth.tmc.edu

D. Amin, H. Marwan (eds.), *Pearls and Pitfalls in Oral and Maxillofacial Surgery*, https://doi.org/10.1007/978-3-031-47307-4_44

- Documentation of MRD1 and MRD2 preoperatively (Fig. 44.1).
- Evaluation of lower lid laxity via lower lid distraction test and snapback test, as it directly relates to postoperative ectropion and retraction. These tests help evaluate the need to perform a lateral canthopexy (Figs. 44.2 and 44.3).

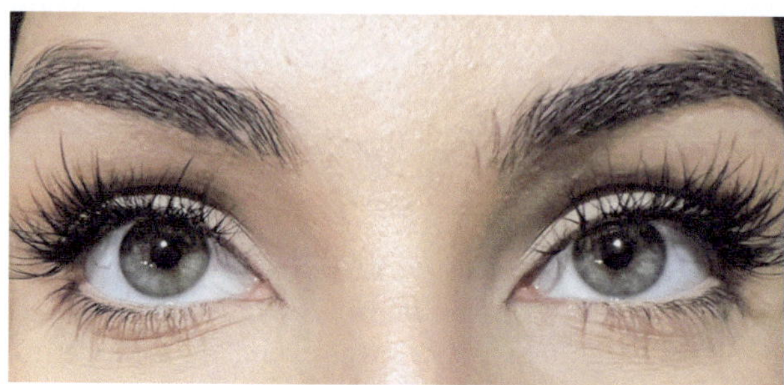

Fig. 44.1 The upper marginal reflex distance (MRD 1) is the distance from the pupillary light reflex to the upper lid margin, normally 4 mm. MRD 2 is the distance from the pupillary light reflex to the lower lid margin, normally 6 mm. An MRD 1 less than 4 mm is diagnostic for ptosis; an MRD 2 less than 6 mm is diagnostic for lower lid retraction

Fig. 44.2 Here, the lower lid distraction test evaluates lower lid laxity

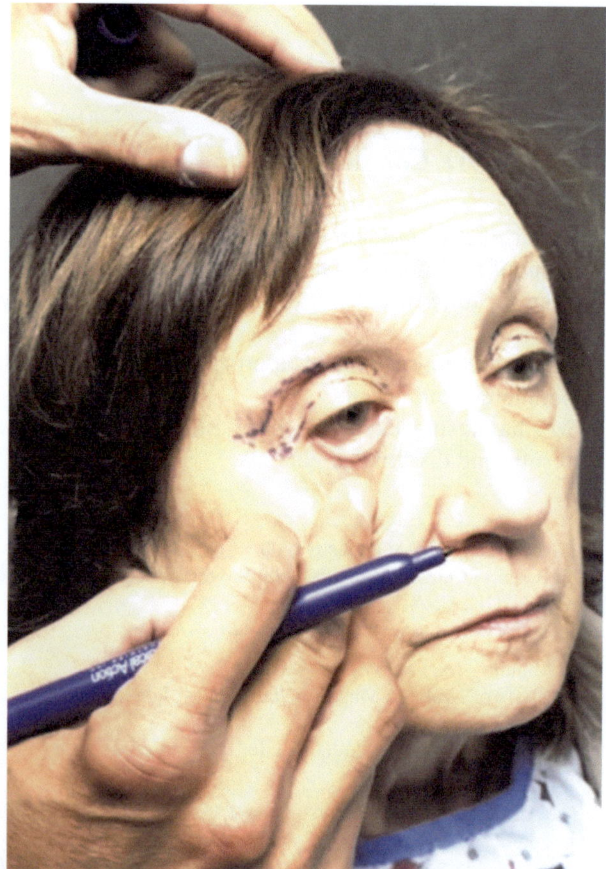

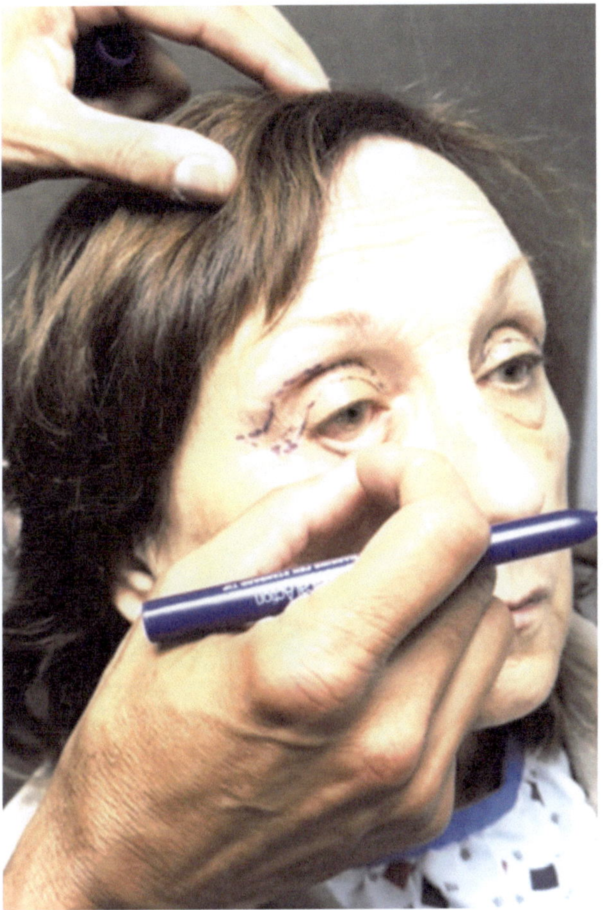

Fig. 44.3 Snapback test is performed to evaluate lower lid integrity

- Proper marking of the patient in a relaxed and upright position prior to injecting local anesthetic to avoid distortion.
- The authors recommend a fine-tip caliper for all measurements.

Intraoperative Consideration

- Conservative approach when first starting out. Revision surgery for a more dramatic effect is always an option, but you cannot go back once the tissue is excised.
- A good rule of thumb is maintaining a minimum of 20 mm of upper eyelid skin for adequate eye closure. This helps prevent lagophthalmos, dry eyes, and vision changes postoperatively (Fig. 44.4).

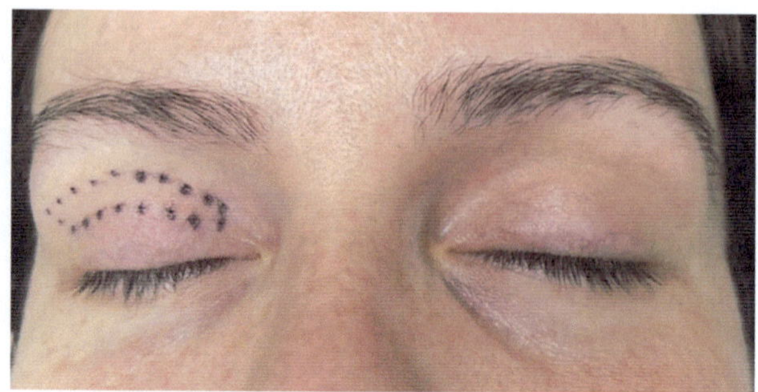

Fig. 44.4 The patient is marked in an upright position

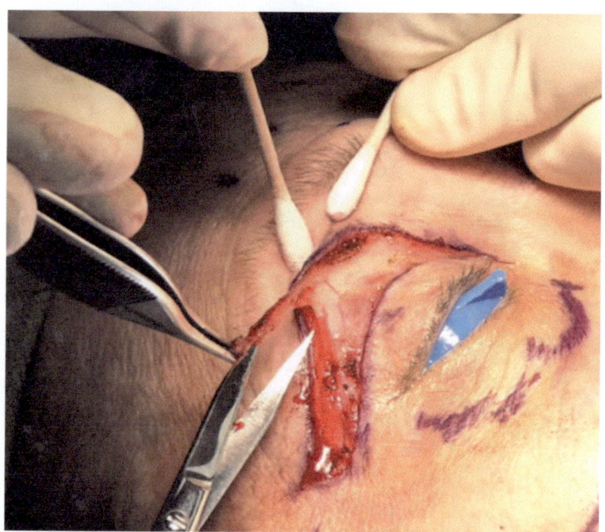

Fig. 44.5 Strip excision of orbicularis oculi muscle with fine iris scissors

- Correct identification and precise marking of the upper eyelid crease. Female creases tend to sit higher than males.
- Constant awareness that asymmetries may be inherently present requiring differential resection.
- The excision of a 4–5 mm strip of orbicularis muscle is commonly indicated; again, this is to be evaluated and modified as needed on a case-by-case basis (Fig. 44.5).
- Applying gentle pressure on the globe will help demarcate the location of fat pads under the orbital septum.
- Do not mistake the lacrimal gland for a fat pad. The upper eyelid has two fat pads.
- Conservative fat reduction is advised, as over-reduction can lead to a hollowing effect around the orbital rims. Keep in mind that fat transfer is a tool to be utilized to revitalize an aging face.

Postoperative Consideration

- Evaluation of postoperative visual acuity. Test with finger count and object identification.
- Close follow-up with patients to help guide them through the recovery period, which can look scary to many patients.
- Managing expectations by reminding them that results are only noticeable once they have completed their healing.
- Clear postoperative care instructions include activity restrictions, sleeping positions, and a pain management regimen.

Pearls

- Preoperative documentation of margin reflex distance 1 (MRD 1) and MRD 2 is necessary.
- Female creases tend to sit higher than males.
- Lower lid laxity directly relates to postoperative ectropion and retraction.

Pitfalls

- Misdiagnosing excessive brow skin for eyelid skin, resulting in suboptimal results and dissatisfied patients.
- Consider a fine-tip caliper for all measurements.
- Do not mistake the lacrimal gland for a fat pad.

Further Readings

Hollander MHJ, Schortinghuis J, Vissink A, Jansma J, Schepers RH. Aesthetic outcomes of upper eyelid blepharoplasty: a systematic review. Int J Oral Maxillofac Surg. 2020;49(6):750–64. Epub 2019 Nov 10. PMID: 31722817. https://doi.org/10.1016/j.ijom.2019.10.014.

Hollander MHJ, Delli K, Vissink A, Schepers RH, Jansma J. Patient-reported aesthetic outcomes of upper blepharoplasty: a randomized controlled trial comparing two surgical techniques. Int J Oral Maxillofac Surg. 2022;51(9):1161–9. Epub 2022 Feb 23. PMID: 35219565. https://doi.org/10.1016/j.ijom.2022.02.007.

Chapter 45
Pearls and Pitfalls of Facelift Surgery

Todd Hanna

Abstract Not all facelifts are for age-related changes. Young individuals with "doughy" or heavy cheeks or after significant weight loss can be appropriate candidates for face and/or neck lifts. Typically, however, a facelift is best suited for skin and soft tissue laxity, most commonly due to aging.

Definition and History

- Cervicofacial rhytidectomy: The excision of wrinkles in the skin of the face and neck (Fig. 45.1a, b).

    - Misnomer: Rhytids are not "excised"; they are redraped.
    - Commonly known as a face and neck lift, comprehensive facelift, or "full" facelift.

- Historically, it included periauricular and coronal incisions, hence the term "full" facelift.

Supplementary Information The online version contains supplementary material available at https://doi.org/10.1007/978-3-031-47307-4_45.

T. Hanna (✉)
Aesthetic Face and Jaw Surgery, Oral and Maxillofacial Surgery, Microvascular Head and Neck Reconstruction, Hanna Face and Jaw, PC, NY, USA

OMFS-Head & Neck Surgery, Mount Sinai Health System, New York, NY, USA
e-mail: dr.hanna@toddhannamddds.com

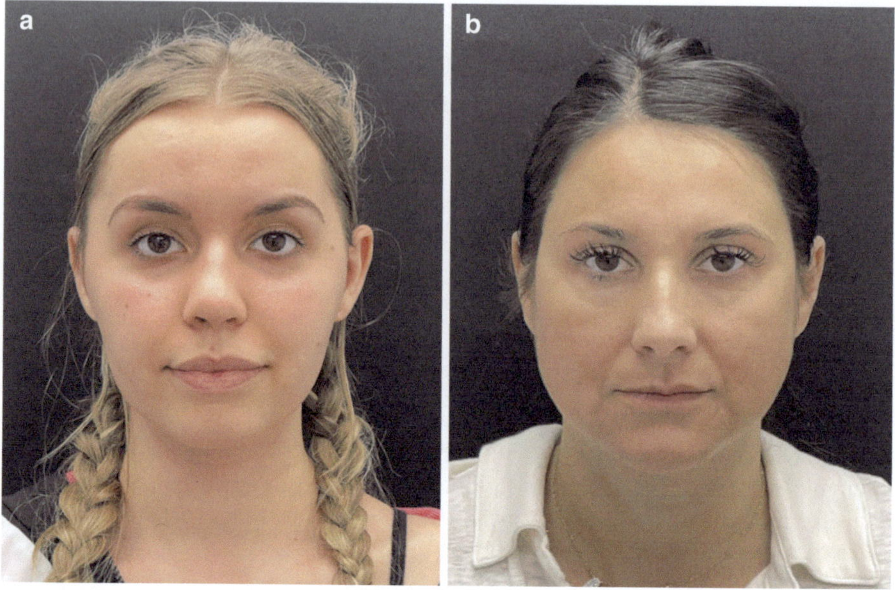

Fig. 45.1 (**a, b**) "Doughy" or heavy cheeks. These cases are best managed with lifting and buccal fat pad reduction procedures

- Modified and related techniques include the mini/short-scar facelift, mid-facelift, neck lift/submentoplasty, deep plane and dual plane face/neck lift, endoscopic facelift, jaw surgery facelift, and many others.
- Throughout the early 1900s, various skin-excision techniques were documented.
- In 1973, Skoog documented the first variation of a "deep plane" technique via elevating within the subplatysmal plane while leaving skin attachments intact.
- In 1976, Peyronie and Mitz presented the SMAS technique, the predecessor of the common facelift performed today.
- Throughout the 1970s–1990s, variations of SMAS management techniques were described, such as plication, imbrication, and SMASectomy.
- In 1990, Hamra described a more formal deep plane technique.
- The extended deep plane, dual plane, and endoscopic procedures have recently become popular.

Anatomy and the Aging Face and Neck

- Evaluation of directly involved areas: cheeks (malar and buccal fat pads), ears and earlobe attachments, jowls, submental region (submandibular glands, digastric muscles, sub- and supra-platysmal fat, platysmal decussation, and banding), nasolabial folds, and marionette lines.

- Evaluate associated areas, skin quality, upper and lower eyelids, upper lip, commissures and perioral region, and brow position.

  - Ignoring associated areas needing treatment will create a disharmonious result, as all areas of the face and neck should relate to one another.

- Common adjunctive procedures done with a face/neck lift are blepharoplasty, brow lift, skin resurfacing (laser or chemical), and upper lip lift.

  - Laser resurfacing should be performed prudently in the periphery of the skin flaps, as this area is more susceptible to necrosis.

- Anatomy layers: skin, lipocutaneous plane, SMAS/platysma, parotidomasseteric fascia, and deep plane structures (parotid gland, facial nerve branches, facial muscles).

Preoperative

- Listen:

  - The majority of the initial consultation should be listening to the patient's goals, desires, and expectations.

- Ask:

  - Get a feel for their understanding of their own anatomy and the requested procedure.
  - Do they have a support system?
  - Can they cope with the postoperative period and healing process?
  - Do they have external motivators?
  - Do they display body dysmorphic signs?
  - How have they fared with prior aesthetic procedures?

- Explain:

  - Review their preoperative photographs. Quality photographs are paramount. Standardize lighting, camera, and angles. It is proper not to use flash.
  - Review cases of patients with similar anatomy. Pay attention to any feedback from patients here.
  - Review different treatment options with pros and cons.
  - Review risks, benefits, and discomforts clearly.

- Illustrate:

  - Mark the incision on a patient's photograph (e.g., on a tablet), or demonstrate with a mirror (Fig. 45.2a, b).

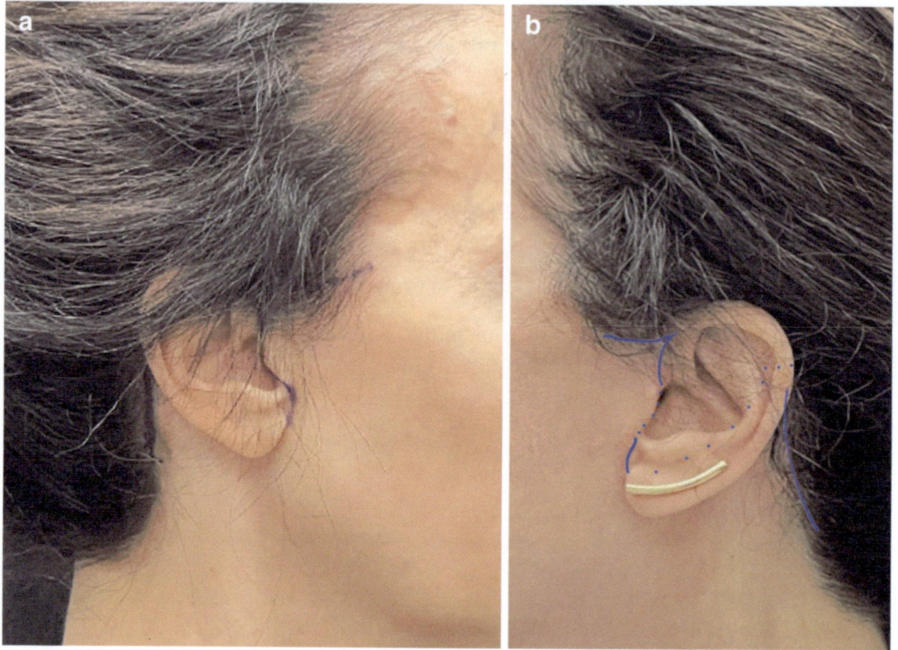

Fig. 45.2 (**a**, **b**) Markings (**a**, on patient; **b**, on a tablet)

- Review:

  - Encourage them to bring a friend or relative before surgery to review the procedure and act as a "second set of ears."
  - Establish home nursing for wound care and drain management if used.
  - Out-of-town patients must stay in town for 10–14 days.
  - Verbalized and written no-smoking prerequisite. Smokers must refrain for 3 weeks pre- and 3 weeks post-surgery.

Setup and Anesthesia

- Instrumentation is variable but commonly includes the following:

  - Head light, rulers and calipers, facial liposuction cannulas (used on wall suction), retractors, skin hooks, periosteal elevator, #11 and #15 blade scalpels, facelift scissors (e.g., Kaye), curved and straight fine scissors (e.g., Iris or Webster), Mayo scissors, Adson and Brown pickups, Cushing pickups, Debakey pickups, radio wave or electrosurgical unit with Colorado fine tip and insulated bipolar, various sized clamps (mosquito, hemostat, Adson, tonsils), needle holder (fine and long), smooth needle holder for holding stabilizing suture under tension during knot placement (e.g., Webster), stapler, sutures (3-0 Monocryl, 4-0 Monocryl, 5-0 gut, 5-0 nylon), gauze, hair comb, various suctions (Yankauer, tonsil, vascular, Frazier), tumescence (lidocaine, epinephrine, normal saline) with 22 gauge spinal needle and 60 mL syringe or Klein pump, 10 French Blake drains, hair wash (H2O2, shampoo, normal saline) and basin, head wrap (Kerlix, Coban, bacitracin, or mineral oil laced gauze around incisions), soft neck collar, and face bra (placed when head wrap is removed).

- Anesthesia will vary per patient and surgeon.

  - General anesthesia can cause elevated intrathoracic pressure during extubation and may provoke bleeding with subsequent hematoma.
  - Local anesthesia may limit the extent of tissue dissection possible.
  - IV sedation offers the most reasonable degree of sedation with less risk of hematoma and DVT, in the author's opinion.

- Markings should be done in a pre-op setting with the patient watching in a mirror and upright.
- Incision design will vary depending on lift type, surgeon preference, and patient anatomy; however, certain elements are ubiquitously accepted. Presented is the author's standard incision(s) with rationale:

  - Temporal tuft preserving with extreme bevel and undulating pattern at the periphery of sideburn to allow transfollicular hair growth (Fig. 45.3a, b).
  - May extend vertically with burrow's triangle for temporal standing cone/ bulge (Fig. 45.4a–e).
  - Preauricular transition begins hidden behind/posterior to the anterior helix.
  - The ear is pushed forward with the back end of a scalpel handle to find the natural delineation of the helical attachment.
  - Tragal edge-type design is typically preferred by the author over pre-tragal, even in male patients (in which case electrolysis for removing beard hair can be employed postoperatively). It is important to carefully dissect the skin of the tragus, leaving some soft tissue over the cartilage. Skeletonized cartilage tends to retract.

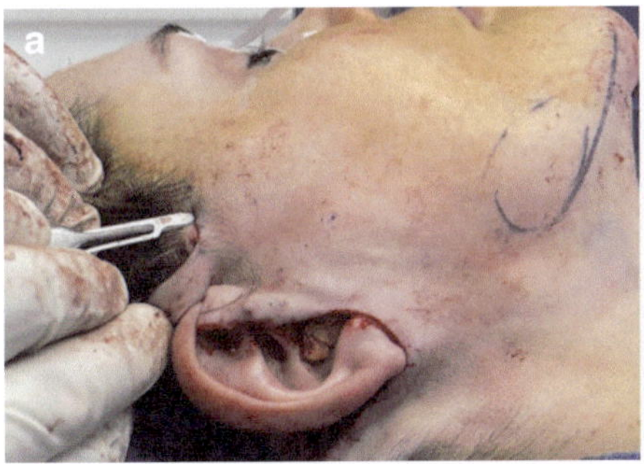
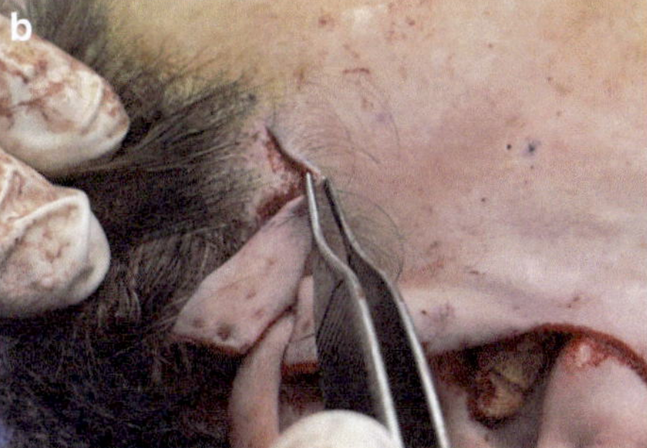

Fig. 45.3 (**a, b**) Extreme bevel (transfollicular) in the hairline

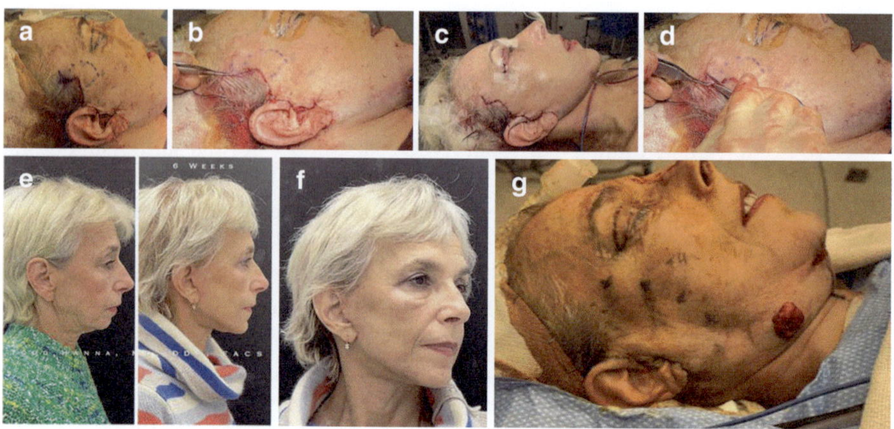

Fig. 45.4 (**a, b, c, d**) Temporal bulge management with Burow's triangle; (**e, f**) at 6 weeks post-op deep plane face and neck lift with submandibular gland reduction, upper and lower blepharoplasty, and genioplasty); (**g**) portion of the submandibular gland below the inferior border removed through the submental incision. Note that only a part of the gland should be removed

- A "notch" just above the lobe can be used, then releasing the lobule into the postauricular crease.
- Staying within the postauricular crease, rather than onto the concha, is preferred as key sutures will prevent retraction of the scar inferiorly.
- At the level where the pinna is closest to the posterior hairline, the incision is carried across the mastoid.

> For short-scar mid-facelifts, the incision stops here.
> For comprehensive face/neck lifts, the author prefers to carry the incision into the posterior cervical hairline, again using an extreme bevel transfollicular approach.
> If a submentoplasty is employed, a 2–3 cm incision made approximately 5 mm posterior to the submental crease is used. Greater distance is used if a chin advancement (genioplasty or chin implant) is done, as this may advance the incision, making it less conspicuous.

- Mark midline lower lip, chin, and neck.

> Helps to confirm equal pull tension bilaterally.
> Outline zones of liposuction: Jowls and submental landmarks (inferior border, SCM muscles, the superior edge of the thyroid cartilage).

Surgical Technique for Standard Comprehensive Cervicofacial Rhytidectomy

- Apply a tumescent solution in the submental zone.

- Allow 5 min for epinephrine to take effect for excellent hemostasis.
- Make stab incision within submentoplasty marking for liposuction cannula.
- Pre-dissect in lipocutaneous plane with dissector or spatulate cannula, not on suction.
- Begin liposuction using sequentially progressive cannulas until a smooth layer of skin and fat can be palpated.
- Avoid liposuction of the jowl from a submental approach, as it will put the marginal branch of the facial nerve at risk of being compressed between the cannula and the inferior border.

- Next, complete the submental incision and dissect it in the lipocutaneous plane with Kaye scissors and a right-angle retractor.

  - Identify the medial border of the platysma and selectively excise minimal subplatysmal fat being mindful to avoid a cobra neck deformity.
  - You can track in the subplatysmal plane laterally to access and reduce the submandibular glands as needed through this incision, as is the author's preferred approach. An alternate approach to the submandibular gland is through the preauricular incision (Fig. 45.4g).
  - The oromandibular ligaments can be released here as well.
  - Plication, or approximation, of the medial platysma is then made using 2–0 Monocryl suture in a corseted fashion.

- Attention is then drawn to the right or left face, and the tumescent solution is administered. It is important to include the mastoid region while injecting as this will help hydro-dissect this tenacious zone making your dissection easier.

  - The incision is made with a #15 blade, and scalpel dissection is used to elevate the first 2–4 cm of the lipocutaneous plane, particularly in the tragal and postauricular zones where the skin is very thin and fixed to deeper layers.
  - The desired extent of dissection is carried out within the lipocutaneous plane with Kaye scissors. Connection should typically be made into the submental dissection to release all retaining ligaments.
  - Liposuction of the jowl is performed from this approach.

- The SMAS should be manipulated to assess laxity and ideal vectors.

  - Incision into the SMAS is made approximately 2 cm anterior to the tragus.
  - The author prefers a "lazy Z-type" SMASectomy pattern that is horizontal below the zygoma, vertical in the preauricular zone, and diagonal along the lateral platysma to allow for ideal vectors of pull (Fig. 45.5).
  - At this point, one can enter the deep plane into the face and neck below the SMAS and lateral platysma if indicated.
  - Caution must be taken to identify and protect the facial nerve branches in deep plane techniques as well as recognize other deep structures such as the parotid gland and master muscle (Fig. 45.6a–d).
  - SMASectomy is performed with scissors or electrocautery, exposing the underlying parotidomasseteric fascia.

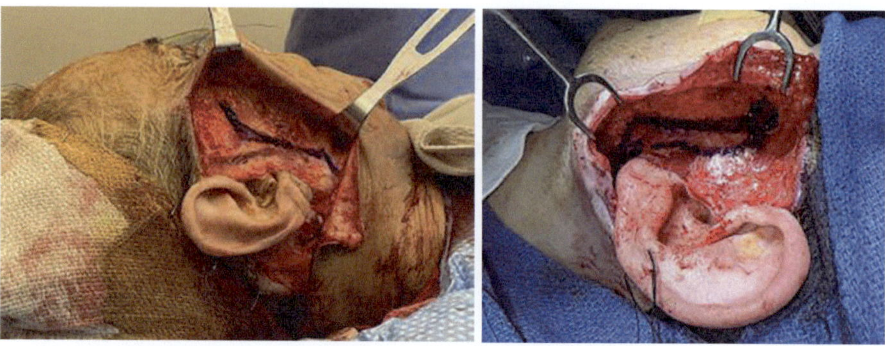

Fig. 45.5 SMASectomy "lazy Z" design

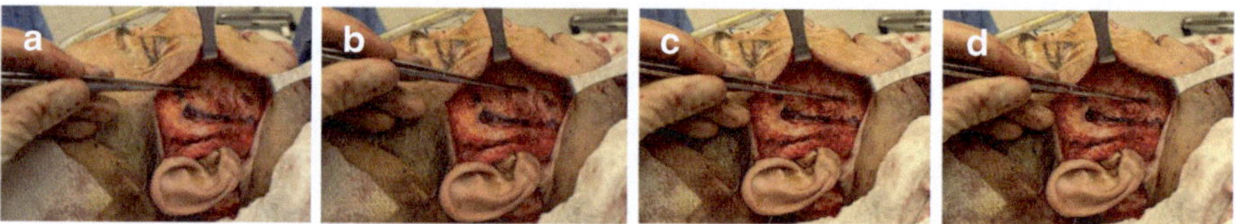

Fig. 45.6 (**a**, **b**, **c**, **d**) Deep plane demonstrating the zygomatic and buccal branch of the facial nerve, the master muscle, and a part of the parotid gland

> – SMAS resuspension sutures, 2-0 Monocryl, are first placed at the jowl and then progressed to the temporal and mastoid regions. Typically 8–10 SMAS sutures are placed in interrupted buried horizontal mattress fashion (Video 45.1).

- The tension of skin redraping should largely be carried by the SMAS sutures.
- The lipocutaneous flap should be passively laid into the ideal vector and position.
- Key sutures, 4-0 Monocryl, are placed on either side of the helix and pinna and above and below the tragus.
- The postauricular vector is typically more vertical than the preauricular vector, cradling the ear.
- The skin is thinned and left in excess at the tragus to avoid a "thick-skinned" appearance at the tragus, which naturally has thinner skin (Fig. 45.7a–c).
- The ear lobe is then passively delivered, and the skin is tailored. The cut end of the ear lobe can be used as a guide for skin excision in this area.

  - Avoid over-resecting here, as the lobe will retract with healing and gravity when upright and can result in a pixie ear deformity.
  - Avoid anterior or posterior lobe position, and refer to preoperative photos here.

- If a more vertical vector is required at the temporal zone, the author prefers a Burow's triangle excision well hidden into the hairline to avoid a dog ear or temporal bulge, as aforementioned.

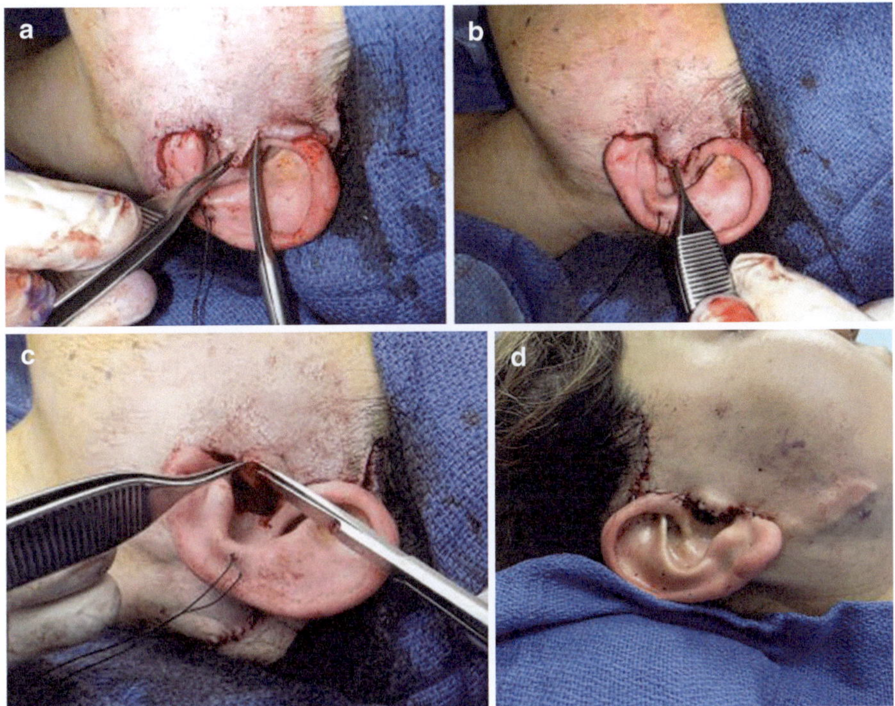

Fig. 45.7 (**a**, **b**, **c**) Trimming and thinning the tragus. (**d**) Final closure

- 10 French Blake or size 3 x 7 mm Jackson-Pratt suction drains extend along the cheek and into the submentum, exiting posteriorly into the hair-bearing scalp.
- Skin closure is performed with 5-0 nylon in running fashion in the preauricular region. One to two interrupted mattress sutures are placed at the lobe as this area is prone to dehiscence from removing a shirt or pulling during sleep (Fig. 45.7d).
- 4-0 Monocryl is used for key and deep sutures.
- 4-0 gut is used in all hair-bearing zones; alternatively, one can use staples.
- The identical procedure is then performed on the contralateral side, being mindful of your midline marking for symmetrical pull.
- The hair is rinsed with H_2O_2 and shampoo and towel-dried.
- Bacitracin, Xeroform gauze, or mineral oil-soaked gauze is placed over the incisions, and a pressure dressing is applied using Kerlix and Coban.
- A soft neck brace is placed to restrict head movement for the first post-op week.
- The suction bulbs are secured to the patient's shirt and monitored in recovery until discharged home with nursing care.

Post-Op Care

- Management of PONV is imperative as retching can result in hematoma formation.

    - Anesthetic methods, as well as post-op steroids and Zofran, are standard.
    - Limiting narcotics is also important.

- Keeping blood pressure low post-op is also imperative to avoid hematoma.
- The pressure dressing is removed on POD 1, and bacitracin is reapplied to the wounds.

    - A face bra is placed and worn along with the soft neck brace for the first week.

- From weeks 2–4, the face bra should be worn at night and, when possible, during the day.
- The drain is removed when output is less than 20 mL in 24 h (typically 2–3 days).

Managing Complications

- Intraoperative:

    - Bleeding.

        Managed with diligent inspection after irrigating the field to find "occult bleeders."

        You can have anesthesia lightened or use Valsalva to increase blood or intrathoracic pressure prior to closure to help identify these.

        Prudent use of bipolar electrocautery, being mindful of nerves and thermal injury to the skin flap.
        Utilize drains and pressure dressing.

    - Injury to the motor or sensory nerves.

        Direct immediate repair if visualized under loupe magnification.
        High-dose steroids and B-complex vitamins postoperatively in case of neuropraxia.
        Some literature supports the use of gabapentin.
        Refer to a facial reanimation specialist as needed.
        Most neuropraxia is temporary and resolves in 60–90 days.
        Can use Botox selectively on the unaffected side for symmetry during the recovery phase.

- Postoperative:

    - Expanding hematoma.

Will present as significant asymmetrical pain, ecchymosis, and firm swelling.
Open and evacuate early to avoid skin flap necrosis.
Compression.

- Seroma.

  Aspiration and compression.
  Commonly redeveloped.

- Neck banding and wash boarding.

  Best prevented by the use of drains.
  Treat with an aspiration of fluid in early stages.
  Dilute steroid injections, warm compresses, and massage in later stages.

- Skin flap necrosis.

  Causes include untreated hematoma, aggressive cautery and thermal injury to the skin flap, aggressive and thin skin flap elevation, excessive tension upon closure, poor patient selection such as smokers, pressure from eyeglasses, and aggressive skin resurfacing at the time of a facelift.
  Manage with wound care.
  Nitric oxide paste and HBO potentially have benefits.
  May require resurfacing or scar revision when healed.

- Hypertrophic or poor scar formation.

  Minimize tension upon closure.
  Gentle soft tissue handling.
  Meticulous skin closure.
  Steroid, 5-FU, or laser treatment as needed.
  Occasionally need surgical scar revision.

- Alopecia.

  Minimize thermal injury to hair follicles.
  Minimize undermining hair-bearing scalp.
  Usually improves within 6 months.
  Follicular unit hair transplants for areas that do not improve.

- Temporal balding.

  Occurs from improper incision design.
  Treat with follicular unit hair transplant.

- Retracted tragus.

  Occurs from undercutting skin flap at tragus, resulting in tension upon closure.
  Prevent by leaving excess skin here.
  Treatment is a revision and redrawing skin flap.

- Pixie ear deformity.

  Occurs from undercutting lobe attachment which retracts with gravity and natural contracture that comes with wound healing.
  Treatment is a revision and redrawing skin flap.

- Residual skin laxity.

  Most commonly seen in the submental area and jowl.
  Small areas may be amenable to excision of skin (at submental incision), radiofrequency, or CO_2 laser for skin retraction.
  Large areas need revision lift.

- Early relapse.

  Usually results from insufficient deep sutures or early and excessive postoperative head/neck movement by the patient.
  A soft neck collar for the first week postoperatively is helpful to prevent the latter.

- Extruded sutures and suture reactions.

  Can be seen several months/years later.
  Can be minimized by burying the knot deep in the SMAS and using slow-resorbable sutures.
  Treatment requires the removal of extruded sutures and wound care.

- Sialocele and salivary gland fistula.

  Most commonly results from partial submandibular gland excision.
  Can also be seen from the parotid gland.
  Placement of drains helps to minimize.
  Treatment includes aspiration, compression, and medications such as Botox and anticholinergics.

Pearls

- Not all facelifts are for age-related changes.
- Preoperative preparation is key for successful results.
- Setting clear expectations and establishing a rapport with the patient are essential.
- Postoperative care is crucial in avoiding complications.
- Management of PONV is imperative, as retching can result in hematoma formation.

Pitfalls

- Learn how to manage complications intraoperatively and postoperatively since they can happen and affect the outcomes of surgery.
- Pay attention to "occult bleeders" intraoperatively.
- Judicious use of drains and compression dressing will minimize postoperative hematoma.
- Expanding hematoma must be drained to avoid skin necrosis.
- Avoid the use of excessive cautery since it will increase the risk of skin flap necrosis.

Typical results of short-scar (mini) lift (Fig. 45.8a–c) and comprehensive face and neck lift (Fig. 45.9a–c).

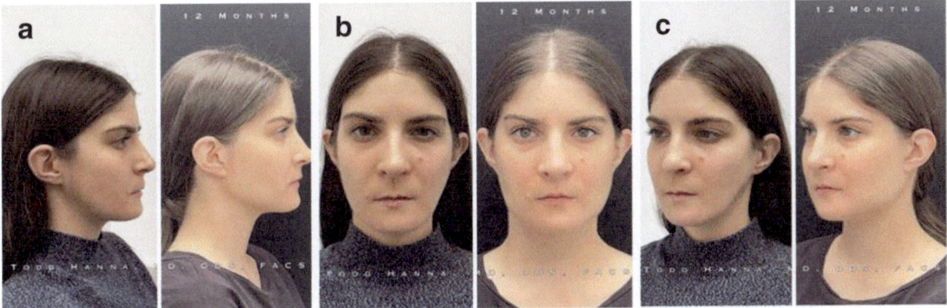

Fig. 45.8 (**a, b, c**) Short-scar mini lift (with custom angle implants and subnasal lip lift)

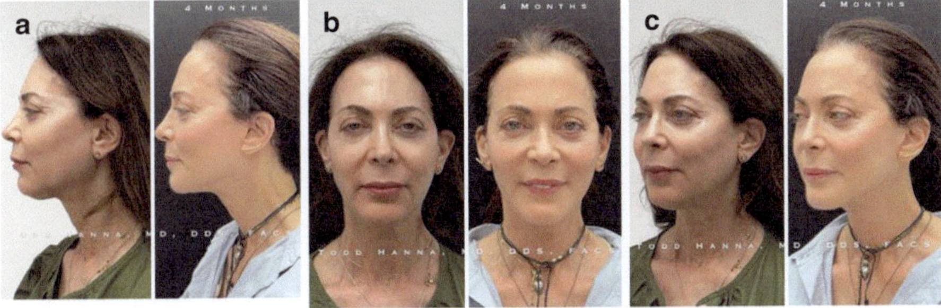

Fig. 45.9 (**a, b, c**) Comprehensive face and neck lift (with chin implant removal and geniotomy, temporal fat grafting, and upper blepharoplasty)

Further Readings

Fedok FG, Lighthall JG. Evaluation and treatment planning for the aging face patient. Facial Plast Surg Clin North Am. 2022;30(3):277–90. PMID: 35934430. https://doi.org/10.1016/j.fsc.2022.03.002.

Kaya KS, Cakmak O. Facelift techniques: an overview. Facial Plast Surg. 2022;38(6):540–5. Epub 2022 Jun 16. PMID: 35709719. https://doi.org/10.1055/a-1877-9371.

Niamtu J III. Cosmetic facial surgery. 2nd ed. New York: Elsevier.

Part VIII
Obstructive Sleep Apnea

Chapter 46
Drug-Induced Sleep Endoscopy

Jessica Jurovich and Ketan Patel

Abstract Drug-induced sleep endoscopy (DISE) is a diagnostic tool to evaluate the dynamic upper airway of patients with sleep-disordered breathing. This procedure is usually a prerequisite for decision-making for a hypoglossal nerve stimulator device. During the procedure, the patient is sedated to mimic sleep, and the upper airway is assessed for obstruction. The information obtained is used to make decisions about further treatment options. The purpose of this chapter is to review pearls and pitfalls for drug-induced sleep endoscopy.

Practical Tips

Preoperative Consideration

- Patients should have all standard sedation monitors during the procedure. It is also recommended to monitor BIS with levels between 50 and 70.
- Use a thin fiber-optic endoscope to evaluate areas of upper airway collapse better.
- To ensure that a dry field is obtained, approximately 0.2 mg of glycopyrrolate is.
- usually given intravenously in the preoperative area before transportation to the operating room. In addition, oxymetazoline spray (Afrin) can also be used to provide vasoconstriction and decongestion to reduce secretions.

J. Jurovich
School of Dentistry, University of Minnesota, Minneapolis, MN, USA

K. Patel (✉)
Head and Neck Oncology and Microvascular Reconstructive Surgery and Oral and Maxillofacial Surgery at North Memorial Health, Adjunct Faculty, North Memorial Hospital Minneapolis, University of Minnesota, Minneapolis, MN, USA
e-mail: ketan.patel@northmemorial.com

D. Amin, H. Marwan (eds.), *Pearls and Pitfalls in Oral and Maxillofacial Surgery*, https://doi.org/10.1007/978-3-031-47307-4_46

Intraoperative Consideration

- After ASA monitors are placed, a nasal cannula is placed. The authors prefer a nasal cannula, which can be placed over the mouth once taken off the nose. A combination of medications is given for sedation. However, propofol delivered via a pump is usually preferred over other agents. The quantity is weight dependent; however, dosing from about 100–150 µg/kg/min is administered to ensure suitable sedation. Additional propofol boluses may be given based on patient history and body habitus.
- Once the patient is sedated and snoring, a fiber-optic scope (pediatric/1.4–1.8 mm diameter) is passed through the nostril. This is typically passed between the middle and inferior turbinates to the posterior nasopharynx. Care must be taken to prevent epistaxis by staying away from the walls during the evaluation.
- The scope is advanced to evaluate the velum, oropharyngeal walls, tongue base, and epiglottis (VOTE analysis) for collapse (Fig. 46.1). It is important to note what type of collapse is observed (anterior, posterior collapse vs. concentric collapse).
- An Esmarch maneuver (jaw thrust) is conducted, and the airway's opening is evaluated. A good opening of the airway at this point is a good indicator for potential airway stimulation treatment. Once the other pharyngeal anatomy is evaluated, the scope is withdrawn.

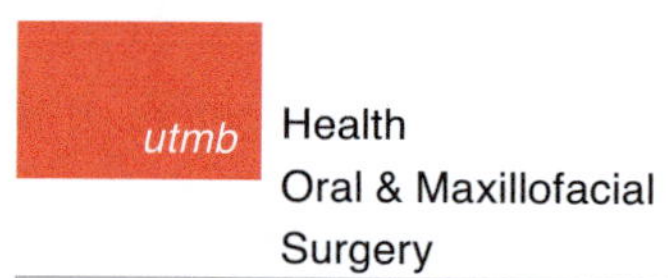

STRUCTURE	DEGREE OF OBSTRUCTION[a]	CONFIGURATION[c]		
		A-P	LATERAL	CONCENTRIC
Velum				
Oropharynx[b]				
Tongue Base				
Epiglottis				

Fig. 46.1 Example of the VOTE analysis chart. Note the level and the direction of the obstruction for each anatomical level

- Although this is a relatively benign procedure, a few risks could be incurred that the surgeon needs to prepare for depending on the level of complexity. Laryngospasm can occur with direct stimulation of the cords with a risk of aspiration. Obstructive sleep apnea more commonly occurs in patients with a higher BMI; therefore, caution must be taken regarding desaturation with subsequent loss and airway and the need for a surgical airway.

Postoperative Consideration

- There are no postoperative considerations for a drug-induced sleep endoscopy, as the entire procedure is completed under sedation.

Pearls

- Obstructive sleep apnea more commonly occurs in patients with a higher BMI.
- Consider ensuring 0.2 mg of glycopyrrolate and oxymetazoline spray (Afrin).
- Pass the fiber-optic scope through the nostril, between the middle and inferior turbinate to the posterior nasopharynx.

Pitfalls

- For sedation, propofol is preferred over other agents.
- Laryngospasm can occur with direct stimulation of the cords with a risk of aspiration.
- Obstructive sleep apnea more commonly occurs in patients with a higher BMI.

Further Reading

Charakorn N, Kezirian EJ. Drug-induced sleep endoscopy. Otolaryngol Clin N Am. 2016;49(6):1359–72.

Kotecha B, De Vito A. Drug-induced sleep endoscopy: its role in evaluation of the upper airway obstruction and patient selection for surgical and non-surgical treatment. J Thorac Dis. 2018;10(Suppl 1):S40–7.

Zapanta P, DeVries G, Singleton A. Sleep endoscopy: overview, periprocedural care, technique. Medscape; 2022. https://emedicine.medscape.com/article/1963060-overview?form=fpf.

Chapter 47
Practical Tips for Pharyngoplasty Procedure

Hisham Marwan and Victoria Manon

Abstract Uvulopalatopharyngoplasty (UPPP) is the most used procedure for treating obstructive sleep apnea (OSA). There are several technique modifications of the procedure to minimize the complications and expedite the recovery. Most of the failures of UPPP happen after surgery, and patients will return with a relapse of their OSA. Recently, the focus was redirected toward the lateral wall collapsibility of the airway at the level of the velum and oropharynx. All pharyngoplasty procedures now aim to minimize the procedure's invasiveness and expand the lateral pharyngeal wall. There is a change in the concept from UPPP to pharyngoplasty regarding the amount of normal tissues to be removed. For instance, the goal of UPPP was to remove the tonsils, part of the anterior tonsillar pillar, and the uvula and suture the anterior and posterior tonsillar pillars. A large amount of the soft palate is usually removed, and the risk of postoperative velopharyngeal insufficiency (VPI) after UPPP is about 2%. This "resective" concept has changed to a "reconstructive" concept with maintaining the normal tissues and instead suspending the pharyngeal muscles to expand the lateral pharyngeal wall. The purpose of this chapter is to review pearls and the pitfalls of using expansion pharyngoplasty (ESP) with barbed sutures.

H. Marwan (✉)
Department of Surgery, The University of Texas Medical Branch, Galveston, TX, USA
e-mail: himarwan@utmb.edu

V. Manon
Oral and Maxillofacial Surgery Department, McGovern Medical School, UTHSC School of Dentistry at Houston, University of Texas, Houston, TX, USA

D. Amin, H. Marwan (eds.), *Pearls and Pitfalls in Oral and Maxillofacial Surgery*, https://doi.org/10.1007/978-3-031-47307-4_47

Practical Tips

Preoperative Consideration

- Drug-induced sleep endoscopy (DISE) is an essential diagnostic tool to identify the area of anatomical obstruction. The ESP is mainly indicated for patients with lateral wall collapsibility at the level of the velum and oropharynx.
- Assess the size of the tonsils using the Friedman staging system. The procedure can be performed for patients who have had tonsillectomy before.
- The procedure is relatively contraindicated in singers and professional speakers.
- Counsel the patient about postoperative dysphagia. In general, normal swallow function comes back after 3 months of surgery.

Intraoperative Consideration (Fig. 47.1)

- The goal is to suspend the palatopharyngeus muscle to the hamulus (superior-lateral direction).
- Use shoulder roll and Dingman mouth gag to provide wide access to the surgical field.
- The first step is to remove the palatine tonsils if present. Use the Coblator device to remove the tonsils and preserve the mucosa of the tonsillar pillar.
- The palatopharyngeus muscle is identified and dissected inferiorly. The muscle should be slightly released inferiorly but kept attached to the mucosa. This will help suspend the muscle without tension and prevent relapse.
- A 1 cm incision is made in the soft palate, as close as possible to the hamulus. Debulking of the supratonsillar fat is recommended to facilitate lateral expansion.
- Three marks are used to direct the suspension, the central palate and the bilateral pterygomandibular raphe.
- The use of V-Loc 90-degree sutures to suspend the muscle to the pterygomandibular raphe and the hamulus.
- Start the suspension by passing the sutures at the soft palate incision toward the pterygomandibular raphe.
- Tunnel the suture toward the palatopharyngeus muscle. The muscle should be imbricated and suspended toward the hamulus and the pterygomandibular raphe.
- Symmetrical lateral expansion bilaterally is required for successful outcomes.
- Remove the uvula tip only if it is long.
- Ensure adequate hemostasis before closure, especially if the palatine tonsils are removed.

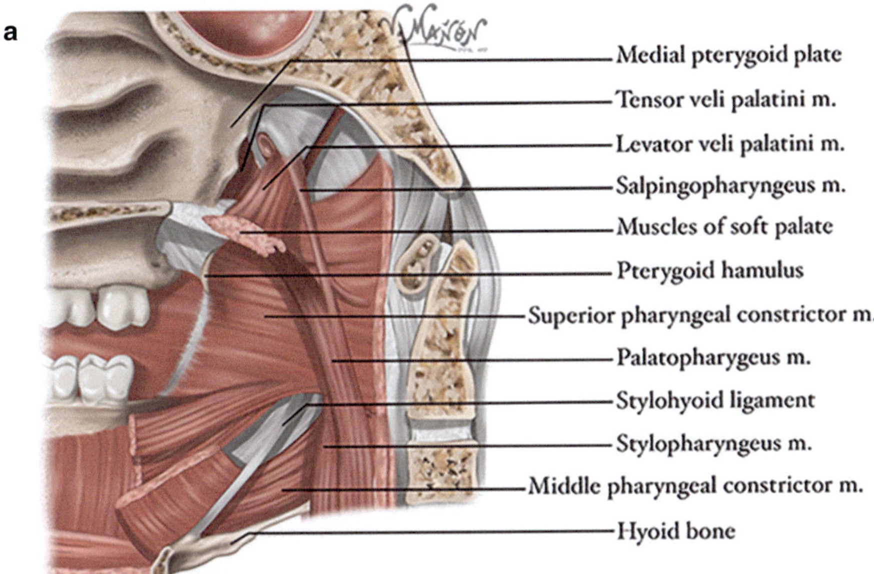

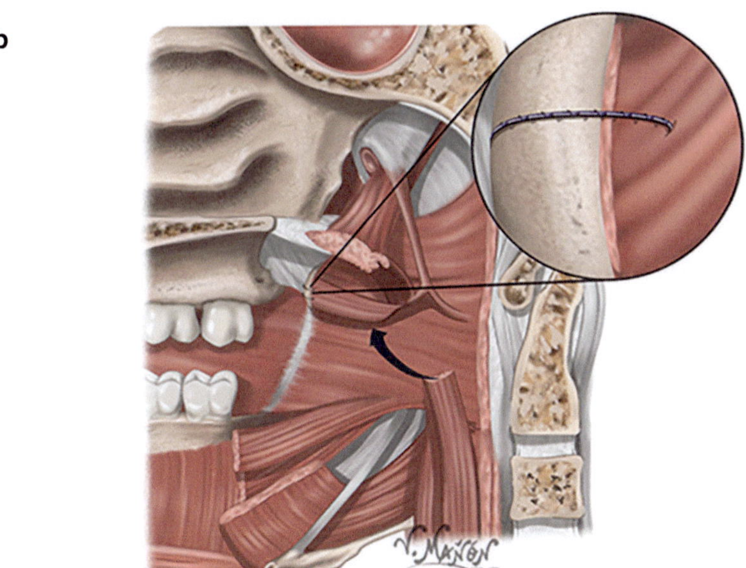

Fig. 47.1 Sagittal sections of the pharynx. (**a**) Detailed anatomy of the pharynx. Note the location of the palatopharyngeus muscle. (**b**) Suspension of the muscle to the hamulus notch

Postoperative Consideration

- The patient can swallow liquid without difficulty; however, regular food might be difficult to swallow during the immediate postoperative period.
- Applying ice inside the mouth will help with the swelling.
- Keep the patient for 23 h observation to monitor the airway.
- Foreign body sensation in the throat is relatively common and usually self-limiting.

Pearls

- Expansion pharyngoplasty is a modification of UPPP that is less invasive with a higher success rate.
- DISE exam should show a dominant lateral wall instability.
- Suspension should always involve the pterygomandibular raphe.
- Removal of the supratonsillar fat will increase the airway dimension and help the palatopharyngeal muscle's suspension.

Pitfalls

- Swallowing dysfunction is common, and swallow therapy would help the patient recover faster.
- The procedure will not give an excellent long-term result in patients with concentric collapse.
- Voice changes can happen after the surgery. Avoid the procedure in singers and professional speakers.

Further Reading

Pang KP, Woodson BT. Expansion sphincter pharyngoplasty: a new technique for the treatment of obstructive sleep apnea. Otolaryngol Head Neck Surg. 2007;137(1):110–4.
Olszewska E, Woodson BT. Palatal anatomy for sleep apnea surgery. Laryngosc Investig Otolaryngol. 2019;4:181. https://doi.org/10.1002/lio2.238.

Chapter 48
Pearls and Pitfalls in the Preoperative Planning for Maxillomandibular Advancement

Brian Kinard

Abstract Obstructive sleep apnea (OSA) is often of multifactorial etiology. When the pathogenesis of OSA is associated with anatomical abnormalities such as retrognathia, bimaxillary retrusion, transverse maxillary deficiency, and clockwise inclination of the occlusal plane, skeletal correction is indicated. The maxillomandibular advancement (MMA) for OSA treatment is a site-specific surgery that enlarges the posterior airway space and increases pharyngeal wall tension at multiple anatomic levels, including the nasopharynx, oropharynx, and hypopharynx. The MMA for airway expansion is carried out through osteotomies of the maxilla, mandible, and chin with available concomitant adjunctive procedures such as nasal septoplasty, bilateral inferior turbinate reductions, uvulectomy, and genial tubercle advancement.

Advancement of the maxilla pulls the soft tissues of the palate forward, including the palatoglossal muscles, and increases tongue support. Advancement of the mandible repositions several muscles forward, including the anterior belly of the digastric, mylohyoid, genioglossus, and geniohyoid muscles. Both maxillary and mandibular surgeries increase available tongue space. The genial tubercle advancement provides additional advancement of the genioglossus and geniohyoid muscles. The MMA is a first-line surgical treatment for patients with pre-existing dentofacial deformities, severe OSA, and/or complete concentric collapse airway pattern (at velum and lateral pharyngeal walls), as demonstrated by drug-induced sleep endoscopy (DISE). Secondary indications for MMA are failure of other forms of therapy. The success rate for MMA ranges between 75% and 100%. In addition to AHI reduction, the MMA also mitigates patient symptoms and comorbid risk.

It is important to clarify the patient's diagnosis of occlusion and facial aesthetic needs in addition to sites of upper airway obstructions. In efforts to maximally treat OSA, treatment planning includes a cosmetically viable maximal skeletal advance-

B. Kinard (✉)
Department of Oral and Maxillofacial Surgery, University of Alabama at Birmingham, Birmingham, AL, USA

Department of Orthodontics, University of Alabama at Birmingham, Birmingham, AL, USA
e-mail: BrianKinard@uabmc.edu

D. Amin, H. Marwan (eds.), *Pearls and Pitfalls in Oral and Maxillofacial Surgery*, https://doi.org/10.1007/978-3-031-47307-4_48

ment for the maxilla, mandible, and chin with maximization of the chin advancement through counterclockwise (CCW) rotation. For most patients, facial aesthetics can be improved or preserved through the MMA. Unpleasant aesthetic changes may result in the perinasal region if strategies are not employed to limit perinasal fullness, such as CCW rotation and recontouring of the nasal floor and aperture. The purpose of this chapter is to review pearls and pitfalls in the preoperative planning for maxillomandibular advancement.

Practical Tips

Preoperative Consideration

- Clarify patient goals; discuss facial aesthetic, occlusal, and OSA concerns.
- Confirm the sleep study is accurate and demonstrates obstructive apneas.
- Complete a thorough history and exam, review polysomnography, and consider fiber-optic nasopharyngoscopy and/or DISE.
- Counsel patient on the increased risk for complications:

  - The OSA population is often with multiple comorbidities.
  - A comprehensive medical review with patient optimization is of value.
  - Comorbidities may contribute to delayed healing.
  - There is an increased risk of unfavorable sagittal ramus splits among adults secondary to decreased marrow space.
  - Counsel on the risk of inferior alveolar nerve paresthesias, which increases with age and larger movements.

- Screen for chronic obstructive nasal breathing and indications for concomitant nasal septoplasty and bilateral inferior turbinate reductions.
- Plan for temporary anchorage devices or orthodontic brackets if considering postoperative orthodontic therapy.

Surgical Treatment Planning and Modifications

- Maximize cosmetically viable advancement:

  - Andrews' analysis for confirmation that maxillary advancement is possible.
  - Soft tissue laxity and a thick soft tissue envelope will aesthetically tolerate a greater advancement.
  - Consider selective extractions to allow for maximal advancement of the maxilla and/or mandible.

- Maximize CCW rotation of the occlusal plane (CCWROP):

  - The amount of CCWROP is based on the patient's occlusion, facial appearance, and OSA severity.

- CCWROP rotated around the maxillary central incisor midpoint, can improve the facial profile by providing a larger advancement of the mandible and chin relative to the maxilla (Fig. 48.1). This reduces the prominence of the ANS and pyriform rims and limits unfavorable aesthetic changes to the nose.
- CCWROP may result in an increased show of the posterior maxillary gingiva and result in a non-consonant smile arc.
- CCWROP maximizes oropharyngeal airway enlargement through basal mandibular advancement in the horizontal dimension. This results in a forward and downward movement of the soft palate with increased retropalatal space. CCWROP maximizes airway muscle tension while balancing facial aesthetics.
- Each degree of CCW rotation of the occlusal plane results in approximately 0.7 mm of chin advancement.

• Genial tubercle advancement:

- Computer aided surgical simulation is helpful to accurately locate the genial tubercle. The genial tubercle advancement can be accomplished through a high genioplasty, a rectangular genial tubercle advancement, or a two-segment osteotomy of the genial tubercle and osseous genioplasty (Fig. 48.2). The genial tubercle advancement pulls genioglossus and geniohyoid muscles forward.

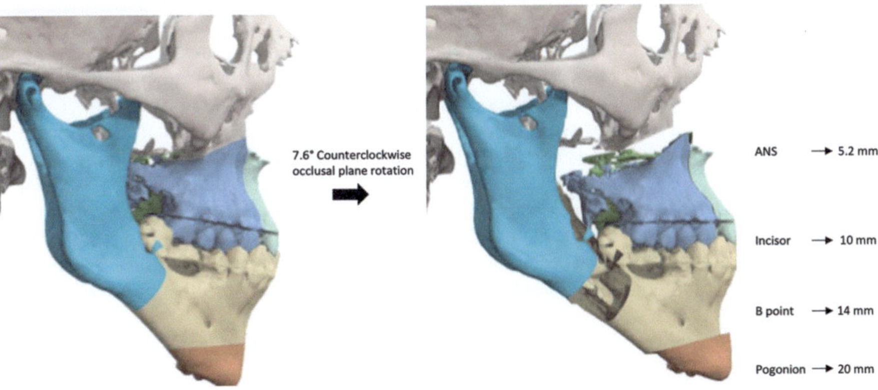

Fig. 48.1 Counterclockwise rotation of the occlusal plane (CCWROP) can improve the facial profile by advancing the mandible and chin more than the maxilla. Computer-aided surgical simulation demonstrates a 10 mm advancement of the maxillomandibular complex, measured as the maxillary central incisor midpoint. 7.6° of CCWROP results in only a 5 mm advancement at the anterior nasal spine, which limits perinasal fullness and decreases the osteotomy gap at the anterior maxillary walls. The CCWROP provides additional advancement of the mandible and chin relative to the maxillary central incisors, maximizing the skeletal advancement for treating OSA

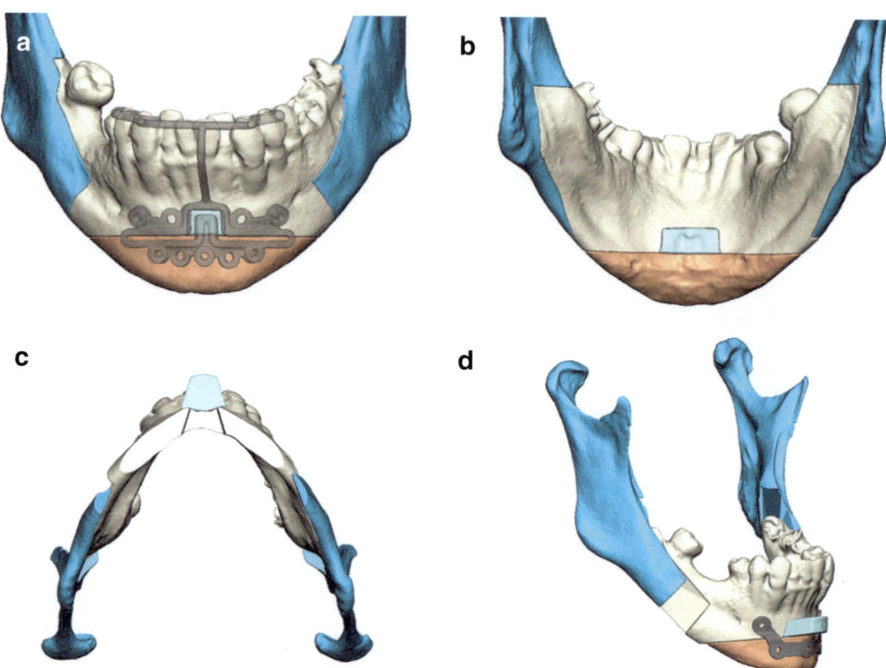

Fig. 48.2 A two-piece genial tubercle advancement and osseous genioplasty are demonstrated. (**a**) Facial view with patient-specific osteotomy guide for the patient-specific plate. (**b**) Lingual view of two-piece genial tubercle segment and osseous genioplasty segment. Computer-aided surgical simulation ensures complete capture of the genial tubercles in the osteotomy. Note that the lingual cortex of the segment is wider than the facial cortex, creating a trapezoidal segment. (**c**) An inferior view of the two-piece osteotomy. The osseous genioplasty segment is hidden from view. The trapezoidal genial tubercle segment is mobilized inferiorly and anteriorly and then locked over the facial surface of the mandibular osteotomy. (**d**) The osseous genioplasty is then positioned through a patient-specific plate, securing the genial tubercle segment. After the genial tubercle is "locked" into position, the outer cortex is reduced with an oval burr to approximate the facial cortex of the mandible. This case demonstrates a 5 mm advancement of the osseous genioplasty segment and a 12 mm advancement of the genial tubercles. Also, note the anterior position of the anterior portion of the sagittal ramus osteotomy to increase postoperative bone overlap

Intraoperative Consideration

- Airway management:
  - Consider temporary tracheostomy when concerning the ability to safely perform nasopharyngeal intubation or where long-term postoperative airway management is required.

- Alter sagittal ramus osteotomy to provide maximal bone overlap:
  - Longer osteotomy (bringing anterior extent to the second premolar) for increased bone overlap and fixation (Fig. 48.3).

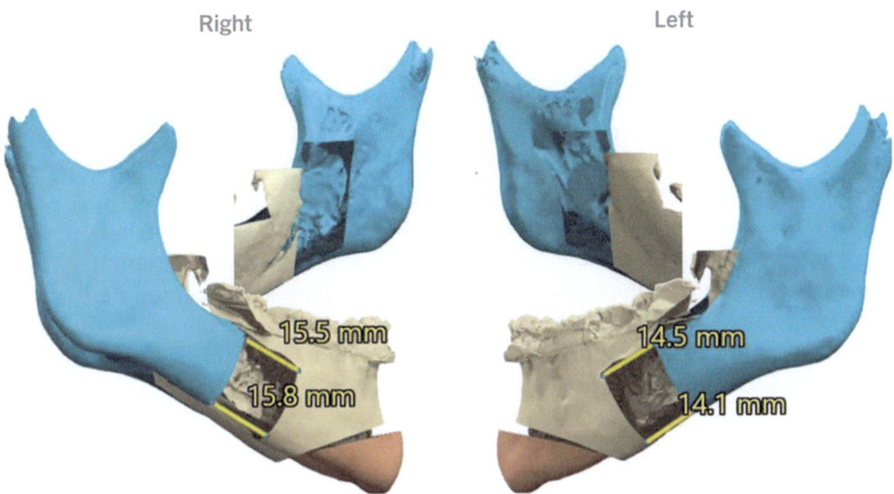

Fig. 48.3 A modified sagittal ramus osteotomy is demonstrated. The anterior extent of the sagittal ramus osteotomy is extended anteriorly to the second premolar region to increase postoperative bone overlap

- Inferior border cut at anterior osteotomy just to 50% of the inferior border (not to be carried past the midline) to maximize the bone overlap of two segments.
- Consider more rigid fixation.

- Rigid maxillary fixation with bone grafting if critical size defect exists.
- Recontouring of the pyriform rims, nasal aperture, and ANS to minimize over-projection and widening of the nasolabial soft tissues that may occur as a result of a large advancement.
- Clarify the role of concomitant procedures such as nasal septoplasty, bilateral inferior turbinate reductions, and uvulectomy. Nasal septoplasty and bilateral inferior turbinate reductions can be safely addressed during the Le Fort I down-fracture. An overly long uvula can contribute to airway collapse during sleep and is amenable to reduction at the time of MMA.

Postoperative Consideration

- Allow for complete emergence from anesthesia before extubation.
- Limit tight intermaxillary elastics to allow patients to breathe orally better.
- Continuous postoperative oxygen monitoring, consider ICU.
- Limit postoperative medications, which may result in excess somnolence.

Pearls

- The maxillomandibular advancement (MMA) for OSA treatment is a site-specific surgery that enlarges the posterior airway space and increases pharyngeal wall tension at multiple anatomic levels, including the nasopharynx, oropharynx, and hypopharynx.
- MMA is indicated for patients with concentric collapse at the level of the velum, patients with multilevel collapse, and patients with dentofacial deformity.
- Counterclockwise rotation of the occlusal plane around the central incisor will help advance the jaw, open the posterior airway, and improve the facial aesthetics.
- Recontouring of the pyriform rims, nasal aperture, and ANS to minimize the over-projection and widening of the nasolabial soft tissues that may occur as a result of a large advancement.

Pitfalls

- Patients with obstructive sleep apnea have multiple comorbidities with an increased risk of complications postoperatively.
- The incidence of postoperative paresthesia of the lower lip is high, and the recovery takes longer, sometimes permanent.
- Bone grafting is often indicated to improve stability and limit long-term relapse.

Further Reading

Christino M. Impact of CCW rotation of the occlusal plane on the MMA. Sleep Breath. 2021;25:2307–13.

Yu W. Combined CCW MMA and uvulopalatopharyngoplasty for OSA. J Craniofac Surg. 2016;28:366–71.

Prinsell JR. MMA surgery in a site-specific treatment approach for obstructive sleep apnea in 50 consecutive patients. Chest. 1999;116:1519–29.

Liu SY, Riley RW, Yu MS. Surgical algorithm for obstructive sleep apnea: an update. Clin Exp Otorhinolaryngol. 2020;13(3):215–24.

Goodday R. Diagnosis, treatment planning, and surgical correction of OSA. J Oral Maxillofac Surg. 2009;67:2183–96.

Liu SYC. MMA: Contemporary approach at Stanford. Atlas Oral Maxillofac Surg Clin N Am. 2019;27:29–36.

Boyd SB. Management of OSA by MMA. Oral Maxillofac Surg Clin N Am. 2009;21:447–57.

Carlo B. Modified genioplasty and bimaxillary advancement for treating OSA. J Oral Maxillofac Surg. 2008;66:1971–4.

Liao YF. Modified maxillomandibular advancement for obstructive sleep apneoa: towards a better outcome for Asians. Int J Oral Maxillofac Surg. 2015;44:189–94.

Chen YF. Optimizing mandibular sagittal split of large MMA for OSA. Clin Oral Investig. 2020;24:1359–67.

Kriwalsky MS. Risk factors for bad splits during sagittal split osteotomy. Br J Oral Maxillofac Surg. 2008;46:177–9.

Melinda P. Maxillomandibular advancement: the Canadian experience. Atlas Oral Maxillofac Surg Clin N Am. 2019;27:37–42.

Wolford LM. Occlusal plane alteration in orthognathic surgery. Part I: effects on function and aesthetics. Am J Orthod Dentofacial Orthop. 1994;106:304–16.

Brevi BC. Counterclockwise rotation of the occlusal plane in the treatment of obstructive sleep apnea syndrome. J Oral Maxillofac Surg. 2011;69:917–23.

Li KK. Obstructive sleep apnea surgery: genioglossus advancement revisited. J Oral Maxillofac Surg. 2001;59:1181–4.

Chapter 49
Hypoglossal Nerve Stimulator

Jessica Jurovich and Ketan Patel

Abstract Hypoglossal nerve stimulators are an effective treatment option for patients with moderate to severe obstructive sleep apnea who have failed treatment with positive airway pressure. An implantable pulse generator is implanted into the right chest, with a lead to the hypoglossal nerve and a respiratory sensing lead. The device generates electrical impulses by detecting respiratory efforts and simulating the hypoglossal nerve. The hypoglossal nerve innervates all extrinsic (genioglossus, hyoglossus, styloglossus) and intrinsic tongue muscles except for the palatoglossus muscle. During the procedure, the surgeon will test the hypoglossal nerve to determine the inclusion and exclusion branches for stimulation cuff electrode placement. The inclusion fibers supply the genioglossus and the geniohyoid muscles, which protrude from the tongue. The exclusion fibers supply the hyoglossus and the styloglossus muscles, which retrude the tongue and should therefore be kept out of the stimulation cuff. During an obstructive event, the sensing lead over the internal intercostal muscle fails to recognize a breath/chest rise and sends a signal to the impulse generator, which then stimulates the protrusive fibers of the hypoglossal nerve, thereby relieving the obstruction.

Hypoglossal nerve stimulation is not for every obstructive sleep apnea patient. Indications for such therapy include adults 18 years or older, obstructive apnea with an AHI range from 15 to 65 events/h, failed CPAP, BMI of less than 36, and appropriate airway anatomy determined by a drug-induced sleep endoscopy. Contraindications for such therapy include concentric airway collapse noted on drug-induced sleep endoscopy, > 25% central and mixed apneas, preexisting compromised neurological control of the upper airway, and patients who cannot operate

J. Jurovich
School of Dentistry, University of Minnesota, Minneapolis, MN, USA

K. Patel (✉)
Head and Neck Oncology and Microvascular Reconstructive Surgery and Oral and Maxillofacial Surgery at North Memorial Health, Adjunct Faculty, North Memorial Hospital Minneapolis, University of Minnesota, Minneapolis, MN, USA
e-mail: ketan.patel@northmemorial.com

D. Amin, H. Marwan (eds.), *Pearls and Pitfalls in Oral and Maxillofacial Surgery*, https://doi.org/10.1007/978-3-031-47307-4_49

the hypoglossal nerve stimulator remotely. The purpose of this chapter is to review pearls and pitfalls in the hypoglossal nerve stimulator procedure.

Practical Tips

Preoperative Consideration

- The authors prefer to complete the surgical markings in the preoperative area in the reclined position to prevent soft tissue movement in the supine position, especially at the chest incision site to prevent superior positioning.
- Inform the anesthesia staff that the patient should not be paralyzed for the procedure and to not interfere with nerve testing.
- Have the patient positioned supine with a shoulder roll and their head turned to the left.

Intraoperative Consideration

- A 3 cm incision is made 2 cm inferior to the inferior border of the mandible on the right side.
- Dissection is made through subcutaneous tissue and platysma to the anterior belly of the digastric muscle.
- Carry the dissection posterior along the muscle to the digastric tendon.
- Identify the mylohyoid muscle, dissect it posteriorly along the muscle until its most extent, and retract it anteriorly.
- With a clear view of the hypoglossal nerve, the nerve can be carefully dissected off the ranine veins. The use of bipolar electrocautery can help with cumbersome ranine vein bleeding to ensure a hemostatic field, as this is paramount for good visualization of nerve fibers.
- Exclusion and inclusion branches are detected with a nerve stimulator. This can be done with various nerve monitors available on the market, including a NIMS Vital Monitoring System or, more recently used, the Checkpoint Gemini bipolar nerve stimulator to isolate the protrusive from the retractive nerve fibers. Our preference for the Checkpoint Gemini bipolar probe is to forgo the use of sharp leads in the tongue and floor of the mouth that are typically used with a NIMS Vital Monitor.
- The nerve stimulator cuff is then placed around the tested inclusion branches.
- The lead is then secured with 3-0 silk suture to the digastric tendon in standard fashion.

- A 5 cm incision is made 3 cm lateral to the manubrium and between the second and third ribs on the right side. The right side is chosen over the left in case the patient needs a cardiac implant.
- Dissect down to the pectoralis fascia.
- A suprafascial pocket is created to accommodate the implantable pulse generator.
- Dissection is carried through the pectoralis fascia and between pectoralis muscle fibers until the subpectoral fat pad is identified.
- Carefully dissect through the subpectoral fat pad until the external and internal intercostal muscles between the second and third ribs are identified.
- Create a pocket between the external and internal intercostal muscles to place the respiratory sensing lead and secure it with a 3-0 silk suture. Typically this area between the muscles has a well-defined plane for the placement of the sensing lead. Fine tonsil forceps dissect this area and lift, and the sensing lead is placed under the pocket with a direct vision to prevent inadvertent displacement into the pleural space.
- A tunneling cannula is then used to connect the two incisions, carefully ensuring the tunnel is superficial to the clavicle. We recommend placing the lead in a deeper tunnel as we have encountered lead/wire exposure when placed in the subcutaneous plane/superficial plane (Fig. 49.1). In addition, tunneling should be done slowly and carefully to prevent injury to the subclavian vessels and the external jugular vein.
- Stimulating leads are drawn into the lower incision with a cannula.
- All leads are connected to the implantable pulse generator.

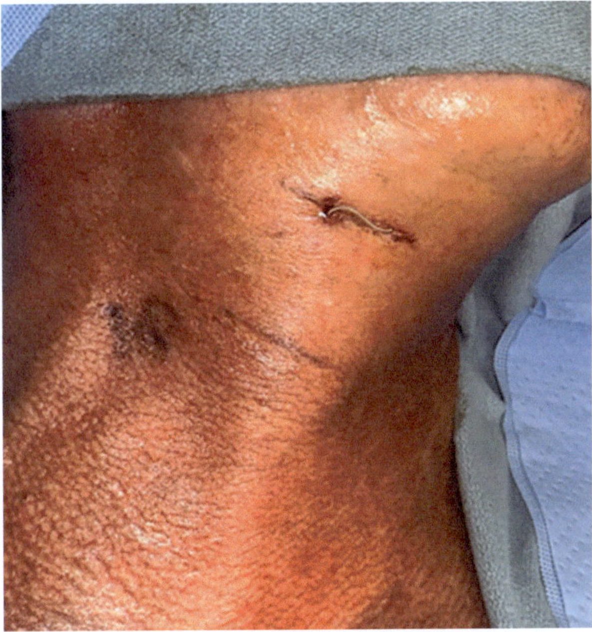

Fig. 49.1 Exposed stimulation lead in the neck

- A telemetry lead is placed over the implantable pulse generator to stimulate the hypoglossal nerve and protrude the tongue.
- The implantable pulse generator is secured to the pectoralis fascia with a 2-0 silk suture. Consideration should be given to patients who hunt as the generator may need to be placed more medially.
- A system check is completed where the nerve is stimulated at different voltages to check the level of protrusion, and the sensing lead is checked for respiratory changes.
- Deep dermis of both incisions is closed with a 3-0 Vicryl suture, and the skin is closed with a 4-0 Monocryl suture in a running subcuticular fashion.

Postoperative Consideration

- Chest X-rays are obtained to document baseline device position and rule out adverse sequelae such as pneumothorax.
- Skull X-ray in a lateral position is also completed to disclude displacement of the stimulation lead.
- The implantable pulse generator needs to heal for about 4 weeks postoperatively for healing/scarring of the device to prevent movement. The neurologist/pulmonologist completes subsequent device activation with present titration over another sleep study.

Pearls

- During the procedure, the surgeon will test the hypoglossal nerve to determine the inclusion and exclusion branches for stimulation cuff electrode placement.
- The inclusion fibers supply the genioglossus and the geniohyoid muscles, which protrude from the tongue.
- The exclusion fibers supply the hyoglossus and the styloglossus muscles, which retrude the tongue and should therefore be kept out of the stimulation cuff.

Pitfalls

- Create a pocket between the external and internal intercostal muscles to place the respiratory sensing lead and secure it with a 3-0 silk suture.
- Consider placing the lead in a deeper tunnel to avoid lead/wire exposure when placed in the subcutaneous plane/superficial plane.
- Chest X-rays are obtained to document baseline device position and rule out adverse sequela, such as a pneumothorax.

Further Reading

Eastwood PR, Barnes M, Walsh JH, Maddison KJ, Hee G, Schwartz AR, Smith PL, Malhotra A, McEvoy RD, Wheatley JR, O'Donoghue FJ, Rochford PD, Churchward T, Campbell MC, Palme CE, Robinson S, Goding GS, Eckert DJ, Jordan AS, Catcheside PG, Tyler L, Antic NA, Worsnop CJ, Kezirian EJ, Hillman DR. Treating obstructive sleep apnea with hypoglossal nerve stimulation. Sleep. 2011;34(11):1479–86.

Mashaqi S, Patel SI, Combs D, Estep L, Helmick S, Machamer J, Parthasarathy S. The hypoglossal nerve stimulation as a novel therapy for treating obstructive sleep apnea—a literature review. Int J Environ Res Public Health. 2021;18(4):1642.

Olson MD, Junna MR. Hypoglossal nerve stimulation therapy for the treatment of obstructive sleep apnea. Neurotherapeutics. 2021;18(1):91–9.

Whelan R, Soose RJ. Implantable Neurostimulation for treatment of sleep apnea: present and future. Otolaryngol Clin North Am. 2020;53(3):445–57.

Chapter 50
Practical Tips for Hyoid Suspension Surgery

Hisham Marwan

Abstract Hyoid suspension and myotomy is one of the procedures performed to treat obstructive sleep apnea. The main indication for the procedure is tongue base obstruction during drug-induced endoscopic (DISE) evaluation. Regardless of the technique used, hyoid suspension and myotomy can be categorized into two main techniques: hyoidthyroidpexia, where the hyoid bone is fixated to the thyroid cartilage, and hyomandibular suspension, where the hyoid is suspended to the mandible. Both aim to widen the hypopharyngeal airway and open the retrolingual space. The outcomes and risk of complication are generally better with hyomandibular suspension than the hyoidthyroidpexia. This chapter will discuss the pearls and pitfalls of hyoid suspension using the hyomandibular suspension technique.

Preoperative Assessment

- The procedure is indicated for the full base of tongue obstruction diagnosed during DISE.
- The procedure is contraindicated for severe OSA with AHI of more than 60 and in patients who had a Sistrunk procedure.
- For severe OSA with a complete base of tongue obstruction, hyoid suspension can be combined with other procedures (multilevel surgery).
- Counsel the patient about possible voice changes after the procedure.

Intraoperative Procedure

- Positioning: Keep the patient's head extended and place a shoulder roll.

H. Marwan (✉)
Department of Surgery, The University of Texas Medical Branch, Galveston, TX, USA
e-mail: himarwan@utmb.edu

D. Amin, H. Marwan (eds.), *Pearls and Pitfalls in Oral and Maxillofacial Surgery*, https://doi.org/10.1007/978-3-031-47307-4_50

- Two incisions should be planned, a superior incision underneath the chin and the inferior incision on the top of the hyoid.
- Make the superior incision one finger breadth below the inferior border of the mandible to hide the scar.
- Always stay in the midline. Once the hyoid is reached, use the cricoid hook to lift the hyoid superiorly.
- Avoid overzealous maneuvering and pulling on the hyoid to avoid fracturing the bone.
- If the hyoid is fractured during the procedure, you can use a miniplate to fixate the bone or suspend each segment of the fracture separately.
- Minimally released the suprahyoid muscles from the hyoid. Do not release the infrahyoid muscle, as this is unnecessary during the procedure and will reduce the complication rate.
- Do not dissect the hyoid beyond the lesser horns to prevent injury to the superior laryngeal nerve.
- When reflecting the lingual surface of the mandible, be careful with the periosteal blood supply. Careful use of cautery will help prevent bleeding and possible hematoma formation.
- Use a large hemostat to create a tunnel and connect the two incisions. The tunnel should be as small as possible. Creating a large tunnel between the two incisions might collect a hematoma underneath.
- The author uses the AIRLIFT system to perform the procedure. The system has all the required sutures and screws to do the hyomandibular suspension easily and efficiently.
- During the suspension of the hyoid to the mandible anchor, always remove the shoulder roll to help advance the hyoid bone more superiorly closer to the mandible.
- Achieve proper hemostasis before closure. Drain is optional if good hemostasis is achieved.

Postoperative

- Patients can be discharged home the same day.
- Mild dysphagia is expected for 5 days after surgery.
- Applying ice to the surgical site will help reduce the swelling and discomfort.

Further Reading

Tassel V, et al. Hyoid suspension with UPPP for the treatment of obstructive sleep apnea. Ear Nose Throat J. 2023;102:NP212–9.
Siesta Medical Whitepaper—Hyoid suspension to the mandible is more effective than to thyroid cartilage (LS0034).

Part IX
Craniofacial and Orthognathic Surgery

Chapter 51
Minimizing the Risk of Complications in Sagittal Split Osteotomies

Carolyn Brookes

Abstract Sagittal split osteotomies of the mandible are used to address skeletal malocclusions and obstructive sleep apnea. This approach can also provide access to the inferior alveolar nerve for micro-neurosurgical procedures. This versatile procedure is used frequently.

In addition to complications inherent to surgery, such as pain, swelling, bleeding, and infection, potential complications include malocclusion, TMJ dysfunction, need for hardware removal, temporary or permanent altered sensation in the lingual and inferior alveolar nerve distributions, and unfavourable fractures. Strategies to minimize the risk of complications will be reviewed.

Minimizing Altered Sensation

- When dissecting the medial aspect of the mandible to facilitate the medial osteotomy, remain subperiosteal. Begin dissection above the anticipated level of the mandibular foramen. Protect the soft tissue with a narrow retractor while making your medial cut; while doing this, avoid excessive soft tissue retraction and remove the medial retractor once your cut is complete.
- Be mindful of nerve position at your planned osteotomy sites, referencing 3-D planning images. While making the lateral osteotomy, take care to transect the cortex but avoid damage to the bundle by going beyond the cortex. Consider ultrasonic devices if proximity to the nerve is high or if you prefer this instrumentation.
- Minimize manipulation of the neurovascular bundle, releasing only enough to minimize neuropraxia with the patient's specific planned jaw movements if the bundle remains with the proximal segment.

C. Brookes (✉)
Oral and Maxillofacial Surgery Associates, Waukesha, WI, USA
e-mail: carolynbrookes@omsawaukesha.com

© The Author(s), under exclusive license to Springer Nature
Switzerland AG 2024
D. Amin, H. Marwan (eds.), *Pearls and Pitfalls in Oral and Maxillofacial Surgery*, https://doi.org/10.1007/978-3-031-47307-4_51

- Smooth sharp areas of bone that may abut/impinge upon the nerve.
- If using bicortical positional screws to secure the segments, be mindful of nerve position when placing screws. Use a depth gauge to assess the appropriate screw length to avoid discomfort and to minimize the risk of lingual nerve injury. Palpate lingually before closure to verify screw length is not excessive.
- Witnessed transection of the inferior alveolar nerve is rare. If this occurs, immediate direct repair of the nerve using fine sutures under magnification is ideal.

Preventing Malocclusion

- Avoid over- or under-seating the condyles – it can be helpful to create a notch near the inferior aspect of the proximal segment to enhance control of this segment while seating.
- Applying torque to the condyle should be avoided. To facilitate seating the condylar segment without interferences, assess sites of interference with manual manipulation. Protecting the soft tissue, address these interferences with your instrument of choice – hand or reciprocating rasps, rongeurs, and/or rotary drills such as a barrel bur. If using plates and non-locking screws for fixation, ensure excellent plate adaptation to avoid movement of the segment during screw tightening. It can be helpful for one surgeon or assistant to maintain the proximal segment in a seated fashion while the other adapts the plate. If using bicortical screws, watch both segments during screw placement to ensure the screw does not alter the segment relationship during final tightening.
- If you note a malocclusion, remove fixation and address the malocclusion before moving on.
- If centric relation is difficult to repeat, consider mandible-first surgery.

Avoiding Unfavorable Fractures

- While creating your osteotomies, avoid sharp angles that create stress points.
- Get through the cortex completely. This can be accomplished with a saw or drill per surgeon preference and is often verified with osteotomes.
- While completing the split, ensure you can see the entire osteotomy well. You should see the lateral osteotomy widening with the application of pressure along the length of the cut. You should see the sagittal split separating both proximally and distally during initial spreading; a v-shaped opening typically indicates an area of incomplete separation. When separating, use gentle pressure so you can detect areas of increased resistance and address them before they result in aberrant fracture patterns. If you note a point of resistance, recapitulate the osteotomy

with an osteotome. If this site is inferior to the neurovascular bundle, identify the bundle, and then use an osteotome to gently tap the site of resistance and apply local force (i.e., twisting with an osteotome or blunt instrument) to advance the osteotomy. If using an osteotome at the sagittal osteotomy, rotate it so the pressure is applied proximally on the proximal segment (Figs. 51.1 and 51.2).

Fig. 51.1 The use of osteotome to complete the fracture

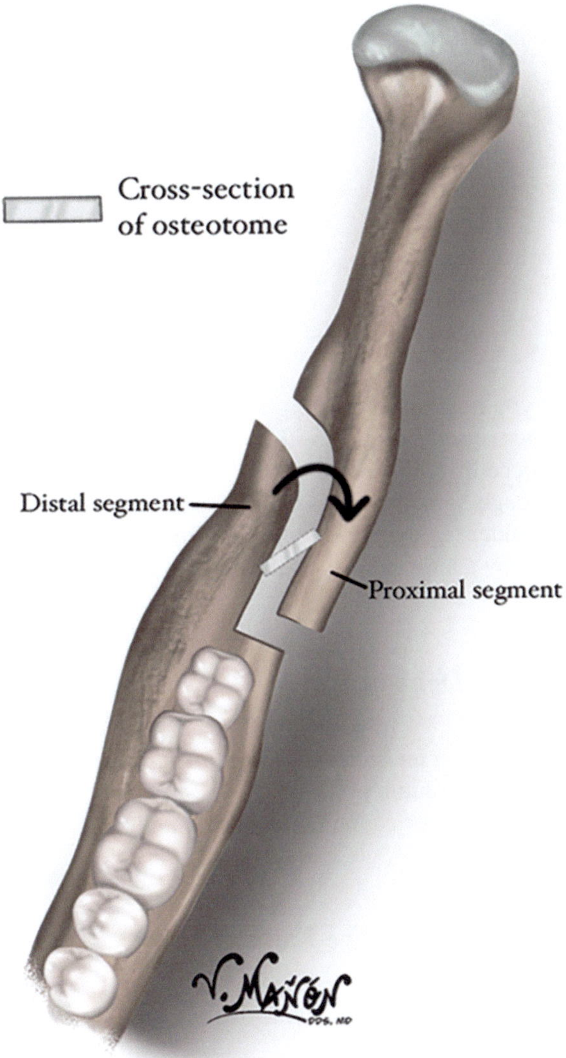

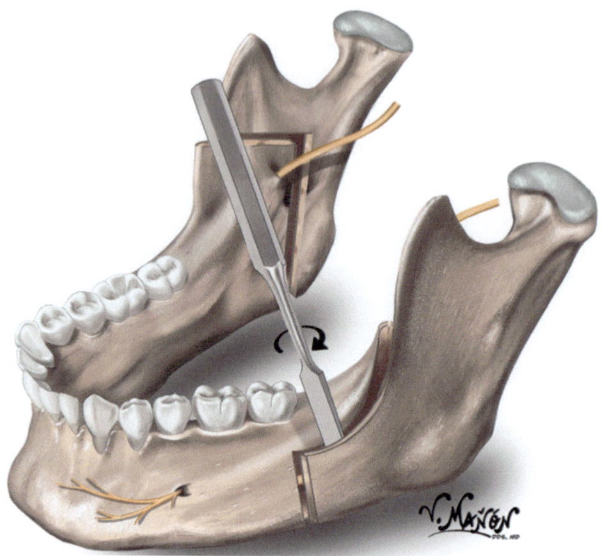

Fig. 51.2 The cross-sectional position of the osteotome during the osteotomy procedure

- If you note an impending fracture, pause and assess the site or sites of resistance contributing to the impending fracture. Address as above before proceeding.
- Though some surgeons always remove third molars in advance, at a minimum consider removing difficult impacted third molars or impacted third molars that occupy a large portion of the mandible 6–9 months before BSSO.

Avoiding Dehiscence

- Design your incision to allow an adequate cuff of tissue (after elastic contraction) to which to suture.
- Consider a horizontal mattress closure to enhance water tightness posteriorly.

Avoiding Hardware Failure

- Use copious irrigation while drilling.
- Adapt hardware carefully.
- Consider locking screws if purchase or plate adaptation is poor.

Avoiding Facial Nerve Injury

- Use protective retractors (such as a channel retractor) when creating the lateral and inferior border osteotomies.
- Minimize soft tissue traction/aggressive retraction.

Pearls

- BSSO is a versatile procedure used for multiple interventions.
- Create a notch near the inferior aspect of the proximal segment to enhance control while seating the condyle.
- If centric relation is difficult to repeat, consider mandible-first surgery.
- Consider removing difficult impacted third molars or impacted third molars that occupy a large portion of the mandible 6–9 months before BSSO.

Pitfalls

- Transection of the IAN will require immediate micro-neural repair to achieve complete sensory recovery.
- In case of malocclusion, remove and repeat all the fixations before continuing the procedure.

Further Readings

Mensink G, Verweij JP, Frank MD, Eelco Bergsma J, Richard van Merkesteyn JP. Bad split during bilateral sagittal split osteotomy of the mandible with separators: a retrospective study of 427 patients. Br J Oral Maxillofac Surg. 2013;51(6):525–9. https://doi.org/10.1016/j.bjoms.2012.10.009. Epub 2013 Jan 8

Steenen SA, van Wijk AJ, Becking AG. Bad splits in bilateral sagittal split osteotomy: systematic review and meta-analysis of reported risk factors. Int J Oral Maxillofac Surg. 2016;45(8):971–9. https://doi.org/10.1016/j.ijom.2016.02.011. Epub 2016 Mar 12. PMID: 26980136

Steenen SA, Becking AG. Bad splits in bilateral sagittal split osteotomy: systematic review of fracture patterns. Int J Oral Maxillofac Surg. 2016;45(7):887–97. https://doi.org/10.1016/j.ijom.2016.02.001. Epub 2016 Feb 28

Chapter 52
How to Avoid Complications in Le Fort 1 Osteotomy

Shadi Alzahrani

Abstract Le Fort 1 osteotomy is one of the most commonly used osteotomies in craniofacial surgery. It can be used to change horizontal and vertical deformity in the midface. In addition, Le Fort 1 osteotomy can be used for correcting asymmetry, occlusal plane abnormalities, and obstructive sleep apnea cases. Avoiding complications during osteotomy is critical to the successful management of such deformities. The purpose of this chapter is to review pearls and pitfalls on how to avoid complications in Le Fort 1 osteotomy.

Practical Tips

Preoperative Consideration

- Medical comorbidities should be evaluated preoperatively to ensure the safe management of facial deformity. Airway evaluation should be conducted to document the initial airway evaluation, such as Mallampati classification, nasal septum deviation, and large tonsils. In addition, exceptions for the postoperative changes in the skeletal support of the airway should be discussed.
- Accurate preoperative diagnosis is essential, dictating the plane for the facial deformity.
- Collecting all required databases, such as facial analysis, facial photographs, dental casts, and others, will help to reach the appropriate diagnosis and ensure accurate transfer to the operating room.
- If a traditional model surgery is planned, a model mounted using a facebow on an articulator is used.
- With a virtual plan, a cone-beam computed tomography with an intraoral scan is enough for proper planning.

S. Alzahrani (✉)
Department of Oral and Maxillofacial Surgery, King Abdulaziz University, Jeddah, Saudi Arabia

D. Amin, H. Marwan (eds.), *Pearls and Pitfalls in Oral and Maxillofacial Surgery*, https://doi.org/10.1007/978-3-031-47307-4_52

- Detailed discussion regarding the surgery and complication should be conducted with the patient or the patient's family.
- Communicating with the orthodontist ensures the patient is ready for surgery. Surgical wires and hooks should be placed before taking the final record for planning. Also, adequate space between roots should be created to ensure safe interdental osteotomy.

Intraoperative Consideration

- Communication with the anesthesia team is crucial in Le Fort 1 osteotomy, and hypotensive anesthesia is requested to minimize the bleeding, especially during the down-fracture of the maxilla.
- Using a reference, either external or internal, to determine the vertical distance is essential to avoid any discrepancy in the vertical distance. A non-threaded Kirschner wire can be placed in the bridge of the nose as an external reference. Then a measurement is recorded using a Boley gauge to the upper part of the braces in the central incisors and the incisors' edges for confirmation after removing the splint.
- A maxillary vestibular incision is made with a blade or electrocautery from molar to molar through the mucosa, 1 cm above and parallel to the mucogingival line to facilitate the closure afterward. Then the incision is deepened to subcutaneous tissue, muscle, and periosteum. Then subperiosteal dissection is created to expose the piriform aperture, the infraorbital nerves, and the zygomatic buttresses. This will minimize the bleeding, avoid recession, especially in the anterior teeth, and protect the infraorbital nerve. The last area to expose is the junction of the maxillary tuberosity with pterygoid plates through a tunnel, considering to stay subperiosteal to avoid expelling the buccal fat pad, which may obliterate the surgical field.
- Carefully reflect and protect the nose mucoperiosteum floor using a #9 periosteal elevator and an angled Freer elevator. This will minimize the mucosal tear during the maxilla down-fracture. In addition, a Seldin retractor is placed in the nose to protect the mucoperiosteum and nasotracheal tube during the osteotomy.
- An Obwegeser toe-out retractor is placed behind the pterygomaxillary junction. The horizontal osteotomy is initiated above the apices of the maxillary teeth to avoid any dental trauma, posterior to the maxillary tuberosity heading to the midline, superior to the nasal floor, with a reciprocating saw. Pulpal necrosis is not usual after Le Fort osteotomy, and endodontic treatment is not indicated even with the loss of pulp vitality unless there *are clinical symptoms or radiographic evidence of infection.*
- The surgical field should be visualized carefully to avoid any injury, laceration, or injury to the soft tissue, which *leads to necrosis of the soft tissues and possibly vascular compromise of the bone.*
- Attention should be directed to separating the nasal septum and vomer bone from the nasal crest of the maxilla. The index finger is placed at the end of the hard

palate, and a double guarded vomer osteotome is advanced until feeling that with the index finger.

- A curved pterygoid osteotome is used and directed medially and inferiorly, away from the pterygoid plexus and internal maxillary artery to divide the pterygo-maxillary junction. A finger is placed at the hamular notch to palpate the advancement of the osteotome and the separation of the junction.
- A single guarded osteotome separates the lateral nasal wall. Changes in the sound should be considered during the advancement of the osteotome once engaging the thicker perpendicular plate of the palatine bone. It is essential to ensure the palatal bone's osteotomy is completed before the down-fracture of the maxilla to avoid unfavorable fractures that may extend to the orbital and cranial bone.
- A digital pressure is used to down-fracture the maxilla. If any resistance is encountered, all osteotomies should be checked before completing the down-fracture.
- A descending palatine artery is ligated or preserved at the surgeon's preference, but it can be safely ligated to prevent bleeding while manipulating the maxilla.
- In the case of the third molars, they can be removed at this stage.
- The use of Rowe's disimpaction forceps should be minimized to prevent any damage to the palatal mucosa during the mobilization of the maxilla.
- The splint is placed, and intermaxillary fixation is applied. Then, while correctly seating the condyle in the glenoid fossa, the complex is placed in the desired vertical position using the vertical reference. Any bony interference from the nose floor is removed until the maxilla is passively positioned.
- The nasal septum is reduced to prevent buckling, which leads to nasal deformity. Especially for maxillary impaction, the inferior turbinate is trimmed at this point if it is indicated before fixating the maxilla in the final position.
- Fixation of the maxilla is performed after carefully checking all the parameters with two plates on each side. The first plate is fixated in the piriform area, and the other is in the malar buttress region. Ensuring that the condyle is appropriately seated in the glenoid fossa is crucial.
- Wires are removed, and then verify the occlusion is reproducible in the splint, as planned preoperatively without the splint.
- Suturing is started with an alar cinch suture to prevent the alar flare.
- Resulting from the maxillary surgery. The alar cinch is performed by everting the lip and grasping the fibrous tissue located immediately below the alar cartilage with 0 Vicryl or PDS suture. Pulling the alar region should be visualized on both sides before tying the suture in the midline. The position and tension of the ala are checked carefully afterward.
- The V-Y closure of the anterior part of the wound is initiated to ensure the proper protrusion and length of the upper lip. Then, the wound is closed with 3–0 Vicryl suture in one layer, including mucosa muscle and periosteum.
- A guided elastic may be applied to guide the occlusion to the new position.
- Communicate with the anesthesia team to ensure smooth extubation to minimize increasing blood pressure, which may increase the bleeding.

Postoperative Consideration

- Panoramic and cephalometric X-rays are obtained to verify the planned result and as baseline X-rays for future comparison.
- Postoperative instruction regarding feeding and postoperative care to avoid dehiscence or infection.
- Verify the occlusion to ensure it is stable and reproducible.
- Any significant discrepancy worth returning to OR should be considered at this stage.
- The minor discrepancy can be managed with the elastic.
- The patient can continue his orthodontic treatment between 4 and 6 weeks.

Pearls

- Accurate preoperative diagnosis is essential, dictating the plane for the facial deformity.
- Pulpal necrosis is not usual after Le Fort osteotomy, and endodontic treatment is not indicated even with the loss of pulp vitality unless there *are clinical symptoms or radiographic evidence of infection.*

Pitfalls

- Consider using external or internal reference to determine the vertical distance.
- The descending palatine artery can be safely ligated to prevent bleeding while manipulating the maxilla.

Further Reading

Proffit WR, Turvey TA, Phillips C. Orthognathic surgery: a hierarchy of stability. Int J Adult Orthodon Orthognath Surg. 1996;11(3):191–204.

Bell WH, Fonseca RJ, Kenneky JW, Levy BM. Bone healing and revascularization after total maxillary osteotomy. J Oral Surg. 1975;33(4):253–60.

Bauer RE 3rd, Ochs MW. Maxillary orthognathic surgery. Oral Maxillofac Surg Clin North Am. 2014;26(4):523–37. https://doi.org/10.1016/j.coms.2014.08.005. Epub 2014 Sep 8

Turvey TA, Fonseca RJ. The anatomy of the internal maxillary artery in the pterygopalatine fossa: its relationship to maxillary surgery. J Oral Surg. 1980;38(2):92–5.

Chapter 53
Pearls and Pitfalls in Multipiece Maxillary Osteotomy

Kevin C. Lee, and Michael R. Markiewicz

Abstract The Le Fort I is the workhorse osteotomy for addressing dentofacial deformities involving the maxilla. Segmentation of the maxilla is commonly used to address transverse discrepancies and multiplane occlusions. Original investigations by Bell et al. concluded that maxillary segmentation and pedicle stretch only exhibited transitory effects on revascularization and bone healing even after ligation of the descending palatal vessels. Therefore, the segmental Le Fort I osteotomy is generally a reliable and safe procedure when performed correctly. Still, there are a variety of pitfalls to this procedure that the surgeon should anticipate and attempt to mitigate. The ascending pharyngeal and ascending palatine arteries provide the blood supply to the down-fractured maxilla. The resulting soft tissue pedicle is comprised of the intact palatal and labial/buccal mucosa. The integrity of the palatal mucosa is critical to maintaining the vitality of the maxillary segments. With a conventional three-piece design, the anterior segment is particularly vulnerable to palatal disruptions because there is reduced collateral blood supply from the buccal tissue. Rarely, palatal perforations can result in postoperative fistulas, particularly in the setting of a large transverse expansions and/or unrepaired nasal floor tears overlying the defect. Although devascularization is one of the most feared complications of segmental surgery, injury to the neighboring teeth is much more frequently seen. Roots can be amputated, and the osteotomy can propagate through and violate the

K. C. Lee
Department of Head & Neck and Plastic & Reconstructive Surgery, Roswell Park
Comprehensive Cancer Center, Buffalo, NY, USA

M. R. Markiewicz (✉)
Department of Neurosurgery and Department of Surgery, Roswell Park Comprehensive
Cancer Center, Buffalo, NY, USA

Department of Head & Neck and Plastic & Reconstructive Surgery, Roswell Park
Comprehensive Cancer Center, Buffalo, NY, USA

Cleft and Craniofacial Team, Craniofacial Center of Western New York, Buffalo, NY, USA
e-mail: mrm25@buffalo.edu

D. Amin, H. Marwan (eds.), *Pearls and Pitfalls in Oral and Maxillofacial
Surgery*, https://doi.org/10.1007/978-3-031-47307-4_53

periodontal ligament. Disruptions to the periodontal ligament can cause ankylosis or, in the case of root delamination, reduced bony support. Finally, even afterward, there is a heightened risk of surgical relapse. Maxillary transverse expansion is considered an unstable movement as the elasticity of the palatal tissues works to pull the segments together. Likewise, the three-piece closure of an anterior open bite is prone to reopening. The purpose of this chapter is to review pearls and pitfalls in the multipiece maxillary osteotomy.

Practical Tips

Palatal Osteotomy

- It is important to segment the palate in a parasagittal axis where the mucosa is the thickest and the bone is the thinnest.
- For large transverse expansions, a U-shaped osteotomy can be used to island the palate and distribute the tension. A single paramedian osteotomy should only be reserved for smaller expansions.
- Transverse lacerations are more disruptive to the blood supply than sagittal ones. If the palate is perforated or lacerated, care should be taken to free the mucosal edges and repair the defect primarily. The nasal floor should also be carefully restored to avoid communication. An interpositional barrier membrane, gel foam, or fibrin glue can be placed to facilitate healing.
- When small oronasal fistulas occur, they can occasionally resolve spontaneously with conservative measures.
- If the blood supply to the maxillary segments is compromised and the gingiva appear pale/ischemic, then hypotensive anesthesia should be reversed, any palatal stretch should be relaxed, and warmed irrigation should be applied. Fixation should be released, and consideration for a lesser maxillary advancement and a mandibular setback should be given.

Interdental Osteotomy

- Dorfman and Turvey advise a minimum of 3 mm root separation for periodontal safety. When less than 2.5 mm of interdental bone exists, higher dental injury rates are known to occur with a free-handed approach.
- For spaces <2 mm, discussing options for flaring the roots with the treating orthodontist is advisable. Cutting guides can be used to avoid intraoperative guesswork. A very thin sagittal saw or ultrasonic cutting instrument can be used to start these cuts.

- The interdental cut should be completed before the down-fracture. This allows the surgeon to work on a stable platform. A finger on the palate can give tactile verification that the cut is complete.

Relapse

- Any transverse discrepancy greater than 6 mm should ideally be addressed first with distraction osteogenesis in the transverse plane (surgically assisted rapid palatal expansion with either a tooth-borne or bone-borne expander). The authors prefer a bone-borne expander.
- It is often possible to obtain more than 6 mm of stretch in the operating room. This can be done with careful dissection of the palatal mucosa and stretching for soft tissue creep.
- The passive fit of the segments into the maxillary splint is imperative to avoid excess torque on the cusps. A clamp or other instrument can be used to stretch and spread the segments gently. A palatal splint, trans-palatal arch, or combination of those with a splint may be used for added support.
- Gaps in the maxilla larger than 2–3 mm should be grafted.
- The palatal splint should still be maintained postoperatively for 4–6 weeks, even if the fixation spans the segments. Consideration for a longer consolidation phase should be done for cleft patients.
- Following the correction of an open bite, box elastics can be placed anteriorly to close the gap if there is evidence of early relapse.

Pearls

- It is important to segment the palate in a parasagittal axis where the mucosa is the thickest and the bone is the thinnest.
- When small oronasal fistulas occur, they can occasionally resolve spontaneously with conservative measures.
- It is often possible to obtain more than 6 mm of stretch in the operating room.

Pitfalls

- Consider distraction osteogenesis in the transverse plane for transverse discrepancies >6 mm.
- A minimum of 3 mm root separation for periodontal safety is recommended for interdental osteotomies.
- Consider using cutting guides when the interdental space is <2 mm.

Further Reading

Bell WH, You ZH, Finn RA, Fields RT. Wound healing after multisegmental le fort i osteotomy and transection of the descending palatine vessels. J Oral Maxillofac Surg. 1995;53:1425.

Dorfman HS, Turvey TA. Alterations in osseous crestal height following interdental osteotomies. Oral Surg Oral Med Oral Pathol. 1979;48:120.

Chapter 54
Pearls and Pitfalls of the Intraoral Vertical Osteotomy

Shahid R. Aziz

Abstract The vertical ramus osteotomy was originally developed at Walter Reed Medical Center by Jack Caldwell and George Letterman in 1954.2 It was initially performed from an extraoral approach and used to treat mandibular prognathism. Its novelty was that it was an osteotomy that minimized injury to the mandibular nerve. In 1970, Jon Kent and Ed Hinds (from the University of Texas—Houston) designed an intraoral 90-degree saw to osteotomize the ascending ramus of the mandible from a purely intraoral approach. During the 1970s and 1980s, David Hall (from Vanderbilt University) further refined the VRO procedure and demonstrated that it could treat mandibular prognathism and mild mandibular retrognathia (advancement of 2 mm or less). In addition, Hall and McKenna championed VRO as a treatment for temporomandibular joint dysfunction. The purpose of this chapter is to review the pearls and pitfalls of intraoral vertical osteotomy.

Practical Tips

Preoperative Consideration

- The primary indication for VRO is the treatment of mandibular prognathism. VRO can be used for anterior jaw repositioning of 2 mm or less.

S. R. Aziz (✉)
Oral and Maxillofacial Surgery, Hackensack University Medical Center, Hackensack, NJ, USA

Smile Bangladesh, Dhaka, Bangladesh

New Jersey Society of Oral and Maxillofacial Surgeons, Hillsborough, NJ, USA

Oral & Maxillofacial Surgery, Rutgers University, New Brunswick, NJ, USA

D. Amin, H. Marwan (eds.), *Pearls and Pitfalls in Oral and Maxillofacial Surgery*, https://doi.org/10.1007/978-3-031-47307-4_54

387

Intraoperative Consideration

- Approach: The approach for VRO is via an intraoral technique. The incision starts on the anterior border of the ramus 1 cm posterior to the third molar region and sweeps forward into the buccal vestibule while leaving an adequate cuff of mucosa superiorly to allow easy closure. The anterior extent of the incision is to the area adjacent to the first molar.
- Dissection: Dissection of the lateral ramus is started by detaching the insertion of the temporalis muscle on the anterior border of the ramus. The Hargis anterior border stripper is recommended. The temporalis should be stripped to the tip of the coronoid process. The dissection then proceeds to stripping the lateral border of the ramus and identifying the sigmoid notch and the posterior border of the ramus.

  - Dissect laterally only—do not strip on the medial aspect of the ascending ramus to avoid sagging of the proximal segment (condylar sag). Landmarks to be identified at this time are the sigmoid notch, the posterior border of the ramus, the angle, and the inferior border of the mandible. Identifying the area of the antilingula, a bump on the lateral cortex helps localize the point of entry of the mandibular nerve into the medial ramus.
  - Bauer retractors are placed in the sigmoid notch superiorly and at the antegonial notch inferiorly. Using fiber-optic Bauer retractors is also helpful for illuminating the surgical cavity and maximizing visualization. Additionally, a posterior border retractor, the Merrill-LeVasseur retractor, can be used as well. Once the surgical cavity is adequately exposed and illuminated, the VRO saw is used.
  - The VRO saw typically comes in two blade sizes—7- and 12-mm length—and is angled to allow the operator to create the osteotomy away from the neurovascular bundle. The vast majority of osteotomies can be completed with the 7-mm blade. A score mark is placed 5 mm behind the antilingula and checked with a dental mirror. If there is no prominent antilingula, the osteotomy can be started by placing the saw 5–7 mm anterior to the posterior border in the mid-ramus area. The osteotomy is scored from a position posterior to the antilingula, inferior to the posterior aspect of the antegonial notch, and superior to the midportion of the sigmoid notch. Once the score mark has been completed and determined to be in a proper position, the osteotomy can be started at the antilingula and walked down the lateral ramus to the antegonial angle with the aid of a Bauer retractor. Once the inferior aspect of the ramus osteotomy has been completed, the VRO saw is then walked back up the ramus superiorly. After the saw has passed the antilingula, it should be directed slightly anteriorly to complete the osteotomy into the sigmoid notch.
  - Care should be taken not to run the saw into the contents of the sigmoid notch, specifically the masseteric artery or the IMA. Injury to the masseteric artery close to its takeoff from the IMA or damage to the IMA itself can cause significant bleeding that is impossible to control locally and may require

embolization. Injury to the masseteric artery 1–2 cm away from its takeoff from the IMA can usually be controlled by pressure. Completing the osteotomy at the superior aspect last, if bleeding occurs, the osteotomy can be completed quickly, and more effective pressure applied.

- Once bilateral VROs are completed, the mandible should be passively positioned posteriorly and placed into the predetermined final occlusal relationship.

  - If unable to set mandible posteriorly, coronoidotomies may be needed as the coronoid process may be in the way. In general, for setbacks of more than 8 mm, a coronoidotomy should be performed.
  - Other areas of interference may be in osteotomy around the sigmoid notch requiring trimming.

- After the mandible has been set back and the ideal occlusion achieved, the mandible is wired to the maxilla. Once MMF is completed, the proximal segments of the osteotomies should be checked to ensure that they are laterally positioned with adequate bone overlap and contact, and the proximal segment's vertical position should be determined. The incision is closed in a single layer with combinations of interrupted sutures in the posterior aspect of the incision and a running suture anteriorly. Remember to remove the throat pack before placing the patient in MMF.

Pearls

- Dissect laterally only—do not strip on the medial aspect of the ascending ramus to avoid sagging of the proximal segment (condylar sag).
- Bauer retractors are placed in the sigmoid notch superiorly and at the antegonial notch inferiorly.
- Using fiber-optic Bauer retractors is also helpful for illuminating the surgical cavity and maximizing visualization.

Pitfalls

- The VRO saw typically comes in two blade sizes—7- and 12-mm length—and is angled to allow the operator to create the osteotomy away from the neurovascular bundle. The vast majority of osteotomies can be completed with the 7-mm blade.
- Care should be taken not to run the saw into the contents of the sigmoid notch.
- Consider coronoidotomies if unable to set mandible posteriorly.
- Other areas of interference may be in osteotomy around the sigmoid notch requiring trimming.

Further Reading

Caldwell JB, Letterman GS. Vertical osteotomy in the mandibular rami for the correction of prognathism. J Oral Surg (Chic). 1954;12:185202.

Hebert JM, Kent JN, Hinds EC. Correction of prognathism by an intraoral vertical subcondylar osteotomy. J Oral Surg. 1970;28:651–3.

Hall HD, McKenna S. Further refinement and evaluation of the intraoral vertical ramus osteotomy. J Oral Maxillofac Surg. 1987;45:684–8.

Aziz SR, Dorfman B, Ziccardi VB, et al. Accuracy of using the antilingula as a sole determinant of vertical ramus osteotomy position. J Oral Maxillofac Surg. 2007;65:859–62.

Chapter 55
Pearls and Pitfalls in Pediatric Mandibular Distraction

Ashley Manlove and Shelly Abramowicz

Abstract Pediatric mandibular distraction osteogenesis (MDO) is commonly utilized to treat neonatal airway obstruction in Robin sequence (RS) patients. Newborns with RS have a triad of findings, including the posterior position of the tongue, which obstructs the airway making breathing and feeding difficult. These patients are often managed conservatively; however, if conservative modalities fail, then the neonates may require more invasive treatments such as tongue-lip adhesion, intubation, MDO, or tracheostomy. When the obstruction is from the tongue, at the level of the hypopharynx above the level of the vocal cords, MDO is a highly successful treatment for neonatal airway compromise because it addresses the etiology of the obstruction. By lengthening the mandible slowly, the body's own healing mechanisms are utilized to create bone under the incremental traction, and the tongue is pulled forward, relieving the obstruction. Numerous studies have shown that with MDO the need for tracheostomy or supplemental airway support is low.

Practical Tips

Preoperative Consideration

- Diagnosis.

  - Prenatal history.

    History of polyhydramnios.

A. Manlove (✉)
Division of Oral and Maxillofacial Surgery, Carle Illinois College of Medicine, Carle
Foundation Hospital, Urbana, IL, USA
e-mail: ashley.manlove@carle.com

S. Abramowicz
Division of Oral and Maxillofacial Surgery, Department of Surgery, Emory University School
of Medicine, Children's Healthcare of Atlanta, Atlanta, GA, USA

D. Amin, H. Marwan (eds.), *Pearls and Pitfalls in Oral and Maxillofacial
Surgery*, https://doi.org/10.1007/978-3-031-47307-4_55

  – Common syndromes requiring mandibular distraction osteogenesis (MDO).

    Treacher Collins.
    Craniofacial microsomia.
    Pierre Robin sequence.
    Goldenhar syndrome.

  – Physical exam.

    Vitals (desaturation/bradycardia when supine, desaturation/bradycardia when feeding, improvement in oxygenation with side-lying or prone positioning).
    Difficulty with feeding.
    Presence of cleft palate.
    Mandibular micrognathia and retrognathia.
    Glossoptosis.
    Improvement with jaw thrust/prone positioning.

  – Imaging may be obtained to evaluate bone and virtually plan surgery.

    Computerized tomography (CT) facial bones (optional).

  – Polysomnography.

    Confirm obstructive apneas rather than central apnea.
    Optional—not always possible to obtain in neonates.

- Treatment timeline.

  – Position side-lying or prone (Fig. 55.1a).
  – May use nasopharyngeal airway or high flow nasal cannula (HFNC) to maintain oxygenation and ventilation (Fig. 55.1b, c).
  – Nasogastric tube feeds if cannot tolerate oral feeding (Fig. 55.1a, c).
  – Monitor for tachypnea and hypercapnia, as this will lead to fatigue and respiratory failure with a potential need for emergent intubation.

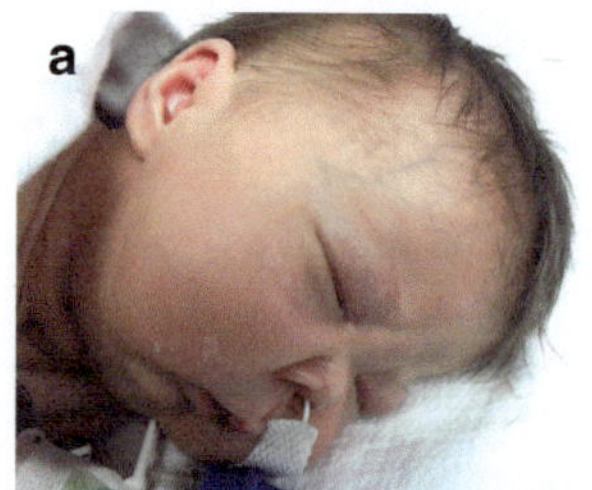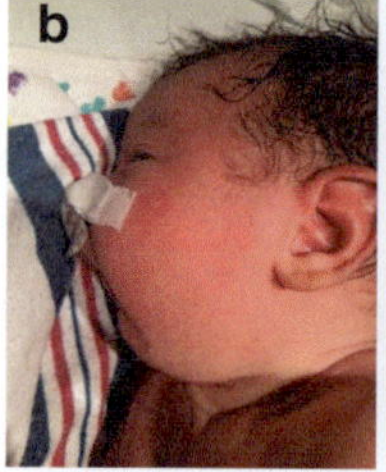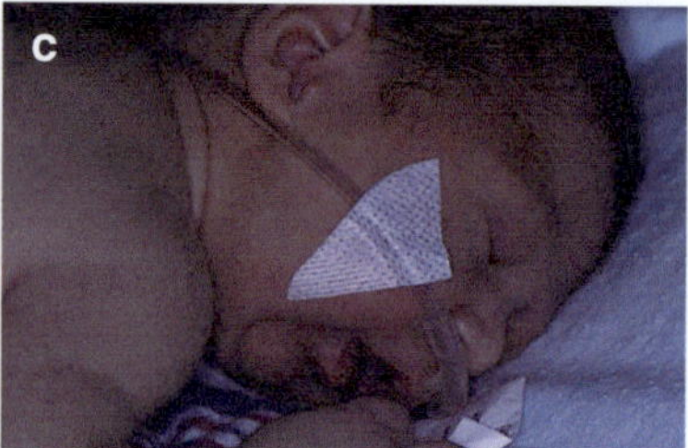

Fig. 55.1 Neonates with RS, pre-surgical. (**a**) RS babies are prone with head to side to maintain oxygenation. NG is in place for feeding. (**b**) RS baby side-lying with nasopharyngeal airway taped in place. (**c**) RS baby prone with head to side with HFNC in place

- Postpone surgery for as long as (safely) possible to allow the mandibular bone to ossify, as this will allow for better retention of the distraction hardware. Neonatal bone is very soft.

- Surgical execution.

  - Preoperative preparation.

    Virtual surgical planning.

    - Optional.
    - CT facial bones without contrast at the surgeon's discretion.
    - CMF plating companies can fabricate custom mandibular cutting guides and/or distractor devices.

    Types of distraction devices.

    - External, uni- and multivector.
    - Internal, uni- and multivector, curvilinear.

Intraoperative Consideration

- Perioperative steps.

  - The patient is intubated orally with a tube midline.

    Anticipate leaving the patient intubated following surgery for 4–7 days, depending on the severity of retrognathia.

  - Surgical steps.

    A small incision just below the inferior border/angle of the mandible 1–1.5 cm in length parallel to the inferior border. The incision is through the skin only.
    Bluntly dissect to the inferior border of the mandible using a hemostat.
    Expose the angle of the mandible via subperiosteal dissection with a mucoperiosteal elevator or freer (Fig. 55.2a).
    Keeping the distraction vector *parallel* to the inferior border of the mandible, seat the distraction footplates on the angle of the mandible and mark the bone where the proximal and distal footplates meet with a pencil. This will be the *osteotomy* (Fig. 55.2b).
    Remark the incision in a "C" fashion so that the curvature of the arc is *posterior* to preserve the tooth buds.
    Use a fine fissure bur or piezoelectric bur to make the osteotomy through the buccal cortex only.
    Use the bur to make a bicortical osteotomy at the superior and inferior borders of the mandible.

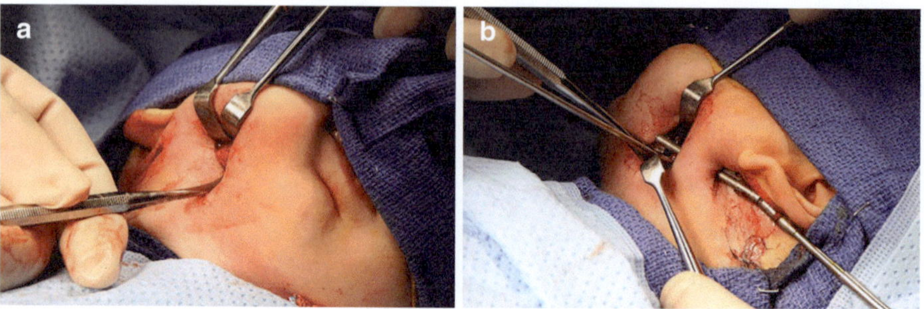

Fig. 55.2 Surgical approach. (**a**) Expose the mandible via subperiosteal dissection. (**b**) Maintain the distraction vector parallel to the inferior border of the mandible

Place mandibular distractor footplates on the angle of the mandible, straddling the osteotomy, and mark the approximate location of the distraction arm.

- Arm can exit anteriorly toward the chin or posteriorly under the ear.
- Use #15C blade to make a stab incision.
- Dissect bluntly with a hemostat.
- Use the hemostat to hold the end of the distraction arm and pull through the incision.

Ensure the proximal and distal footplates are touching (0 mm position) and the distraction arm is parallel to the inferior border.
Secure the *proximal* footplate first. Engage as many screw holes as possible along the inferior portion of the footplate, as the superior screws are more difficult to remove.

- If the bone is very soft, engage all screw holes to prevent the distraction footplates from pulling off the bone.

Secure the distal footplate engaging as many screw holes as possible.
Distract the mandible to open osteotomy.
Use a small osteotome to complete the osteotomy.

- As the distractor is activated, the lingual cortex must separate.
- The inferior alveolar nerve will be intact.

Once the osteotomy is confirmed, rewind the distractor to the 0 mm position.
Repeat on the opposite side.
At the completion of the case, immediately activate the distractors bilaterally to ensure the mandible is moving symmetrically.
Rewind the distractors to the 0 mm position and lock the distractors, so they only turn in one direction. Irrigate and close incisions bilaterally.

- Recovery.

  - Wrap distractor arm sites with Xeroform.
  - Wound care: distractor arms should be cleaned with dilute hydrogen peroxide and sterile water or antibacterial soap and water.
  - Latency phase: allows callus formation, which is the first phase of bone healing.

    Shorter period of time for neonates and infants (24–48 h).
    Longer period of time for children and adolescents (5–7 days).

  - Activation phase: incrementally separates the bone placing traction on the callus.

    Activate 2 mm per day.

    - Divided equally between AM and PM sessions.

    Activate until the mandible is 3–5 mm past the ideal position.

    - There will be a relapse as bone consolidates.

  - Consolidation phase.

    Once the ideal position is reached, the device is left in place for 4–8 weeks, depending on age.

    - Allows the callus to ossify.
    - Distractors provide rigid stability of the segments.

  - The patient typically remains intubated for 5–7 days after surgery to allow for stabilization and initial healing.
  - Extubate with a team ready to re-intubate if necessary.
  - If indicated, patients can be evaluated postoperatively by polysomnography, lateral cephalograms, and computerized tomography of the head and neck.

- Removal of distractors.

  - The distractors remain 4–8 weeks after activation to allow for bone consolidation depending on the age of the patient.
  - External devices are removed by removing the external fixation pins.
  - Internal devices are accessed through the previous submandibular incisions.

    Require general anesthesia.
    Usually, less than 24-hour stay.
    The airway is no longer as difficult since distraction was completed.
    Scar revision can be performed at the time of device removal.

Pearls

- Common syndromes requiring mandibular distraction osteogenesis (MDO) .

  - Treacher Collins.
  - Craniofacial microsomia.

-   – Pierre Robin sequence.
-   – Goldenhar syndrome.

- • Confirm obstructive apneas rather than central apnea.

    -   – The patient is intubated orally with a tube midline.
    -   – Anticipate leaving the patient intubated following surgery for 4–7 days, depending on the severity of retrognathia.

- • Continue to activate the device and advance the mandible until the mandibular arch is more anterior than the maxillary arch (Fig. 55.3).

    -   – There will be a relapse during consolidation.

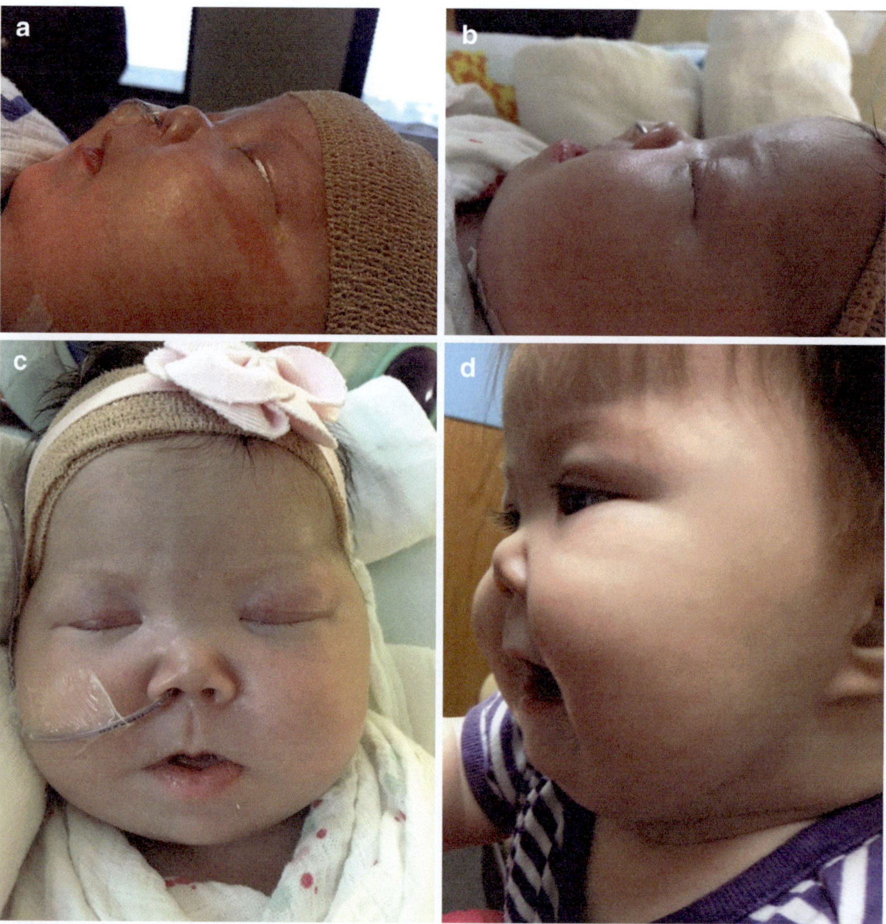

Fig. 55.3 Progression photos. (**a**) Profile photo 7 days following surgery, advancement of 7 mm. (**b**) Profile photo at the conclusion of activation, advancement total 14.5 mm. (**c**) Frontal photo at the conclusion of activation. (**d**) Profile photo at 2 years following distraction

Pitfalls

- Diagnosis.

  - Glossoptosis without micrognathia (Fig. 55.4).

    Mandibular distraction will not have the same benefit, and the baby may only need tongue-lip adhesion or tracheostomy.

  - Patients with abnormal mandibular morphology, such as Treacher Collins or craniofacial microsomia.

    Distraction osteogenesis will not provide a benefit without a definitive condylar stop, such as in Kaban IIb or III.
    The vertical distraction of the ramus can lead to ankylosis.

- Treatment timeline.

  - Too early—bone is very soft.
  - Too long—baby may decompensate and require prolonged intubation or tracheostomy.

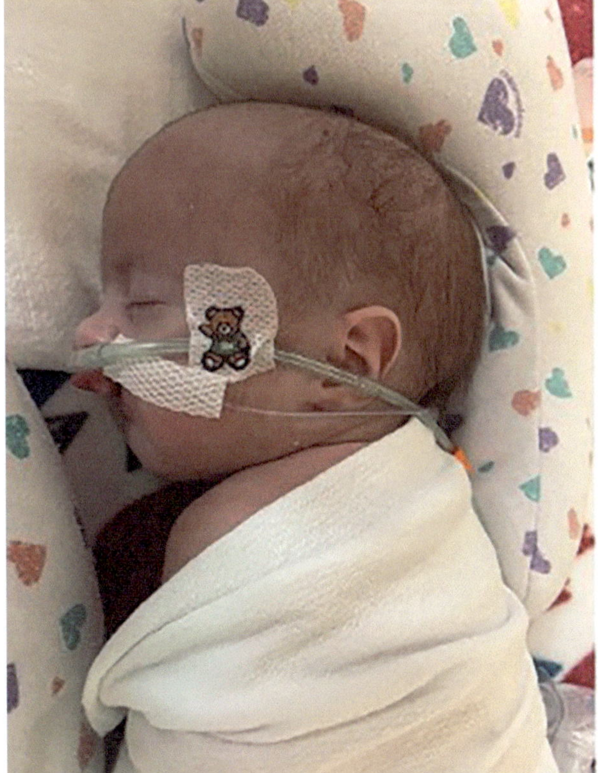

Fig. 55.4 Baby with glossoptosis (hypotonia due to 1p36 deletion) *without* micrognathia. Baby does appear mildly micrognathic due to protuberance of premaxilla secondary to bilateral complete cleft lip and palate

- Surgical execution.

  - Injury to tooth buds.

    Straight osteotomy rather than curvilinear.
    Bicortical rather than monocortical osteotomy.
    Aggressive osteotomy at the superior border.

  - Damage to facial or inferior alveolar nerves.
  - Device failure.
  - Device extrusion.
  - Ankylosis.

    Vertical distraction rather than anterior-posterior can cause too much force on the temporomandibular joint (TMJ), causing ankylosis.

  - Surgical site infection.

    Oral antibiotics and local hygiene can treat superficial infections around the pin sites.
    Deep infection is usually caused by the device pulling off of the bone (Fig. 55.5a, b).

    - May require IV antibiotics.

- Recovery.

  - Malocclusion.
  - Infection.
  - Relapse.

    Expect 3–5 mm during the consolidation phase.

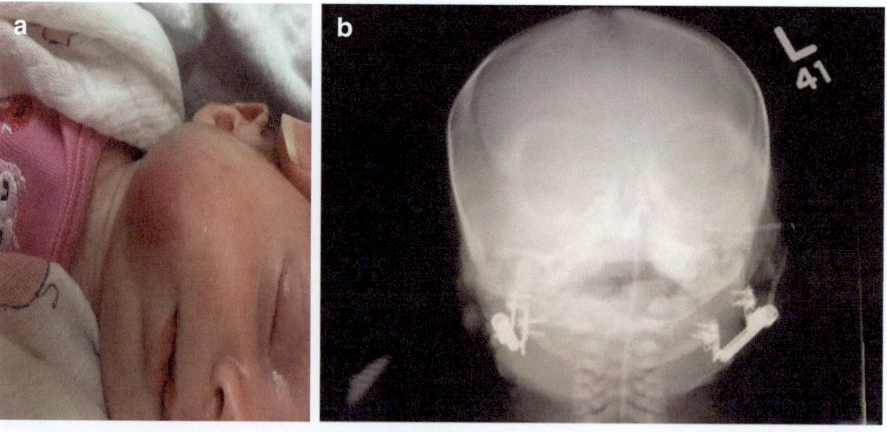

Fig. 55.5 Deep infection related to distal footplate pulling off the bone. (**a**) Clinical photograph, soft tissue infection on the R. (**b**) An AP radiograph showing the right distal footplate is no longer fixated to the mandible

- Scarring.

  External distractors: scarring at the pin sites.
  Internal distractors: scarring at the distraction arm site.

- Noncompliance with distraction can lead to inadequate mandibular distraction lengths.

  Parent education is of the utmost importance as the procedure's success relies heavily on at-home compliance.

Further Reading

Rhee ST, Buchman SR. Pediatric mandibular distraction osteogenesis: the present and the future. J Craniofac Surg. 2003;14(5):803–8.

Brody-Camp S, Winters R. Craniofacial distraction osteogenesis. [Updated 2022 Jul 1]. In: StatPearls [Internet]. Treasure Island (FL): StatPearls Publishing; 2022 Jan-. Available from: https://www.ncbi.nlm.nih.gov/books/NBK560915/

Index